RAPID REVIEW SERIES

Series Editor

Edward F. Goljan, MD

W0009119

USMLE STEP 1

Mosby

An Imprint of Elsevier Science

St. Louis   London   Philadelphia   Sydney   Toronto

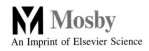
Mosby
An Imprint of Elsevier Science

The Curtis Center
Independence Square West
Philadelphia, PA 19106

NOTICE

Pharmacology is an ever-changing field. Standard safety precautions must be followed, but as new research and clinical experience broaden our knowledge, changes in treatment and drug therapy may become necessary or appropriate. Readers are advised to check the most current product information provided by the manufacturer of each drug to be administered to verify the recommended dose, the method and duration of administration, and contraindications. It is the responsibility of the licensed prescriber, relying on experience and knowledge of the patient, to determine dosages and the best treatment for each individual patient. Neither the publisher nor the editor assumes any liability for any injury and/or damage to persons or property arising from this publication.

The Publisher

International Standard Book Number 0-323-00841-0

Acquisitions Editor: Jason Malley
Managing Editor: Susan Kelly
Publishing Services Manager: Patricia Tannian
Project Manager: John Casey
Senior Designer: Kathi Gosche
Cover Designer: Melissa Walter

GW/CCW

Printed in the United States of America

Last digit is the print number: 9   8   7   6   5   4   3   2   1

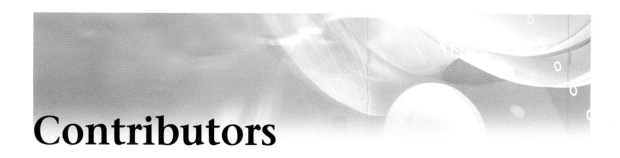

Contributors

Paul H. Brand, PhD
Associate Professor
Department of Physiology and Molecular Medicine
Medical College of Ohio
Toledo, Ohio

E. Robert Burns, PhD
Professor and Course Director
Department of Anatomy and Neurobiology
University of Arkansas for Medical Sciences
Little Rock, Arkansas

Barbara A. Cubic, PhD
Associate Professor
Department of Psychiatry and Behavioral Sciences
Eastern Virginia Medical School
Norfolk, Virginia

Bernell K. Dalley, PhD
Associate Professor
Department of Cell Biology and Biochemistry
Assistant Dean of Admissions School of Medicine
Texas Tech University Health Sciences Center
Lubbock, Texas

Craig W. Davis, PhD
Associate Professor
Department of Pharmacology and Physiology
University of South Carolina School of Medicine
Columbia, South Carolina

Mary Ann Emanuele, MD
Professor of Medicine and Cellular and Molecular Biochemistry
Department of Endocrinology and Metabolism
Loyola University of Chicago
Stritch School of Medicine
Maywood, Illinois

Çağatay H. Erşahin, MD, PhD
Postdoctoral Fellow
Molecular Pharmacology and Biological Chemistry and Drug Discovery
  Program
Northwestern University Medical School
Chicago, Illinois

Edward F. Goljan, MD
Professor and Chairman
Department of Pathology
Oklahoma State University Center for Health Sciences
College of Osteopathic Medicine
Tulsa, Oklahoma

Richard L. Gregory, PhD
Professor
Departments of Oral Biology and Pathology and Laboratory Medicine
Indiana University School of Medicine
Indianapolis, Indiana

James A. Hightower, PhD
Associate Professor
Department of Cell Biology and Neuroscience
University of South Carolina School of Medicine
Columbia, South Carolina

Margaret W. Hougland, PhD
Associate Professor
Department of Anatomy and Cell Biology
East Tennessee State University College of Medicine
Johnson City, Tennessee

Glenn J. Merkel, PhD
Associate Professor
Department of Microbiology and Immunology
Indiana University School of Medicine
Fort Wayne, Indiana

Alya Nayvelt, DMD
Assistant Professor
Department of Anatomy and Cell Biology
University of Illinois Medical Center College of Medicine
Chicago, Illinois

Gary M. Peterson, PhD
Professor
Department of Anatomy and Cell Biology
East Carolina University School of Medicine
Greenville, North Carolina

Balbina J. Plotkin, PhD
Professor of Microbiology
Department of Microbiology
Chicago College of Osteopathic Medicine
Midwestern University
Downers Grove, Illinois

Glen W. Sizemore, MD
Emeritus Professor of Medicine
Division of Endocrinology
Loyola University of Chicago
Stritch School of Medicine
Maywood, Illinois

Roger L. Sopher, MD
Former Professor and Chairman
Department of Pathology
University of North Dakota School of Medicine and Health Sciences
Grand Forks, North Dakota

Mary K. Vaughan, PhD
Medical Neuroscience Task Force Chairman
Department of Cellular and Structural Biology
University of Texas Health Science Center
San Antonio, Texas

Charles L. Webber, Jr., PhD
Professor of Physiology
Department of Physiology
Loyola University of Chicago
Stritch School of Medicine
Maywood, Illinois

Preface

The *Rapid Review Series* is designed for today's busy medical student who has completed basic science courses and has only a limited amount of time to prepare for the United States Medical Licensing Examination (USMLE) Step 1. With a commitment to meeting the needs of these students, we conducted numerous focus groups throughout the United States, trying to learn what would better prepare students for the Step 1 exam. Each book in the *Rapid Review Series* offers a visually integrated approach to review and is packaged with a CD-ROM to help students practice for the actual USMLE Step 1.

Special Features

BOOK

- **Seven practice tests**: each test includes 50 multiple-choice questions emphasizing both basic and clinical sciences in current USMLE Step 1 format. Some questions require the ability to interpret graphs and charts and to identify gross and microscopic pathologic and normal specimens.
- **Answers and discussions (rationales):** each question set is followed by a section with answers and discussions for all options

CD-ROM

- **Full color: 1050 multiple-choice questions** simulating the current USMLE Step 1 in format and content, with emphasis on integration of basic and clinical sciences
- **Color images** included for pathologic and histologic specimens and color schematics
- **Discussions** (rationales) for the correct answer and all incorrect options
- **Test mode:** 60-minute timed test of 50-question block by science, system, or random selection
- **Tutorial (review) mode:** customize your review by science, system, or random selection; get immediate feedback and discussions
- **Bookmark capability**
- **Table of common laboratory values**
- **Scoring function:** instant statistical analysis showing your strengths and weaknesses; print capability

Acknowledgment of Reviewers

The publisher wishes to express sincere thanks to the medical students and the resident physician who reviewed both the text and the questions for the book and CD-ROM and provided us with many useful comments and helpful suggestions for improving this product. Our publishing program will continue to benefit from the combined insight and experience provided by your reviews. For always encouraging us to focus on our target, the USMLE Step 1, we thank the following:

Thomas A. Brown
West Virginia University School of Medicine

Natasha L. Chen
University of Maryland School of Medicine

John D. Cowden
Yale University School of Medicine

Patricia C. Daniel, PhD
University of Kansas Medical Center

John A. Davis
Yale University School of Medicine

Steven J. Engman
Loyola University of Chicago
Stritch School of Medicine

Mark D. Fisher
University of Virginia School of Medicine

Dane Hassani
Rush Medical College

Caron Hong
University of Hawaii School of Medicine at Manoa

Ellen W. King
University of Iowa College of Medicine

Joan Kho
New York Medical College

Katie L'Armand
Medical College of Pennsylvania
Hahnemann School of Medicine

Michael W. Lawlor
Loyola University of Chicago
Stritch School of Medicine

Christopher Lupold
Jefferson Medical College

Erica L. Magers
Michigan State University

Tracey A. McCarthy
Loyola University of Chicago
Stritch School of Medicine

Mrugeshkumar K. Shah, MD, MPH
Tulane School of Medicine
Harvard Medical School/Spaulding Rehabilitation Hospital

Stephanie H. Shah, MD
Harvard Medical School/Massachusetts General Hospital

John K. Su, MPH
Boston University School of Medicine

Table of Contents

COMMON LABORATORY VALUES

Test	Conventional Units	SI Units
Blood, Plasma, Serum		
Alanine aminotransferase (ALT, GPT at 30° C)	8-20 U/L	8-20 U/L
Amylase, serum	25-125 U/L	25-125 U/L
Aspartate aminotransferase (AST, GOT at 30° C)	8-20 U/L	8-20 U/L
Bilirubin, serum (adult) Total // Direct	0.1-1.0 mg/dL // 0.0-0.3 mg/dL	2-17 μmol/L // 0-5 μmol/L
Calcium, serum (CA^{2+})	8.4-10.2 mg/dL	2.1-2.8 mmol/L
Cholesterol, serum	Rec: <200 mg/dL	<5.2 mmol/L
Cortisol, serum	8:00 AM: 6-23 μg/dL // 4:00 PM: 3-15 μg/dL	170-630 nmol/L // 80-410 nmol/L
	8:00 PM: ≤50% of 8:00 AM	Fraction of 8:00 AM: ≤0.50
Creatine kinase, serum	Male: 25-90 U/L	25-90 U/L
	Female: 10-70 U/L	10-70 U/L
Creatinine, serum	0.6-1.2 mg/dL	53-106 μmol/L
Electrolytes, serum		
Sodium (Na^+)	136-145 mEq/L	135-145 mmol/L
Chloride (Cl^-)	95-105 mEq/L	95-105 mmol/L
Potassium (K^+)	3.5-5.0 mEq/L	3.5-5.0 mmol/L
Bicarbonate (HCO_3^-)	22-28 mEq/L	22-28 mmol/L
Magnesium (Mg^{2+})	1.5-2.0 mEq/L	1.5-2.0 mmol/L
Estriol, total, serum (in pregnancy)		
24-28 wk // 32-36 wk	30-170 ng/mL // 60-280 ng/mL	104-590 // 208-970 nmol/L
28-32 wk // 36-40 wk	40-220 ng/mL // 80-350 ng/mL	140-760 // 280-1210 nmol/L
Ferritin, serum	Male: 15-200 ng/mL	15-200 μg/L
	Female: 12-150 ng/mL	12-150 μg/L
Follicle-stimulating hormone, serum/ plasma (FSH)	Male: 4-25 mIU/mL	4-25 U/L
	Female: premenopause 4-30 mIU/mL	4-30 U/L
	midcycle peak 10-90 mIU/mL	10-90 U/L
	postmenopause 40-250 mIU/mL	40-250 U/L
Gases, arterial blood (room air)		
pH	7.35-7.45	[H^+] 36-44 nmol/L
P_{CO_2}	33-45 mm Hg	4.4-5.9 kPa
P_{O_2}	75-105 mm Hg	10.0-14.0 kPa
Glucose, serum	Fasting: 70-110 mg/dL	3.8-6.1 mmol/L
	2 hr postprandial: <120 mg/dL	<6.6 mmol/L
Growth hormone–arginine stimulation	Fasting: <5 ng/mL	<5 μg/L
	provocative stimuli: >7 ng/mL	>7 μg/L
Immunoglobulins, serum		
IgA	76-390 mg/dL	0.76-3.90 g/L
IgE	0-380 IU/mL	0-380 kIU/L
IgG	650-1500 mg/dL	6.5-15 g/L
IgM	40-345 mg/dL	0.4-3.45 g/L

Continued

COMMON LABORATORY VALUES—cont'd

Test	Conventional Units	SI Units
Blood, Plasma, Serum—cont'd		
Iron	50-170 µg/dL	9-30 µmol/L
Lactate dehydrogenase, serum (LDH)	45-90 U/L	45-90 U/L
Luteinizing hormone, serum/plasma (LH)	Male: 6-23 mIU/mL	6-23 U/L
	Female: follicular phase 5-30 mIU/mL	5-30 U/L
	midcycle 75-150 mIU/mL	75-150 U/L
	postmenopause 30-200 mIU/mL	30-200 U/L
Osmolality, serum	275-295 mOsm/kg	275-295 mOsm/kg
Parathyroid hormone, serum, N-terminal	230-630 pg/mL	230-630 ng/L
Phosphatase (alkaline), serum (p-NPP at 30° C)		
Phosphorus (inorganic), serum	3.0-4.5 mg/dL	1.0-1.5 mmol/L
Prolactin, serum (hPRL)	<20 ng/mL	<20 µg/L
Proteins, serum		
Total (recumbent)	6.0-8.0 g/dL	60-80 g/L
Albumin	3.5-5.5 g/dL	35-55 g/L
Globulin	2.3-3.5 g/dL	23-35 g/L
Thyroid-stimulating hormone, serum or plasma (TSH)	0.5-5.0 µU/mL	0.5-5.0 mU/L
Thyroidal iodine (^{123}I) uptake	8%-30% of administered dose/24 hr	0.08-0.30/24 hr
Thyroxine (T_4), serum	4.5-12 µg/dL	58-154 nmol/L
Triglycerides, serum	35-160 mg/dL	0.4-1.81 mmol/L
Triiodothyronine (T_3), serum (RIA)	115-190 ng/dL	1.8-2.9 nmol/L
Triiodothyronine (T_3) resin uptake	25%-38%	0.25-0.38
Urea nitrogen, serum (BUN)	7-18 mg/dL	1.2-3.0 mmol urea/L
Uric acid, serum	3.0-8.2 mg/dL	0.18-0.48 mmol/L
Cerebrospinal (CSF) Fluid		
Cell count	0-5 cells/mm^3	0-5 × 10^6/L
Chloride	118-132 mEq/L	118-132 mmol/L
Gamma globulin	3%-12% total proteins	0.03-0.12
Glucose	50-75 mg/dL	2.8-4.2 mmol/L
Pressure	70-180 mm H_2O	70-180 mm H_2O
Proteins, total	<40 mg/dL	<0.40 g/L
Hematology		
Bleeding time (template)	2-7 min	2-7 min
Erythrocyte count	Male: 4.3-5.9 million/mm^3	4.3-5.9 × 10^{12}/L
	Female: 3.5-5.5 million/mm^3	3.5-5.5 × 10^{12}/L
Erythrocyte sedimentation rate (Westergren)	Male: 0-15 mm/hr	0-15 mm/hr
	Female: 0-20 mm/hr	0-20 mm/hr

COMMON LABORATORY VALUES—cont'd

Test	Conventional Units	SI Units
Hematology—cont'd		
Hematocrit (Hct)	Male: 40%-54%	0.40-0.54
	Female: 37%-47%	0.37-0.47
Hemoglobin A_{IC}	≤6%	≤ 0.06%
Hemoglobin, blood (Hb)	Male: 13.5-17.5 g/dL	2.09-2.71 mmol/L
	Female: 12.0-16.0 g/dL	1.86-2.48 mmol/L
Hemoglobin, plasma	1-4 mg/dL	0.16-0.62 mmol/L
Leukocyte count and differential		
Leukocyte count	4500-11,000/mm^3	4.5-11.0 × 10^9/L
Segmented neutrophils	54%-62%	0.54-0.62
Bands	3%-5%	0.03-0.05
Eosinophils	1%-3%	0.01-0.03
Basophils	0%-0.75%	0-0.0075
Lymphocytes	25%-33%	0.25-0.33
Monocytes	3%-7%	0.03-0.07
Mean corpuscular hemoglobin (MCH)	25.4-34.6 pg/cell	0.39-0.54 fmol/cell
Mean corpuscular hemoglobin concentration (MCHC)	31%-37% Hb/cell	4.81-5.74 mmol Hb/L
Mean corpuscular volume (MCV)	80-100 μm^3	80-100 fl
Partial thromboplastin time (activated) (aPTT)	25-40 sec	25-40 sec
Platelet count	150,000-400,000/mm^3	150-400 × 10^9/L
Prothrombin time (PT)	12-14 sec	12-14 sec
Reticulocyte count	0.5%-1.5% of red cells	0.005-0.015
Thrombin time	<2 sec deviation from control	<2 sec deviation from control
Volume		
Plasma	Male: 25-43 mL/kg	0.025-0.043 L/kg
	Female: 28-45 mL/kg	0.028-0.045 L/kg
Red cell	Male: 20-36 mL/kg	0.020-0.036 L/kg
	Female: 19-31 mL/kg	0.019-0.031 L/kg
Sweat		
Chloride	0-35 mmol/L	0-35 mmol/L
Urine		
Calcium	100-300 mg/24 hr	2.5-7.5 mmol/24 hr
Creatinine clearance	Male: 97-137 mL/min	
	Female: 88-128 mL/min	
Estriol, total (in pregnancy)		
30 wk	6-18 mg/24 hr	21-62 μmol/24 hr
35 wk	9-28 mg/24 hr	31-97 μmol/24 hr
40 wk	13-42 mg/24 hr	45-146 μmol/24 hr
17-Hydroxycorticosteroids	Male: 3.0-9.0 mg/24 hr	8.2-25.0 μmol/24 hr
	Female: 2.0-8.0 mg/24 hr	5.5-22.0 μmol/24 hr
17-Ketosteroids, total	Male: 8-22 mg/24 hr	28-76 μmol/24 hr
	Female: 6-15 mg/24 hr	21-52 μmol/24 hr
Osmolality	50-1400 mOsm/kg	
Oxalate	8-40 μg/mL	90-445 μmol/L
Proteins, total	<150 mg/24 hr	<0.15 g/24 hr

Test 1

TEST 1

DIRECTIONS: Each numbered item or incomplete statement is followed by options arranged in alphabetical or logical order. Select the best answer to each question. Some options may be partially correct, but there is only **ONE BEST** answer.

1. A 30-year-old woman who complains of diplopia, bilateral ptosis, and fatigue states that she has difficulty climbing stairs and raising her arms over her head, and often regurgitates ingested fluids. There is a nasal quality to her speech. Edrophonium results in a brief but striking improvement in her condition. The most likely cause of these findings is

○ A. Duchenne muscular dystrophy
○ B. lesion in the basal ganglia
○ C. lesion in the cerebellum
○ D. myasthenia gravis
○ E. tardive dyskinesia

2. While observing a child talking to his parents, the pediatrician notes that the child understands that water and ice are different forms of the same object. The child also recognizes that pouring water from a short, round container into a tall, slim container does not change the amount of water present. According to Piaget's stages of cognitive development, this child is most likely to be in which of the following age groups?

○ A. 2–4 years
○ B. 4–7 years
○ C. 7–11 years
○ D. 11–13 years
○ E. 13–18 years

3. A 22-year-old man who has undergone an appendectomy without complications has markedly reduced bowel sounds and an absence of flatus or defecation during the immediate postoperative period. Which of the following mechanisms best explains this decrease in bowel sounds?

○ A. Decreased sympathetic activity to the gut
○ B. Increased activity of the gastrocolic reflex
○ C. Increased parasympathetic activity to the gut
○ D. Increased plasma acetylcholine concentration
○ E. Increased plasma norepinephrine concentration

4. A 68-year-old woman has developed spastic paralysis of the left arm and leg. Her face appears asymmetrical; the loss of symmetry is most apparent on the left side of her mouth when she smiles. When she raises her eyebrows, the wrinkles on her forehead remain symmetrical. This patient most likely has a lesion in the

○ A. left basilar pons
○ B. left facial nerve
○ C. left precentral gyrus
○ D. right caudal medulla
○ E. right internal capsule

5. A 62-year-old man has smoked two packs of cigarettes a day for 30 years. He states that almost every morning during this time, he has coughed up a tablespoon or more of yellow-green sputum. Physical examination shows cyanosis of the skin and mucous membranes and an increased anteroposterior diameter of the chest. On auscultation, scattered sibilant rhonchi and rales are heard in both lung fields. Referring to the figure below, which of the following letters, labeled A through F on the curves, represents the expected arterial blood gases in this patient?

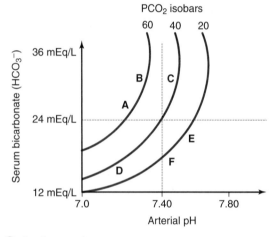

- ○ A. Letter A
- ○ B. Letter B
- ○ C. Letter C
- ○ D. Letter D
- ○ E. Letter E

6. The mother of a 6-month-old boy says that her child has been having choking spells for 10 days. Each spell begins with repetitive coughing, and then he turns red or blue, gasps for breath, and makes a strange sound when he inhales. He has also been vomiting. His pulse is 160/min, and respirations are 72/min. Blood studies show a white blood cell count of 15,500/mm^3 with 70% lymphocytes. A nasal swab specimen is cultured on Bordet-Gengou agar, and a small, encapsulated, gram-negative coccobacillus is isolated. The causative organism's ability to induce many of the clinical manifestations of this patient's disease is attributable to which of the following?

- ○ A. Capsule that activates complement
- ○ B. Cytotoxin that causes the lysis of red blood cells
- ○ C. Enterotoxins that increase the level of intracellular cyclic guanosine monophosphate (cGMP)
- ○ D. Exotoxins that increase the synthesis of cyclic adenosine monophosphate (cAMP)
- ○ E. Exotoxins that inhibit the synthesis of proteins

7. A 49-year-old man with a history of chronic alcoholism suddenly develops severe pain in the midabdominal area, that radiates to the back. Within 24 hours, he goes into shock and develops hypocalcemia. His serum amylase is markedly increased. Despite appropriate care, he dies. Which of the following morphologic changes may account for the hypocalcemia?

- ○ A. Hemorrhagic fat necrosis of the pancreas with yellow soap deposits on adjacent adipose tissue
- ○ B. Impacted gallstones in the ampulla of Vater with acute ascending cholangitis
- ○ C. Perforation of a gastric ulcer with hemorrhage into the peritoneal cavity and marked chemical peritonitis
- ○ D. Rupture of the aorta with exsanguination into the retroperitoneal space
- ○ E. Swollen kidneys with a marked degree of necrosis of the proximal renal tubular epithelium

8. A 35-year-old woman has an 8-year history of back pain and has had only limited relief from treatment with narcotic agents. No organic cause has been determined despite extensive medical examinations, and there is no evidence that the pain is feigned. She acknowledges mild frustration, but denies symptoms of depression or other psychiatric problems. Based on this limited information, the most likely diagnosis is

- ○ A. factitious disorder
- ○ B. major depressive disorder
- ○ C. malingering
- ○ D. somatization disorder
- ○ E. somatoform pain disorder

9. A 43-year-old man who works as a crop duster is brought to the emergency department suffering from weakness and profuse sweating. He is wheezing and has abdominal cramps and diarrhea. Physical examination shows miosis, bradycardia, and muscle fasciculations. The patient says that he was spraying a local cornfield with malathion and accidentally flew through his back-draft. Treatment aimed at correcting the patient's weakness and labored breathing would include

○ A. atropine
○ B. ipecac
○ C. nicotine
○ D. physostigmine
○ E. pralidoxime

10. Which of the following would directly lead to impaired cellular amino acid uptake from the extracellular space?

○ A. Defect in Ca^{2+} ATPase
○ B. Defect in gap junctions
○ C. Defect in Na^+, K^+-ATPase
○ D. Defective antiport system
○ E. Defective symport system

11. A 50-year-old woman is undergoing cardiac catheterization to determine the cause of exertional shortness of breath accompanied by chest pain. During catheterization, blood gas measurements and the following hemodynamic data are obtained:

Systolic blood pressure	144 mm Hg
Diastolic blood pressure	92 mm Hg
Heart rate	80/min
Arterial O_2 content	0.15 mL O_2/mL blood
Mixed venous O_2 content	0.10 mL O_2/mL blood
Hematocrit	32%
Left ventricular end-diastolic volume	30 mL
Left ventricular end-systolic volume	100 mL

Which of the following factors is most likely to contribute to shortness of breath in this patient?

○ A. Abnormally low arterial O_2 content
○ B. Depressed cardiac ejection fraction
○ C. Increased extraction of O_2 by peripheral tissues
○ D. Increased metabolic demand as reflected in the heart rate
○ E. Systemic hypertension

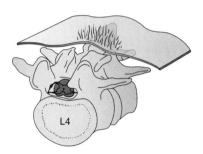

12. A 6-month-old infant is diagnosed with the embryologic anomaly shown in the figure above. No neurologic deficits are evident. The mother's prenatal care was poor, with no vitamin supplements. Which of the following is the most likely explanation for this embryologic defect?

○ A. Lentigo melanoma
○ B. Myelomeningocele
○ C. Rachischisis
○ D. Spina bifida occulta

13. A 16-year-old high school student develops pharyngitis with fever, cervical lymphadenopathy, and erythema and edema of the posterior pharynx. His tonsils are inflamed, enlarged, and covered with a nonadherent exudate. Blood cultures yield negative results, and pharyngeal swab cultures grow a predominance of small β-hemolytic colonies. Gram stains of the pharyngeal exudate show numerous gram-positive cocci occurring in pairs and chains. Which of the following substances is a virulence factor found on the causative bacterium's surface and exerts its effects by inhibiting activation of the alternative complement pathway?

- ○ A. F protein
- ○ B. Group-specific carbohydrate
- ○ C. Hyaluronic acid
- ○ D. Lipoteichoic acid
- ○ E. M protein

14. A 51-year-old man with type 2 diabetes mellitus is treated with glipizide. This drug's efficacy is due to its ability to

- ○ A. block ATP-dependent K^+ channels in the pancreatic beta cells
- ○ B. decrease hepatic production of glucose and improve insulin sensitivity
- ○ C. directly open voltage-dependent Ca^{2+} channels in the pancreatic beta cells
- ○ D. increase transcription of insulin-responsive genes that control glucose uptake
- ○ E. inhibit 5α-glucosidase activity in the brush border of the small intestine

15. A 54-year-old woman with severe right upper quadrant pain, fever, and jaundice is in shock when brought to the emergency department. A blood culture grows *Escherichia coli*. The presumptive diagnosis is acute cholecystitis. The most likely cause of shock is

- ○ A. anaphylactic reaction
- ○ B. cardiogenic shock
- ○ C. endotoxemia
- ○ D. hemorrhage
- ○ E. neurogenic shock

16. A 12-year-old boy returned from summer camp with linear vesicular lesions on his legs. The lesions cause intense itching, but they are not accompanied by fever. The rash spreads over the next few days, but it eventually resolves with the use of a topical over-the-counter medication. Which cells are primarily involved in the development of this type of rash?

- ○ A. Keratinocytes
- ○ B. Keratocytes
- ○ C. Langerhans' cells
- ○ D. Melanocytes
- ○ E. Merkel cells

17. A 60-year-old man has left hemiparesis and right ptosis. He cannot adduct, elevate, or depress his right eye. The most likely cause of these findings is a lesion in which of the following sites?

- ○ A. Cavernous sinus
- ○ B. Cerebral cortex
- ○ C. Left genu of the internal capsule
- ○ D. Mesencephalon
- ○ E. Midline of the medulla

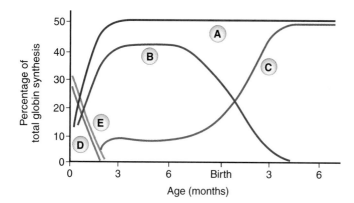

18. The figure above depicts the developmental changes seen in globin chain synthesis in the fetus and newborn infant (from conception to 6 months of age). A defect in one of the globin chains accounts for the death of a 3-year-old black child who had a history of sickle cell anemia and died of intractable infection and renal failure. Which of the following curves (labeled A–E in the figure) best illustrates the synthesis of this chain?

○ A. Curve A
○ B. Curve B
○ C. Curve C
○ D. Curve D
○ E. Curve E

19. A 9-year-old girl is brought to the pediatrician because she has recently reverted to wetting her bed at night and is demonstrating clinging behavior. While performing a physical examination, the pediatrician notices bruises and contusions in the vaginal and pelvic region and immediately suspects sexual abuse. Which of the following is the most appropriate action?

○ A. The child must admit to being sexually abused before child protective services can be contacted
○ B. The pediatrician must find additional evidence of deprivation and neglect to assume sexual abuse
○ C. The pediatrician should ask the parents if sexual abuse occurred, and if they reply in a negative manner, nothing should be reported
○ D. The pediatrician should contact child protective services immediately and ask for an investigation
○ E. The pediatrician should contact child protective services only if there is additional evidence of physical abuse

20. A 50-year-old man has a fever, malaise, anorexia, chest pains, and a productive cough with purulent sputum. He says that his symptoms began about 7 days ago, after he attended a business convention, and have gotten progressively worse. Serologic studies using the indirect fluorescent antibody technique are positive for *Legionella pneumophila.* The most appropriate drug for treating this patient acts by

○ A. binding to the 30S ribosomal subunit, thereby preventing the initiation of protein synthesis

○ B. binding to the 50S ribosomal subunit, thereby preventing translocation of peptidyl tRNA from the acceptor site to the donor site

○ C. inhibiting DNA-dependent RNA polymerase, thereby preventing RNA synthesis

○ D. inhibiting peptidoglycan synthase (transglycosylase), thereby preventing elongation of the peptidoglycan backbone of the bacterial cell wall

○ E. inhibiting transpeptidase, thereby preventing the cross-linking of the bacterial cell wall

21. A 30-year-old woman is taken to the emergency department suffering from excruciating abdominal cramps and vomiting. She says that she and several other family members have suffered from angioedema of the skin and upper respiratory tract. This patient most likely has a deficiency of which of the following complement regulatory proteins?

○ A. Anaphylatoxin inactivator
○ B. C1 esterase inhibitor
○ C. C4 binding protein
○ D. Properdin
○ E. Vitronectin

22. A 76-year-old woman has ataxia, areflexia, and impaired posterior column function. Living on a fixed income often makes it difficult for her to afford to buy groceries. An MRI shows no abnormalities. Which of the following vitamins would most likely improve this patient's neurologic problems?

○ A. Vitamin A
○ B. Vitamin C
○ C. Vitamin D
○ D. Vitamin E
○ E. Vitamin K

23. A 6-week-old male infant developed swelling on the right side of the lower abdomen near the area where the abdomen becomes continuous with the thigh. The swelling is particularly evident when the infant cries or strains. Evaluation confirms a hernia resulting from persistence of the processus vaginalis of parietal peritoneum following the path of the descent of the testis to the scrotum. Which of the following types of hernias is the correct diagnosis?

○ A. Direct inguinal hernia
○ B. Femoral hernia
○ C. Indirect inguinal hernia
○ D. Obturator hernia
○ E. Umbilical hernia

24. A 30-year-old black woman who resides in North Carolina develops increasing shortness of breath. A physical examination shows lymphadenopathy in the axillae and groin. X-ray film of the chest shows a marked degree of hilar lymph node enlargement. A biopsy of an enlarged axillary lymph node shows numerous noncaseating granulomas. No organisms are identifiable, and acid-fast stains are negative. These findings are most likely caused by which of the following?

○ A. Coccidioidomycosis
○ B. Cryptococcosis
○ C. Histoplasmosis
○ D. Sarcoidosis
○ E. Tuberculosis

25. A 9-year-old boy has a deep epidermal inflammatory lesion, accompanied by hair loss in the temporal region of the scalp. A hair sample examined with a Wood's lamp shows green fluorescence. A potassium hydroxide (KOH) preparation of hair from the periphery of the boggy lesion (kerion) shows the presence of an ectothrix fungal infection. This infection is an isolated incident, and the infectious agent is presumed to be zoophilic. Which of the following fungi is the most likely cause of the infection?

○ A. *Candida albicans*
○ B. *Microsporum canis*
○ C. *Trichophyton mentagrophytes*
○ D. *Trichophyton rubrum*
○ E. *Trichophyton verrucosum*

26. One month after a 55-year-old woman begins diuretic therapy for the management of mild essential hypertension, routine blood studies show a low serum potassium level and high levels of serum calcium, uric acid, and glucose. The woman was most likely treated with

○ A. acetazolamide
○ B. furosemide
○ C. hydrochlorothiazide
○ D. mannitol
○ E. triamterene

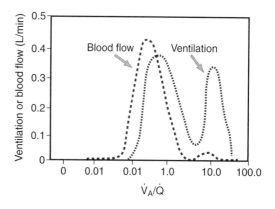

27. A 74-year-old woman has a history of increasing shortness of breath. The distribution of ventilation/perfusion ratios ($\dot{V}_A/\dot{Q}$) is measured by the multiple inert gas elimination technique. The results (shown in the figure above) indicate that shortness of breath in this patient developed because

○ A. a large area of the lung is neither ventilated nor perfused
○ B. a large area of the lung is perfused but not ventilated
○ C. a large area of the lung is ventilated but not perfused
○ D. ventilation and perfusion are well balanced but depressed in all pulmonary units

28. A 1-month-old neonate has failure of separation of the umbilical cord. Histologic sections of the surgically removed cord show an absence of neutrophil pavementing and emigration into the interstitial tissue. The clinical and histologic findings in this case are most closely associated with a defect in

○ A. activation of the complement system
○ B. microtubule polymerization
○ C. respiratory burst mechanism
○ D. synthesis of adhesion molecules
○ E. synthesis of myeloperoxidase

29. A 23-year-old man has had a sore throat, fever, malaise, and joint pain for 6 days. When asked if he has had any other recent medical problems, he says that 4 weeks ago he noticed a painless, round, pink lesion on his penis, and the lesion later ulcerated. Now he has lesions on the palms and soles. Microscopic examination of exudate from a lesion shows the presence of motile spirochetes. Serologic tests are positive for reagin. The patient's medical records indicate that he is allergic to penicillin. The most appropriate drug for the treatment of this patient acts by

- ○ A. binding to the 30S ribosomal subunit, thereby preventing attachment of the aminoacyl tRNA to the acceptor site
- ○ B. binding to the 30S ribosomal subunit, thereby preventing formation of the initiation complex
- ○ C. inhibiting DNA gyrase, thereby preventing the synthesis of DNA
- ○ D. inhibiting peptidoglycan synthase (transglycosylase), thereby preventing elongation of the peptidoglycan backbone of the bacterial cell wall
- ○ E. inhibiting transpeptidase, thereby preventing the cross-linking of the bacterial cell wall

30. A cDNA fragment encoding a fusion protein is constructed by molecular techniques. The fusion protein consists of a signal sequence attached to the amino terminus of a cytoplasmic protein. The signal sequence is composed of amino acids that form a positively charged amphipathic α-helix. The constructed cDNA encoding the fusion protein is used to transfect mammalian cells. After subcellular fractionation of transfected cells is performed, the subcellular fractions are tested for the fusion protein. This protein is most likely to be localized in the

- ○ A. mitochondrion
- ○ B. nucleus
- ○ C. peroxisome
- ○ D. plasma membrane
- ○ E. secretory vesicle

31. A 51-year-old man has severe pain at the base of his left great toe, around the forward portion of the arch. The first metatarsophalangeal joint of his left foot is tender, markedly inflamed, and erythematous. Laboratory studies show a serum uric acid level of 10.4 mg/dL; serum creatinine value and other serum values are within the normal range. A 24-hour urine specimen contains 550 mg of uric acid. Light microscopy of a synovial aspirate shows the presence of monosodium urate crystals. The most appropriate treatment for this patient's arthritic pain is

- ○ A. allopurinol
- ○ B. aspirin
- ○ C. colchicine
- ○ D. methotrexate
- ○ E. probenecid

32. A 26-year-old woman complains of pain and stiffness in the neck. Her temperature is 38.2° C (100.8° F). Because meningitis is suspected, the physician will perform a lumbar puncture (spinal tap) and collect cerebrospinal fluid (CSF), which will be cultured and examined. To perform this diagnostic procedure, the physician will insert the needle

- ○ A. between T12 and L1
- ○ B. into the dura mater but not the arachnoid layer
- ○ C. into the vertebral canal inferior to the conus medullaris of the spinal cord
- ○ D. into the vertebral canal through the intervertebral foramen

33. A 25-year-old man who recently returned from a vacation in the Caribbean develops chills, fever, splenomegaly, and signs of anemia. During the examination, he experiences an attack of chills that lasts for about 30 minutes. His temperature then rises to 40.5° C (105° F). The fever subsides, and he begins to sweat profusely. Another febrile paroxysm occurs within a few hours. A stained blood smear shows the presence of numerous schizonts. The most likely diagnosis is

- ○ A. cryptosporidiosis
- ○ B. leishmaniasis
- ○ C. malaria
- ○ D. mucormycosis
- ○ E. trypanosomiasis

34. A 76-year-old woman is diagnosed with osteoporosis based on height loss, wedging of vertebral bodies, and kyphosis. Dual energy x-ray absorptiometry shows decreased bone density. Which of the following mechanisms is likely to contribute to the decreased bone density in this patient?

- ○ A. Decreased renal production of 1,25-(OH)2D (dihydroxyvitamin D)
- ○ B. Gradually decreasing level of serum parathyroid hormone (PTH)
- ○ C. Increased osteoblastic activity
- ○ D. Increased renal production of dihydroxyvitamin D
- ○ E. Lack of the usual effect of PTH on net renal phosphate secretion

35. An 18-year-old college student who was seen drinking heavily at a party is found in his room completely unresponsive. When he is admitted to the emergency department, his blood alcohol level is 325 mg/dL. In a nonhabituated drinker, this level of blood alcohol is associated with

- ○ A. coma and respiratory collapse
- ○ B. congestive cardiomyopathy
- ○ C. development of acute yellow atrophy of the liver
- ○ D. Korsakoff's syndrome
- ○ E. Wernicke's encephalopathy

36. A physician makes several unsuccessful attempts to encourage a 52-year-old man to take his medication for hypertension and adhere to the regimen of taking the drug twice a day. Which of the following strategies is most likely to increase this patient's willingness to adhere to the prescribed drug regimen?

- ○ A. Adopting an authoritarian style with the patient
- ○ B. Dividing the dose so the patient takes the drug four times a day
- ○ C. Providing written instructions for the patient
- ○ D. Refusing to serve as the patient's physician if the patient does not comply
- ○ E. Using medical jargon to illustrate the seriousness of the issue

37. A 29-year-old woman suffering from a fever, chills, fatigue, headache, and nausea for 2 days develops hepatomegaly and bilirubinuria. Blood studies show an elevated alanine aminotransferase level (ALT) and hypocomplementemia. Bacterial and fungal cultures yield negative results, but a picornavirus is isolated from a fecal specimen. Which of the following viruses is the most likely cause of the disease?

- ○ A. Hepatitis A virus
- ○ B. Hepatitis B virus
- ○ C. Hepatitis C virus
- ○ D. Hepatitis D virus
- ○ E. Hepatitis E virus

38. A 14-year-old boy has become totally deaf in his left ear after a motor vehicle accident. Hearing in his right ear is normal. A lesion at which of the following sites is the most likely cause of this finding?

- ○ A. Left dorsal and ventral cochlear nuclei
- ○ B. Left inferior colliculus
- ○ C. Left superior colliculus
- ○ D. Right medial geniculate nucleus
- ○ E. Right temporal lobe

39. A 54-year-old woman has arthritis, nephritis, fever, and a butterfly rash across her nose and cheeks. She complains of weight loss and fatigue. Immunofluorescence studies show the presence of autoantibodies to U1 snRNP. Which of the following processes is most likely to be impaired in this patient?

○ A. Assembly of the spliceosome
○ B. Binding to the branch site
○ C. Cytoplasmic transport of RNA
○ D. Recognition of the 3′ splice site
○ E. Recognition of the 5′ splice site

40. A 26-year-old man has had Crohn's disease of the ileum for 10 months and has been treated with several drugs. He now suffers from muscle weakness, centripetal obesity, and a round, plethoric face. These side effects are most likely associated with the long-term use of

○ A. azathioprine
○ B. cyclosporine
○ C. olsalazine
○ D. prednisone
○ E. sulfasalazine

41. A 42-year-old woman complains of steadily worsening pain and discomfort on the right side of the head. A CT scan shows a discrete tumor just lateral to the atlas and axis of the vertebral column and involves the superior cervical ganglion. The loss of sympathetic innervation provided by this ganglion may lead to which of the following deficits?

○ A. Dilated pupil on the affected side
○ B. Dry eye
○ C. Dry mouth
○ D. Partial ptosis of the upper eyelid on the affected side
○ E. Persistent sweating from the skin overlying the parotid salivary gland

42. During a routine physical examination of a 13-year-old boy, the physician notices bilaterally enlarged, nontender testicles that do not transilluminate. Additional physical findings include a long face with prominent jaw, high arched palate, and protruding ears. The child has a speech disability and is in a special educational program at school. Which of the following studies would most likely be abnormal in this patient?

○ A. Buccal smear
○ B. Chromosome study of the father
○ C. DNA analysis of the X chromosome
○ D. Serum gonadotropins
○ E. Testicular biopsy

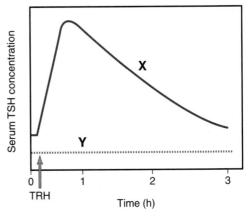

43. Two patients (X and Y) are being evaluated to determine the cause of thyroid dysfunction. They undergo a 3-hour thyrotropin-releasing hormone (TRH) stimulation study in which TRH is administered (see arrow in figure above) and serum thyroid-stimulating hormone (TSH) concentration is measured. Based on the results of the study, which of the following conclusions can be made about these two patients?

○ A. Patient X has a pituitary TSH-secreting tumor
○ B. Patient X has hypothyroidism
○ C. Patient Y has hyperthyroidism
○ D. Patient Y shows a normal response to TRH

44. A 24-year-old woman has just been told that she has an advanced stage of Hodgkin's disease with a poor prognosis. Based on the stages of death described by Elisabeth Kübler-Ross, which of the following stages is this patient most likely to exhibit first?

○ A. Acceptance
○ B. Anger
○ C. Bargaining
○ D. Denial
○ E. Depression

45. A 47-year-old man is admitted to the hospital with marked abdominal distention and edema in the lower extremities. His symptoms are due to a low plasma oncotic pressure. The most likely diagnosis is a disease of which organ?

○ A. Liver
○ B. Pancreas
○ C. Parotid gland
○ D. Spleen
○ E. Thyroid gland

46. A 9-year-old girl has a fever, lymphadenopathy, dysphagia, and pharyngitis with an adherent pseudomembrane (exudate) covering the tonsils and portions of the oral pharyngeal mucosa. Gram stains of the oropharyngeal exudate show gram-positive pleomorphic rods arranged in palisades. The pharyngeal exudate is cultured on potassium tellurite agar, and numerous black colonies develop. Despite the initiation of penicillin therapy, systemic toxemia develops and the girl dies. The clinical manifestations of this patient's disease were mediated by an exotoxin that

○ A. directly disrupts cell membrane integrity
○ B. directly disrupts microtubules
○ C. directly inhibits nucleic acid synthesis
○ D. directly inhibits protein synthesis
○ E. directly lyses mitochondria

47. Investigators are studying the regulation of glycolytic pathway enzymes in a culture of hepatocytes. After citrate is added to the culture, a substrate of which of the following enzyme-catalyzed reactions will accumulate in the hepatocytes?

○ A. 1,3-Bisphosphoglycerate → 3-phosphoglycerate
○ B. Fructose 6-phosphate → fructose 1,6-bisphosphate
○ C. Glucose → glucose 6-phosphate
○ D. Glucose 6-phosphate → fructose 6-phosphate
○ E. Phosphoenolpyruvate → pyruvate

48. A 58-year-old man with a 35-year history of cigarette smoking complains of weight loss and cough. Physical examination shows absence of sweating on the left forehead and face and ipsilateral lid lag and constriction of the pupil. On auscultation, sibilant rhonchi that clear with coughing are heard in all lung fields. The anteroposterior diameter of the chest is increased. Which of the following mechanisms best explains the clinical findings in this patient?

○ A. Destruction of the brachial plexus by a primary lung cancer
○ B. Destruction of the cervical sympathetic plexus by a primary lung cancer
○ C. Extension of a primary lung cancer into the anterior mediastinum
○ D. Uncal herniation secondary to metastatic disease originating in the lung

49. A 21-year-old woman who has had several relapses of acute lymphocytic leukemia now has evidence of another relapse. She begins remission induction treatment with a combination of prednisone, asparaginase, vincristine, and daunorubicin (which was successful on two previous occasions). After remission is induced and she begins weekly maintenance therapy with vincristine and cyclophosphamide, she complains of muscle weakness. Neurologic examination shows evidence of bilateral footdrop and loss of deep tendon reflexes. The cancer chemotherapeutic agent most likely responsible for this patient's neurotoxicity is

○ A. asparaginase
○ B. cyclophosphamide
○ C. daunorubicin
○ D. prednisone
○ E. vincristine

50. A 53-year-old man who works on the hog-slaughtering floor of a pork-processing plant complains that he has been losing weight for 4 weeks and is suffering from a fever, chills, night sweats, fatigue, and myalgia. Physical examination shows lymphadenopathy and splenomegaly. Granulomas are seen in a liver biopsy specimen. Blood and bone marrow cultures grow a gram-negative coccobacillus that is urease-positive and oxidase-positive but does not ferment carbohydrates. A member of which of the following genera is the most likely cause of the disease?

○ A. *Bordetella*
○ B. *Brucella*
○ C. *Francisella*
○ D. *Pasteurella*
○ E. *Yersinia*

ANSWERS AND DISCUSSIONS

1. **D** (myasthenia gravis) is correct. Myasthenia gravis is a disorder of neuromuscular function caused by the presence of antibodies to acetylcholine receptors at the neuromuscular junction. This patient is within the median age range of onset in women (15–30 years) and has many signs and symptoms of the disease, including fatigue and eye muscle weakness. Edrophonium is a short-acting anticholinesterase that improves signs and symptoms of the disease, which helps to confirm the diagnosis.

   A (Duchenne muscular dystrophy) is incorrect. Duchenne muscular dystrophy is a chronic and progressive form of muscular dystrophy that begins during childhood. It is inherited as an X-linked recessive trait and affects only males.
   B (lesion in the basal ganglia) is incorrect. The basal ganglia "fine tune" motor signals before they project to the corticospinal tract. Damage to the basal ganglia results in the "poverty of movement" (subtle tremors) characteristic of Parkinson's disease.
   C (lesion in the cerebellum) is incorrect. The cerebellum projects to the brain stem and thalamus to help control balance, posture, and voluntary movement. A cerebellar lesion could make it difficult to raise the arms or walk up stairs. It would not interfere with the activity of the ocular muscles, which are innervated by the oculomotor nerve (CN III), which originates in a higher region of the brain.
   E (tardive dyskinesia) is incorrect. Tardive dyskinesia is an extrapyramidal disorder characterized by abnormal and stereotypical involuntary movements. It is triggered by certain drugs.

2. **C** (7–11 years) is correct. The concepts of conservation and reversibility imply an understanding of how different objects can simultaneously be similar. According to Piaget's stages of cognitive development, these concepts should be learned between the ages of 7–11 years. A child who recognizes that water and ice are different forms of the same object, and that the shape of the container does not change the amount of liquid it contains, exhibits the level of thought referred to as concrete operations.

   A (2–4 years) and B (4–7 years) are incorrect. From ages 2–7 years, a child is typically in the preoperational thought phase. During this phase, the child is able to use symbols and language and understand the permanence of objects. Children in this age range also demonstrate egocentrism and a belief that events that occur together cause one another.
   D (11–13 years) and E (13–18 years) are incorrect. Formal operations should begin by 11 years of age and continue throughout adolescence and adulthood. During this phase of cognitive devel-

opment, an individual displays abstract thinking and the ability to complete both deductive and inductive reasoning.

3. *E* (increased plasma norepinephrine concentration) is correct. Pain commonly occurring after surgery causes increased blood levels of norepinephrine and increased sympathetic activity to the gut. Both of these factors decrease gut motility and therefore decrease bowel sounds.

A (decreased sympathetic activity to the gut) is incorrect. Sympathetic activity to the gut decreases motility and bowel sounds. Decreased sympathetic activity will remove the inhibitory effect on motility.
B (increased activity of the gastrocolic reflex) is incorrect. The gastrocolic reflex increases gut motility and bowel sounds in the presence of food in the stomach.
C (increased parasympathetic activity to the gut) is incorrect. Increased parasympathetic activity to the gut will increase motility and increase bowel sounds. Painful stimulation of the abdomen will decrease parasympathetic activity.
D (increased plasma acetylcholine concentration) is incorrect. Acetylcholine is metabolized so rapidly that it is not present in plasma in significant quantities. Acetylcholine, as a parasympathetic mediator, will increase motility and bowel sounds.

4. *E* (right internal capsule) is correct. The internal capsule contains upper motor neurons, which terminate on cranial nerve motor nuclei and alpha motor neurons in the spinal cord. Damage to upper motor neurons that synapse on spinal nuclei can result in contralateral spastic paralysis in the arm and leg. Some of the upper motor neurons traveling through the genu of the internal capsule innervate the nucleus of the facial nerve (CN VII). CN VII fibers that innervate the lower face receive input only from the contralateral cortex; those that innervate the upper face receive bilateral innervation. Thus, if the right internal capsule is destroyed, input to the facial nucleus will be differentially affected. The patient would not be able to move the muscles of facial expression below the eyes on the left side of the face, but would be able to move muscles of facial expression above the eyes on both sides of the face. This effect is reflected in the patient's inability to move the left side of the mouth when she smiles, while contracting the frontalis muscle symmetrically when she raises her brow.

A (left basilar pons) is incorrect. A lesion in the basilar pons may damage CN VII, which exits from the pontomedullary border. A lesion in the left basilar pons would damage the facial nerves serving the left side of the face. This could explain the patient's asymmetrical smile, but not the symmetrical wrinkles on her brow. A lesion in the left basilar pons could also damage local corticospinal fibers and cause spastic paralysis in the limbs. However, this would affect the right side of the body, not the left.

B   (left facial nerve) is incorrect. A lesion affecting CN VII motor fibers could cause the patient to have difficulty smiling, but would not affect her arms or legs. Additionally, both the upper (e.g., the frontalis) and lower (e.g., "smiling") muscles of facial expression would be affected.

C   (left precentral gyrus) is incorrect. The precentral gyrus projects to the medullary pyramids, where upper motor neurons cross to innervate anterior horn neurons on the opposite side of the body. Damage to fibers descending from the left precentral gyrus would cause paralysis on the right side of the body, not the left. Corticonuclear fibers descending from the same gyrus would project to the right facial nucleus, causing asymmetry on the right side of the mouth, not the left.

D   (right caudal medulla) is incorrect. A lesion in the corticospinal tract, as it descends through the right caudal medulla, could cause spastic paralysis in the left arm and leg, but not in the face. The muscles of facial expression are controlled by CN VII, the nuclei of which lie rostral to this lesion (specifically, the pontomedullary junction).

5. *B*   (decreased arterial pH; increased arterial PCO_2; increased serum HCO_3^-) is correct. The patient has chronic obstructive pulmonary disease (COPD) with cyanosis secondary to hypoxemia (decreased arterial PO_2). Chronic bronchitis is the primary type of COPD in a patient who has had a productive cough for the majority of the time he has smoked. Obstruction to airflow secondary to inflammation and increased mucus production is at the level of the terminal bronchioles. Therefore, during expiration, air with high concentrations of CO_2 is trapped behind the obstruction. Retention of CO_2 in the alveoli increases the arterial PCO_2, causing respiratory acidosis. Point B on the graph depicts an acid arterial pH, a PCO_2 close to the 60 mm Hg isobar, and an HCO_3^- level above the normal of 24 mEq/L. Because the patient has had COPD for most of his life, there has been ample time for the kidneys to reclaim and synthesize HCO_3^-, producing metabolic alkalosis to compensate for the respiratory acidosis. Compensation for all acid-base disorders brings the pH close to, but not into, the normal range for arterial pH. This describes a partially compensated acid-base condition. Full compensation rarely occurs because it implies that the arterial pH is brought back into the normal range. The absence of compensation indicates that there has not been enough time for the lungs to compensate for primary metabolic conditions or for the kidneys to compensate for primary respiratory conditions.

A   (decreased arterial pH; increased arterial PCO_2; increased serum HCO_3^-) is incorrect. These findings are most consistent with a partially compensated acute respiratory acidosis. When compared with B (a patient with chronic respiratory acidosis), the lack of adequate compensation has done little to raise the arterial pH. Examples of acute respiratory acidosis include depression of the medullary respiratory center (e.g., patient taking barbiturates); paralysis of the muscles of respiration (e.g., polio, Guillain-Barré syndrome); and severe pneumonia.

C   (increased arterial pH; increased arterial PCO_2; increased serum HCO_3^-) is incorrect. These findings are most consistent with a partially compensated primary metabolic alkalosis (compensation is respiratory acidosis). Examples include diuretics (patient taking primarily loop diuretics and thiazides), vomiting, and mineralocorticoid excess (e.g., primary aldosteronism).

D   (decreased arterial pH; decreased arterial PCO_2; decreased serum HCO_3^-) is incorrect. These findings are most consistent with a partially compensated primary metabolic acidosis (respiratory alkalosis is compensation). Examples include renal failure, lactic acidosis, ketoacidosis, and renal tubular acidosis.

E   (increased arterial pH; decreased arterial PCO_2; decreased serum HCO_3^-) is incorrect. These findings are most consistent with a partially compensated primary acute respiratory alkalosis (metabolic acidosis is compensation). Examples include anxiety, a pulmonary embolus, and restrictive lung disease (e.g., sarcoidosis).

F   (increased arterial pH; decreased arterial PCO_2; decreased serum HCO_3^-) is incorrect. These findings are most consistent with a partially compensated chronic respiratory alkalosis. Living at high altitudes is the best example of this condition.

6. **D**   (exotoxins that increase the synthesis of cyclic adenosine monophosphate) is correct. The patient's clinical and laboratory findings are consistent with the diagnosis of whooping cough (pertussis), a disease caused by *Bordetella pertussis*. The bacterium produces two important exotoxins, the pertussis toxin and the adenylate cyclase toxin. Both toxins increase cAMP levels, but they do so by different mechanisms. The actions of these exotoxins lead to an increase in respiratory secretions and mucus production and to the inhibition of phagocytic activity.

A   (capsule that activates complement) is incorrect. Although fresh isolates of *B. pertussis* are encapsulated, the capsule is not considered to be a virulence factor for *B. pertussis*.

B   (cytotoxin that causes the lysis of red blood cells) is incorrect. *B. pertussis* produces tracheal cytotoxin. This cytotoxin does not lyse red blood cells; it kills ciliated epithelial cells.

C   (enterotoxins that increase the level of intracellular cyclic guanosine monophosphate) is incorrect. *B. pertussis* does not produce enterotoxins and does not cause gastrointestinal manifestations.

E   (exotoxins that inhibit the synthesis of proteins) is incorrect. *B. pertussis* does not produce an exotoxin that directly inhibits protein synthesis.

7. **A**   (hemorrhagic fat necrosis of the pancreas with yellow soap deposits on adjacent adipose tissue) is correct. With the massive release of enzymes during the necrosis of the pancreas, the triglycerides stored in adipose tissue are digested into free fatty

acids, which can react with cations to form soap. Calcium and magnesium soaps are insoluble; as they are formed, they complex calcium removing it from circulation. If sufficient calcium soap is formed, the serum calcium level can be significantly diminished.

B (impacted gallstones in the ampulla of Vater with acute ascending cholangitis) is incorrect. Impacted gallstones with acute cholangitis would be a source of pain and shock due to gram-negative infection but would not account for the hypocalcemia.
C (perforation of a gastric ulcer with hemorrhage into the peritoneal cavity and marked chemical peritonitis) is incorrect. A perforated gastric ulcer is certainly a catastrophic event that can cause severe pain and sometimes shock, but it would not be expected to cause hypocalcemia.
D (rupture of the aorta with exsanguination into the retroperitoneal space) is incorrect. This condition would indeed be a source of shock, but it would not be expected to cause hypocalcemia.
E (swollen kidneys with a marked degree of necrosis of the proximal renal tubular epithelium) is incorrect. If the patient had been in shock for a sufficient length of time, he might have exhibited the changes associated with acute tubular necrosis. Although this would cause the electrolyte disturbance, it would not be a cause of acute hypocalcemia.

8. *E* (somatoform pain disorder) is correct. Chronic pain symptoms that occur in the absence of organic pathology and respond only partially to narcotics suggest that a somatoform pain disorder may be present. Pain disorders are most prominent in women in their 30s and 40s.

A (factitious disorder) is incorrect. The cardinal feature of a factitious disorder is deliberate production of symptoms in order to assume the sick role. Additional external incentives do not motivate the behavior. A patient with factitious disorder might intentionally inject feces into her body to create an infection that would lead to hospitalization.
B (major depressive disorder) is incorrect. Although depressed patients often present somatic complaints to their physicians, the disorder most prominently impacts mood. To diagnose a major depressive disorder, a seriously depressed mood or anhedonia must be present for at least 2 weeks in conjunction with three or four more symptoms of depression, and functional impairment must be displayed.
C (malingering) is incorrect. Malingering implies a deliberate attempt to produce symptoms because of external incentives (e.g., money, avoidance of responsibilities).
D (somatization disorder) is incorrect. Individuals with somatization disorder report multiple somatic complaints across various systems (e.g., gastrointestinal, cardiovascular, neurologic). This chronic disorder begins before age 30 and the prognosis is guarded.

9. *E*   (pralidoxime) is correct. The cholinergic syndrome caused by malathion is sometimes referred to as the **SLUDGE-BAM** syndrome and is characterized by the following:

> S = salivation, sweating, and secretions
> L = lacrimation
> U = urination
> D = defecation
> G = gastrointestinal upset
> E = emesis
> plus
> B = bronchoconstriction and bradycardia
> A = abdominal cramps
> M = miosis and muscle fasciculations

Muscle weakness, fasciculations, and labored breathing represent the nicotinic effects of malathion intoxication, while the other manifestations represent the muscarinic effects. Malathion is an irreversible organophosphate cholinesterase inhibitor. Its covalent binding with cholinesterase is stabilized through an "aging" process. If pralidoxime (2-PAM) is administered before the acetylcholinesterase has been irreversibly bound ("aged"), the drug will reverse the patient's skeletal muscle weakness and fasciculations.

A   (atropine) is incorrect. In this case, atropine would be used to reverse the muscarinic effects of malathion intoxication. Atropine would not reverse the nicotinic effects.
B   (ipecac) is incorrect. Ipecac is an emetic agent that acts by stimulating the chemoreceptor trigger zone. It is used in the early management of patients who have swallowed one of a variety of poisonous agents, but it is not helpful in patients who have inhaled poisonous agents.
C   (nicotine) is incorrect. In cases of malathion intoxication, nicotine would worsen the symptoms. Nicotine patches are used in smoking cessation programs.
D   (physostigmine) is incorrect. Physostigmine inhibits cholinesterase and would worsen the symptoms of malathion intoxication. Physostigmine is used to treat glaucoma and to treat severe intoxication with anticholinergics.

10. *E*   (defective symport system) is correct. Not all transport processes are directly driven by the hydrolysis of adenosine triphosphate (ATP). Instead, some are driven by the energy stored in ion gradients. These processes are coupled to the flow of an ion down its electrochemical gradient and are called secondary active transporters. In eukaryotes, Na^+ is usually the cotransported ion. The coupled transporters are divided into symporters and antiporters. A symporter carries two substances in the same direction, while an antiporter carries two substances in opposite

directions. Amino acids are transported by symporters, so impaired amino acid uptake from the extracellular space would be attributable to a defective symport system.

A (defect in Ca^{2+} ATPase) is incorrect. Ca^{2+} ATPase is found in the sarcoplasmic reticulum membrane of skeletal muscles, where it plays an important role in muscle contraction. It is also found in the plasma membrane, where it acts to maintain low cytoplasmic levels of calcium.
B (defect in gap junctions) is incorrect. Gap junctions are large aqueous channels for passive transport of small hydrophilic molecules and ions. Gap junctions are cell-to-cell channels that serve as passageways between contiguous cells. Amino acids can flow through gap junctions, but they flow only from cell to cell (not from extracellular space to cell).
C (defect in Na^+, K^+-ATPase) is incorrect. Na^+, K^+-ATPase maintains the sodium and potassium concentration difference and is an integral part of the Na^+,K^+ pump. The concentration of K^+ is much higher inside cells than outside. For Na^+, the reverse is true. The splitting of ATP provides the energy needed for the active transport of these ions.
D (defective antiport system) is incorrect. As discussed in E, an antiporter carries two substances in the opposite direction. An example is the Na^+,Ca^{2+} antiporter that works in parallel with Ca^{2+} ATPase to maintain a low concentration of Ca^{2+} in the cytosol. Calcium ions are pumped out of the cell while sodium ions enter the cell.

11. *A* (abnormally low arterial O_2 content) is correct. Normal arterial O_2 content is 0.2 mL O_2/mL blood. It is likely that this patient's low arterial O_2 content is related to the reduced hematocrit, indicating that the O_2-carrying capacity of the blood is reduced. The reduced hematocrit might be a result of either occult bleeding or inadequate production of red cells.

B (depressed cardiac ejection fraction) is incorrect. Ejection fraction is normal ($100 - 30/100 = 0.7$).
C (increased extraction of O_2 by peripheral tissues) is incorrect. The O_2 extraction is normal or below normal.
D (increased metabolic demand as reflected in the heart rate) is incorrect. Activity or anxiety that increases metabolic demand also increases heart rate, but this patient's heart rate is within the normal range for her age.
E (systemic hypertension) is incorrect. The patient's blood pressure is borderline elevated. Systemic hypertension is not a cause of shortness of breath.

12. *D* (spina bifida occulta) is correct. The infant has a 3-cm, slightly elevated patch of skin with coarse hair and pigmentation in the midline of the lumbosacral region, and is diagnosed with spina bifida occulta. Failure of the neural tube to close disrupts the fusion of the overlying vertebral arches, resulting in an

open vertebral canal or spina bifida. Spina bifida occulta, the mildest form of the condition, usually occurs in the lumbosacral region and does not involve neural tissue. This defect in the vertebral arch is frequently indicated by a patch of hair, pigmentation, or an angioma. Studies confirm that folic acid supplements taken during pregnancy significantly reduce the risk of neural tube defects in infants. The US Public Health Service recommends that all women of childbearing age take 0.4 mg of vitamin B_{12} daily to reduce the risk of neural tube defects during pregnancy.

A (lentigo melanoma) is incorrect. Lentigo melanomas are flat, tan lesions typically larger than 3 cm, which occur on sun-exposed areas of skin in older adults. They are the least aggressive of the cutaneous melanomas. Lentigo melanomas occur in about 10%–15% of the melanomas.

B (myelomeningocele) is incorrect. Myelomeningocele, a kind of spina bifida cystica, refers to the condition in which neural tissue is included in the meningeal sac. It occurs more often and is a more severe anomaly than spina bifida cystica with a meningocele.

C (rachischisis) is incorrect. In rachischisis, the most extreme neural tube defect, the neural folds fail to elevate and remain flattened. The spinal cord is represented by an exposed mass of undifferentiated neural tissue. The defect may be extensive, as in craniorachischisis totalis, or restricted to a small area. Cranioschisis is incompatible with life.

13. **E** (M protein) is correct. The clinical and laboratory findings are consistent with the diagnosis of pharyngitis caused by *Streptococcus pyogenes*. M proteins are major virulence factors for *S. pyogenes* because they enable the organism to resist phagocytosis. They do this by binding to factor H, which degrades C3b, the main opsonizing component of the alternative complement pathway.

A (F protein) is incorrect. The F protein functions as an adhesion for epithelial cells. It has no role in the activation of complement components.

B (group-specific carbohydrate) is incorrect. The group-specific carbohydrates are useful for classification purposes but are not major virulence factors.

C (hyaluronic acid) is incorrect. The capsule of *S. pyogenes* is composed of nonimmunogenic hyaluronic acid. It is antiphagocytic but has no role in the inactivation of complement components.

D (lipoteichoic acid) is incorrect. Lipoteichoic acids are proinflammatory (similar to lipopolysaccharide), but they have no role in the inactivation of complement components.

14. *A* (block ATP-dependent K$^+$ channels in the pancreatic beta cells) is correct. Glipizide, chlorpropamide, glyburide, and tolbutamide are examples of orally administered sulfonylurea drugs that act by blocking ATP-dependent K$^+$ channels in beta cells of the pancreas. The resulting depolarization opens voltage-sensitive Ca^{2+} channels. The increase in intracellular Ca^{2+} then causes the release of insulin. The most common side effect of the orally administered sulfonylureas is hypoglycemia. Agents that act by opening (rather than blocking) ATP-dependent K$^+$ channels include diazoxide, thiazide, and loop diuretics. These agents prevent the release of insulin and can cause hyperglycemia.

B (decrease hepatic production of glucose and improve insulin sensitivity) is incorrect. Metformin is an oral antidiabetic drug thought to act by decreasing hepatic production of glucose and improving insulin sensitivity. Because this drug does not cause the release of insulin, its use is not associated with hypoglycemia. Metformin use is associated with lactic acidosis, a rare but serious side effect that is more likely to occur in diabetic patients who have impaired renal function.

C (directly open voltage-dependent Ca^{2+} channels in the pancreatic beta cells) is incorrect. No drug acts by directly opening voltage-dependent Ca^{2+} channels.

D (increase transcription of insulin-responsive genes that control glucose uptake) is incorrect. Rosiglitazone is an oral antidiabetic agent believed to act by increasing transcription of insulin-responsive genes. In target tissue (skeletal muscle and adipose tissue), this causes an increase in sensitivity to insulin and thereby lowers the elevated plasma glucose level. Because rosiglitazone does not cause the release of insulin, its use is not associated with hypoglycemia.

E (inhibit 5α-glucosidase activity in the brush border of the small intestine) is incorrect. Acarbose is an oral antidiabetic agent that inhibits 5α-glucosidase activity, prevents the conversion of starches and disaccharides to absorbable monosaccharides, and limits the postprandial rise in the plasma glucose level. Because acarbose does not cause the release of insulin, its use is not associated with hypoglycemia.

15. *C* (endotoxemia) is correct. Endotoxin (lipopolysaccharide), a component of the cell walls of gram-negative bacteria, binds to CD14 receptors. It causes a cascade of events that result in shock, metabolic failure, disseminated intravascular coagulopathy, and eventually multiple organ failure.

A (anaphylactic reaction) is incorrect. No immunologically mediated event has occurred in this case. Production of an anaphylactic (type I hypersensitivity) reaction requires a history of a prior sensitizing event and then challenge with the sensitizing antigen.

B (cardiogenic shock) is incorrect. Although there is an element of myocardial dysfunction in endotoxemia, cardiogenic shock is not the proximate cause.

D (hemorrhage) is incorrect. Nothing in either the history or presenting physical findings of this patient suggests hemorrhage.

E (neurogenic shock) is incorrect. Neurogenic shock is an uncommon type of shock and is generally the result of central nervous system injury. No such event has occurred in this case.

16. *C* (Langerhans' cells) is correct. The patient's clinical manifestations are consistent with the diagnosis of dermatitis due to contact with poison ivy. Langerhans' cells are a type of antigen-presenting cell located exclusively in the stratum spinosum of the epidermis. These cells play a central role in the pathogenesis of contact dermatitis. Specifically, they recognize and transfer molecules from the surface of the skin to T cells located in the neighboring dermis. T cells migrate to nearby lymph nodes, where they proliferate to produce a clone of cells. The clones then migrate from the lymph nodes to the original area of poison ivy contact, where they play a central role in responding to the allergen. The poison ivy rash is a morphologic manifestation of this response.

A (keratinocytes) and B (keratocytes) are incorrect. Keratinocytes are cells that synthesize keratin, a substance that protects the skin from abrasions. Keratocytes are special fibroblasts that are located in the substantia propria of the cornea. Although the two types of cells have similar spellings, keratocytes in the cornea have nothing to do with keratinocytes in the skin.

D (melanocytes) is incorrect. Melanocytes are cells that synthesize and secrete melanin granules. These granules protect underlying skin tissues from ultraviolet light.

E (Merkel cells) is incorrect. Merkel cells are mechanoreceptors and are not involved in the development of contact dermatitis.

17. *D* (mesencephalon) is correct. A lesion in the midbrain will disrupt the transmission of efferent signals along the corticospinal tract and fibers within brain stem motor programs that control oculomotor (CN III) activity. CN III targets include the striated muscles of the eyelids. Since CN III fibers innervate their targets ipsilaterally, right ptosis (droopy eyelid) indicates damage to the right CN III nucleus or its nerve as it exits through the corticospinal fibers and, therefore, damage to the right mesencephalon. Since most of the fibers in the corticospinal tract cross the midline of the brain within the medulla, a lesion in the right mesencephalon will disrupt motor activity on the left side of the body and, thus, could also be responsible for left hemiparesis. This lesion is sometimes called the superior alternating hemiplegia.

A (cavernous sinus) is incorrect. The cavernous sinus is a space within the dura mater that lies adjacent to the sphenoid bone. Although several cranial nerves course through it, a lesion in the cavernous sinus would not cause hemiparesis.

B (cerebral cortex) is incorrect. A lesion in the right motor cortex could contribute to left hemiparesis by blocking efferent signals descending along the corticospinal fibers, most of which cross at the medullary pyramids. However, it would not account for the lower motor neuron lesion of CN III as exhibited by ptosis.

C (left genu of the internal capsule) is incorrect. The left genu contains descending upper motor neurons that synapse on cranial nerve motor nuclei. A lesion affecting this area alone could result in ptosis. It would not cause hemiparesis, however, because these neurons do not project to motor nuclei in the spinal cord.

E (midline of the medulla) is incorrect. A lesion in the midline of the medulla is more likely to affect axial muscles than muscles in the limbs. It would also damage the brain stem motor program that regulates CN III activity.

18. *C* (curve C) is correct. Sickle cell anemia is a form of hemolytic anemia that occurs almost exclusively in black patients. It is caused by the substitution of valine for glutamine at position 6 of the β chain, resulting in the production of an abnormal hemoglobin, hemoglobin S (HbS). In the figure, curve C represents the β chain.

A (curve A) is incorrect. In the figure, curve A represents the α chain. Decreased synthesis or absence of the α chain leads to α-thalassemia, not to sickle cell anemia.

B (curve B) is incorrect. In the figure, chain B represents the γ chain. Production of this chain diminishes shortly before birth. By the time a child reaches the age of 3 months, γ chains have been replaced by β chains.

D (curve D) and E (curve E) are incorrect. In the figure, curves D and E represent the ε and ζ chains, respectively. Production of these chains is limited to the early embryonic stage.

19. *D* (the pediatrician should contact child protective services immediately and ask for an investigation) is correct. Bruises and contusions in the vaginal and pelvic region of any 9-year-old child should lead the pediatrician to suspect sexual abuse. Regardless of circumstances, any form of suspected abuse, including sexual, must be reported by a physician. This allows further investigation by the state's child protective services.

A (the child must admit to being sexually abused before child protective services can be contacted) is incorrect. This child is too young to understand sexual abuse or to consent to a sexual act. She may have been threatened, or she may be too frightened to disclose the abuse. Questioning her about the abuse must be done cautiously. A child's acknowledgment of abuse is not necessary to report an incident.

B (the pediatrician must find additional evidence of deprivation and neglect to assume sexual abuse) and E (the pediatrician should contact child protective services only if there is additional evidence of physical abuse) are incorrect. Suspicion of sexual abuse warrants investigation regardless of additional signs of neglect, deprivation, or physical abuse.

C (the pediatrician should ask the parents if sexual abuse occurred, and if they reply in a negative manner, nothing should be reported) is incorrect. Parents often are unaware that their child has been sexually abused, and in some cases, they may be the perpetrators. Although the pediatrician may want to talk to the parents, acknowledgment of the abuse or permission to contact child protective services by the parents is not necessary to report the incident.

20. *B* (binding to the 50S ribosomal subunit, thereby preventing translocation of peptidyl tRNA from the acceptor site to the donor site) is correct. The patient's symptoms and serologic test results are consistent with the diagnosis of legionnaires' disease (pneumonia due to *Legionella*). Macrolide antibiotics (such as azithromycin, clarithromycin, and erythromycin) are the drugs of choice for treating this disease. They bind to the 50S subunit of bacterial ribosomes and prevent translocation of the peptidyl tRNA from the acceptor site to the donor site. Alternative agents for treating legionnaires' disease include tetracyclines (such as doxycycline) or fluoroquinolones (such as ciprofloxacin and ofloxacin).

A (binding to the 30S ribosomal subunit, thereby preventing the initiation of protein synthesis) is incorrect. This is a description of the mechanism of action of aminoglycosides, such as amikacin, gentamicin, and streptomycin. These drugs are ineffective for treating legionnaires' disease.

C (inhibiting DNA-dependent RNA polymerase, thereby preventing RNA synthesis) is incorrect. This is a description of the mechanism of action of rifampin. This drug is ineffective for treating legionnaires' disease.

D (inhibiting peptidoglycan synthase [transglycosylase], thereby preventing elongation of the peptidoglycan backbone of the bacterial cell wall) is incorrect. This is a description of the mechanism of action of vancomycin. This drug is ineffective for treating legionnaires' disease.

E (inhibiting transpeptidase, thereby preventing the cross-linking of the bacterial cell wall) is incorrect. This is a description of the mechanism of action of beta-lactam antimicrobials, such as carbapenems, cephalosporins, monobactams, and penicillins. These drugs are ineffective for treating legionnaires' disease.

21. *B* (C1 esterase inhibitor) is correct. The patient's history and clinical manifestations are consistent with the diagnosis of hereditary angioedema. This disease, which is also known as hereditary angioneurotic edema, is caused by a deficiency of C1 esterase inhibitor and is one of the most important complement deficiencies.

A   (anaphylatoxin inactivator) is incorrect. A deficiency of anaphylatoxin inactivator and the consequent failure to inactivate C3a, C4a, and C5a could cause edema. However, reports of anaphylatoxin inactivator deficiency are rare.
C   (C4 binding protein) is incorrect. The C4 binding protein inactivates C3 convertase. A deficiency of this protein is rare.
D   (properdin) is incorrect. An individual with a properdin deficiency would most likely be unable to activate complement in the absence of antibodies and would therefore have difficulty clearing infectious agents and endotoxins from the body. A deficiency of this protein is rare.
E   (vitronectin) is incorrect. Vitronectin is a protein that binds to the C5b,6,7 complex, thereby preventing insertion of the membrane attack complex. A deficiency of this protein is rare.

22. *D*   (vitamin E) is correct. As an antioxidant, vitamin E supports normal peripheral nerve function by preventing damage to Schwann cells and dorsal root ganglia. Damage to Schwann cells would lead to demyelination, which plays a role in ataxia and areflexia. Damage to dorsal root ganglia would impair sensory transmission from primary afferents to secondary afferents (which travel in the posterior columns). Therefore, administration of vitamin E may be a helpful component of treatment for this patient.

A   (vitamin A) is incorrect. Vitamin A prevents night blindness and xerophthalmia by supporting lipids (in the membranous disks of photoreceptors) and epithelial tissue (by maintaining differentiation and mucous production). Vitamin A also supports normal osteoid activity (for bone remodelling during growth) and gonadal activity (for fertility), and it may also support macrophage activity. A role for vitamin A in neuronal activity has not yet been identified.
B   (vitamin C) is incorrect. A deficiency in vitamin C (ascorbic acid) results in scurvy or other evidence of abnormal collagen or connective tissue metabolism. It does not result in peripheral neuropathy.
C   (vitamin D) is incorrect. Vitamin D can influence nerve function through its effect on plasma calcium homeostasis. When plasma calcium levels fall, parathyroid hormone is released and triggers the production of 1,25-dihydroxycholecalciferol (1,25-OH; the active form of vitamin D); this causes plasma calcium levels to rise. Calcium helps determine the rate at which neurotransmitters are released from the axon terminal of nerve cells. However, the amount of damage necessary to cause ataxia, areflexia, or the loss of posterior column activity cannot be accounted for by calcium or vitamin D deficiency alone. Enervation (as is seen in patients with vitamin E deficiency) is a more likely cause of these events.
E   (vitamin K) is incorrect. Vitamin K supports blood clotting through its role in the gamma carboxylation of glutamic acid, which is a step in the production of prothrombin and possibly

other proteins (e.g., proteins that help maintain normal activity in bone, connective tissue, and the kidneys). A specific role for this vitamin in nerve function has not yet been identified.

23. *C* (indirect inguinal hernia) is correct. The testes develop within the abdomen and descend along a predetermined path through the abdominal wall and into the scrotum. The peritoneal cavity is also open along this path via the processus vaginalis. Normally, the defect created by the passage of the testis and the proximal extent of the processus vaginalis closes following descent of the testis. Occasionally, this opening either fails to close or does not close properly. Straining causes the channel to reopen, and viscera follow the course of the processus vaginalis through the deep inguinal ring, inguinal canal, and superficial inguinal ring.

Hernias can extend all the way to the scrotum. A hernia that follows the path of the descent of the testis obliquely through the wall is termed an indirect inguinal hernia. Because both direct and indirect inguinal hernias pass through the superficial inguinal ring of the inguinal canal, the relationship of the origin of the hernial sac to the inferior epigastric vessels is critical to diagnosis of the type of inguinal hernia. When the hernial sac passes lateral to the inferior epigastric vessels, it is an indirect inguinal hernia.

A (direct inguinal hernia) is incorrect. A direct inguinal hernia is a weakness in the anterior abdominal wall between the inguinal ligament, the inferior epigastric vessels, and the lateral border of the rectus abdominis muscle. Damage to a fused area of aponeuroses from the internal abdominal oblique and transversus abdominis muscles (the conjoint tendon) results in the bulging of abdominal viscera through the superficial inguinal ring onto the surface of the inguinal region of the lower abdomen. Because the defect takes the hernial sac directly through the abdominal wall and into the inguinal region, it is termed a direct inguinal hernia.

B (femoral hernia) is incorrect. A femoral hernia, which does not involve descent of the testis in any way, occurs inferior to the inguinal ligament at its medial end. This type of hernia is a defect between the abdominal cavity and the anterior thigh through a space created by the passage of the femoral vessels and lymphatics between the abdomen and thigh. The blood and lymphatic vessels are surrounded by a connective tissue sheath (femoral sheath), with three compartments: a lateral compartment containing the femoral artery, a middle compartment containing the femoral vein, and a medial compartment containing the lymphatics. The medial compartment (or femoral canal) is larger than might be deemed necessary for the passage of the lymphatics. The femoral canal is closed off by fascia superiorly at the femoral ring. If not closed off effectively, abdominal viscera can herniate through the femoral ring and femoral canal and into the anterior thigh.

D (obturator hernia) is incorrect. An obturator hernia, which is not related to descent of the testis, consists of herniation of viscera through a hole (probably related to the hole for the passage of the obturator vessels and nerve) in the obturator foramen and into the medial thigh. The obturator foramen is closed off by the obturator membrane, except at the point of passage of the obturator vessels and nerve from the pelvis into the medial thigh.

E (umbilical hernia) is incorrect. An umbilical hernia, which does not relate to descent of the testis, involves the anterior abdominal wall at the umbilicus. It results from weakness or damage to the area of the umbilicus.

24. *D* (sarcoidosis) is correct. Sarcoidosis typically produces noncaseating ("hard") granulomas, rather than lesions characterized by central caseous necrosis. In addition, multisystem involvement, including skin, lungs, lymph nodes, liver, spleen, eyes, and the small bones of the hand and feet, is typical. Sarcoidosis occurs mainly in individuals between the ages of 20 and 40 years; risk is higher in the black population.

A (coccidioidomycosis) is incorrect. *Coccidioides immitis* generally produces large, easily identifiable spherules. Some caseous necrosis would occur with coccidioidomycosis. The disease is endemic in the southwestern United States, not North Carolina where this patient resides.

B (cryptococcosis) is incorrect. *Cryptococcus neoformans* is a large organism that is usually not difficult to demonstrate. Inflammation associated with *C. neoformans* is often mild.

C (histoplasmosis) and E (tuberculosis) are incorrect. In some affected patients (unlike this woman), central nervous system symptoms may develop. *Histoplasma capsulatum* mimics tuberculosis histologically, and the presence of caseating granulomas is expected. *H. capsulatum* is endemic to the Ohio-Mississippi river valleys and in areas of northern Maryland, southern Pennsylvania, central New York, and Texas.

25. *B* *(Microsporum canis)* is correct. The patient's clinical manifestations are typical of tinea capitis (ringworm of the scalp). Of the fungi listed, *M. canis* is the most likely etiologic agent. *M. canis* grows outside the hair shaft (ectothrix growth), causing a sheath of spores to cover the hair surface. Since the organism is zoophilic, the inflammatory reaction is generally more severe. The treatment of choice is orally administered griseofulvin.

A *(Candida albicans)* is incorrect. *C. albicans* does not cause tinea capitis and does not infect the hair. Hair samples would not fluoresce when examined under a Wood's lamp.

C *(Trichophyton mentagrophytes)* and E *(Trichophyton verrucosum)* are incorrect. Although *T. mentagrophytes* and *T. verrucosum* both cause an ectothrix type of tinea capitis, the affected hair does not fluoresce when examined under a Wood's lamp.

D   *(Trichophyton rubrum)* is incorrect. *T. rubrum* causes tinea corporis and tinea cruris, but it generally does not cause infections of the scalp and hair. Hair samples would not fluoresce when examined under a Wood's lamp.

26. *C*   (hydrochlorothiazide) is correct. Thiazides produce their diuretic effect by acting in the early portion of the distal tubule to inhibit the Na^+,Cl^- symporter. An increase in the amount of Na^+ delivered to the collecting duct causes an increase in the amount of exchange of potassium, and this results in hypokalemia. In addition, by a mechanism not completely understood, thiazides increase proximal tubular reabsorption of Ca^{2+}, and this results in hypercalcemia. Thiazides are actively secreted by the organic acid transporter in the proximal tubule. The competition with uric acid for the organic acid transporter can result in hyperuricemia. Thiazides open ATP-dependent K^+ channels in the beta cells of the pancreas, block the release of insulin, and cause hyperglycemia.

A   (acetazolamide) is incorrect. Acetazolamide and dorzolamide are carbonic anhydrase inhibitors. These drugs produce their diuretic effect by acting in the proximal tubule to inhibit carbonic anhydrase. This results in a loss of bicarbonate and sodium. Usually, these inhibitors are prescribed for the treatment of glaucoma. Less commonly, acetazolamide is given to treat acute mountain sickness or is used to alkalinize the urine and facilitate renal excretion of weak acids taken in overdose.

B   (furosemide) is incorrect. Furosemide and other loop diuretics produce their diuretic effect by acting in the ascending limb of Henle's loop to inhibit the Na^+,K^+,$2Cl^-$ cotransport system. Unlike thiazides, loop diuretics decrease the transepithelial electrical potential, thereby increasing the renal excretion of Ca^{2+} and resulting in hypocalcemia. Because of this action, the loop diuretics can be used to treat hypercalcemia. Like thiazides, loop diuretics will produce hypokalemia, hyperuricemia, and hyperglycemia, and they do so via the same mechanisms (described above). The use of loop diuretics has been associated with hearing impairment.

D   (mannitol) is incorrect. Mannitol produces its diuretic effect by acting primarily in the proximal tubule and descending limb of Henle's loop. The drug creates an osmotic gradient that favors the retention of water within the nephron. Mannitol is indicated for the prevention or treatment of the oliguric phase of acute renal failure and for the reduction of intracranial or intraocular pressure.

E   (triamterene) is incorrect. Triamterene and amiloride are examples of potassium-sparing diuretics. They produce their diuretic effect by acting in the collecting duct to block Na^+ transport through channels in the luminal membrane. Potassium-sparing diuretics are used to offset the potassium loss associated with the use of thiazides and other potassium-wasting diuretics.

27. *C* (a large area of the lung is ventilated but not perfused) is correct. The right-hand peak consists of areas of the lung with high ventilation/perfusion ratios (i.e., areas that are ventilated but not perfused).

A (a large area of the lung is neither ventilated nor perfused) is incorrect. An area of the lung that is neither ventilated nor perfused will not be disclosed using the multiple inert gas elimination technique.
B (a large area of the lung is perfused but not ventilated) is incorrect. If a large area of the lung is perfused but not ventilated, then a large peak for blood flow not associated with a peak for ventilation occurs.
D (ventilation and perfusion are well balanced but depressed in all pulmonary units) is incorrect. The presence of a ventilation peak associated with a very low perfusion peak rules out this option.

28. *D* (synthesis of adhesion molecules) is correct. Neutrophil adhesion to endothelial cells (pavementing) is due to the synthesis of adhesion molecules, which are CD_{11}/CD_{18} complexes of glycoproteins. Both neutrophils and endothelial cells synthesize adhesion molecules. Neutrophil adhesion molecule synthesis is stimulated by the complement component C5a and leukotriene LTB_4. Synthesis of endothelial cell–derived adhesion molecules is stimulated by interleukin-1 and tumor necrosis factor. Congenital adhesion molecule deficiency can be acquired or genetic. A key feature is failure of separation of the umbilical cord and the absence of neutrophil pavementing and emigration into the umbilical tissue. These patients also have problems with wound healing.

A (activation of the complement system) is incorrect. Complement deficiencies are more often associated with susceptibility to infections than with adhesion molecule defects.
B (microtubule polymerization) is incorrect. This describes a rare autosomal recessive disease called Chédiak-Higashi syndrome, which is associated with severe infections related to defects in chemotaxis and phagocytosis.
C (respiratory burst mechanism) is incorrect. This describes chronic granulomatous disease (CGD) of childhood. CGD is a sex-linked recessive disease characterized by an absence of NADPH oxidase in the cell membranes of neutrophils and monocytes. In a normal neutrophil or monocyte, the presence of NADPH oxidase + NADPH causes the conversion of molecular oxygen into superoxide free radicals (FRs) in phagosomes. The energy released by this reaction is called the respiratory burst. Superoxide FRs then are converted by superoxide dismutase into peroxide. The lysosomal enzyme myeloperoxidase (MPO) then combines peroxide with chloride ions to produce bleach, which is bactericidal to bacteria. Hence, in patients with CGD, who are defi-

cient in NADPH oxidase, there is no respiratory burst, superoxide FRs, peroxide, or bleach to kill bacteria.
E (synthesis of myeloperoxidase) is incorrect. The loss of MPO is associated primarily with a microbicidal defect related to the inability to produce bleach in the phagosome. In contrast to CGD, the respiratory burst is intact in MPO deficiency.

29. *A* (binding to the 30S ribosomal subunit, thereby preventing attachment of the aminoacyl tRNA to the acceptor site) is correct. The patient's disease manifestations are consistent with syphilis, an infection caused by *Treponema pallidum*. Although penicillin G is the drug of choice, the patient's allergy to penicillin precludes its use. An alternative drug for the treatment of syphilis in this patient is a tetracycline, such as doxycycline. Tetracyclines inhibit protein synthesis by binding to the 30S subunit of the bacterial ribosome and preventing the attachment of the next aminoacyl tRNA to the acceptor site (A site).

B (binding to the 30S ribosomal subunit, thereby preventing formation of the initiation complex) is incorrect. This is a description of the mechanism of action of aminoglycosides. These drugs are inactive against *T. pallidum*.
C (inhibiting DNA gyrase, thereby preventing the synthesis of DNA) is incorrect. This is a description of the mechanism of action of fluoroquinolones. These drugs are inactive against *T. pallidum*.
D (inhibiting peptidoglycan synthase [transglycosylase], thereby preventing elongation of the peptidoglycan backbone of the bacterial cell wall) is incorrect. This is a description of the mechanism of action of vancomycin. This drug is inactive against *T. pallidum*.
E (inhibiting transpeptidase, thereby preventing the cross-linking of the bacterial cell wall) is incorrect. This is a description of the mechanism of action of beta-lactam antimicrobials. Some beta-lactams, such as penicillins and cephalosporins, are active against *T. pallidum* but should not be used to treat a patient with penicillin allergy. Other beta-lactams, such as carbapenems and monobactams, are not indicated for the treatment of syphilis.

30. *A* (mitochondrion) is correct. Mitochondrial proteins are synthesized by free ribosomes. At the amino terminus, each mitochondrial protein has a signal peptide that is 20–80 residues long. In the signal peptide, positively charged amino acids alternate with hydrophobic ones, and this enables the peptide to form an amphipathic α-helix. The amino-terminal mitochondrial signal peptide placed at the beginning of a cytosolic protein will target this protein to the mitochondrion. In addition to the signal peptide, which directs the protein to the mitochondrial matrix, there are signal sequences that direct proteins to the mitochondrial intermembrane space.

B   (nucleus) is incorrect. A nuclear localization signal directs nuclear proteins to the nucleus. The signal sequence is short (4–8 amino acids) and is rich in positively charged lysine and arginine residues, which can be located almost anywhere in the polypeptide chain. An example is the Pro-Lys-Lys-Lys-Arg-Lys-Val sequence.

C   (peroxisome) is incorrect. Proteins destined for peroxisomes have a specific signal sequence of three amino acids (for example, Ser-Lys-Leu) at their carboxyl terminus. A defect in the ability to import proteins into peroxisomes causes Zellweger syndrome, an inherited disorder that is characterized by severe abnormalities of the brain, liver, and kidneys. Affected patients die soon after birth.

D   (plasma membrane) is incorrect. Integral plasma membrane proteins that are initially found in the endoplasmic reticulum (ER) will move to the plasma membrane unless they carry instructions to the contrary.

E   (secretory vesicle) is incorrect. All proteins destined for secretion and for the plasma membrane are first imported cotranslationally into the lumen of the ER. Soluble proteins in the lumen of the ER emerge in constitutive secretory vesicles and will be exported unless special signals are present to direct them to the contrary. Secretory vesicles are a default destination.

31. C   (colchicine) is correct. The patient's presenting clinical and laboratory findings are consistent with a diagnosis of acute gouty arthritis. Acute attacks of gout can be treated with colchicine, indomethacin, sulindac, or naproxen. Colchicine has several actions. First, it binds to microtubules and thereby prevents the migration of phagocytes. Second, it blocks the release of inflammatory mediators (such as leukotriene B_4, or LTB_4) from granulocytes. Third, it arrests cells in metaphase. This third action of colchicine has nothing to do with its therapeutic effects in gout, but it may explain its toxicity to the gastrointestinal mucosa.

A   (allopurinol) is incorrect. Allopurinol is not effective in the treatment of an acute attack of gout, but it is beneficial for the long-term prevention of attacks in patients with gout. Allopurinol is converted to alloxanthine (oxypurinol), an agent that irreversibly inhibits xanthine oxidase and thereby blocks the synthesis of uric acid. Allopurinol treatment is useful in patients who underexcrete or overproduce uric acid. If allopurinol is given concurrently with drugs that are detoxified by xanthine oxidase (drugs such as azathioprine and mercaptopurine), the dosage of these drugs must be reduced.

B   (aspirin) is incorrect. Aspirin (acetylsalicylic acid, or ASA) would be of no benefit in terminating the patient's acute attack of gout and may even aggravate the condition. ASA has a dose-dependent effect on the renal excretion of uric acid. At low doses, ASA blocks the secretion of uric acid and causes hyperuricemia. At high doses, ASA blocks the reabsorption of uric acid and exerts a uricosuric effect.

D   (methotrexate) is incorrect. Methotrexate is not used for the treatment of gouty arthritis but is an excellent drug for the advanced treatment of rheumatoid arthritis.

E   (probenecid) is incorrect. Probenecid is not effective in the treatment of an acute attack of gout, but it is beneficial for the long-term prevention of attacks. Probenecid acts as a uricosuric agent to competitively block the proximal tubular reabsorption of uric acid. It is most useful in patients who underexcrete uric acid. Its utility is limited in those who overproduce uric acid or have a low glomerular filtration rate (<50 mL/min).

32. *C*   (into the vertebral canal inferior to the conus medullaris of the spinal cord) is correct. CSF is contained in the subarachnoid space, the space between the arachnoid and pia mater, and the procedure used to collect the fluid is by lumbar puncture (spinal tap). The spinal cord ends as a gradual taper, known as the conus medullaris, typically coming to an end at the lower border of L1 or at the upper border of L2. The nerve roots of the cauda equina "sprout" from the conus medullaris and extend caudally within the vertebral canal as far as the caudal end of the sacrum. Although these roots still represent nerve tissue, they are less susceptible to damage if entrance into the subarachnoid space is made by insertion between adjacent lamina below L2, which is the most prudent approach to a lumbar puncture.

A   (between T12 and L1) is incorrect. Insertion of the needle at T12–L1 would risk damaging the spinal cord. To protect against damage to delicate tissue of the central nervous system, the insertion point must be caudal to the termination of the spinal cord. The spinal cord ends at the level of the first and/or second lumbar vertebrae (L1–L2). Thus, spinal taps are typically at the L3 vertebral level or lower.

B   (into the dura mater but not the arachnoid layer) is incorrect. The layers that must be pierced to reach the CSF in the subarachnoid space include both the dura mater and arachnoid mater. On its way to the subarachnoid space, the needle also passes through the skin and fasciae, erector spinae muscles, interspinous ligaments, ligamentum flavum, epidural space, dura mater, subdural space, and the arachnoid mater.

D   (into the vertebral canal through the intervertebral foramen) is incorrect. Use of this route of entry is a poor approach and may prove impossible because of the angle of approach necessary to reach the intervertebral foramen, and because of the risk of damaging the exiting spinal nerve.

33. *C*   (malaria) is correct. The clinical and laboratory findings are consistent with the diagnosis of malaria. This disease can be caused by *Plasmodium falciparum, Plasmodium malariae, Plasmodium ovale,* or *Plasmodium vivax.* Plasmodia are blood- and tissue-dwelling protozoan parasites, and the schizont is part of the organism's erythrocytic asexual cycle. Chloroquine can be taken to prevent malaria in travelers to the Caribbean. The Carib-

bean is one of the few regions of the world in which *P. falcipa-rum* and other *Plasmodium* species are still sensitive to this drug. In regions where chloroquine resistance is reported, malaria can be prevented by taking an alternative drug, such as meflo-quine or doxycycline.

A (cryptosporidiosis) is incorrect. Infection with *Cryptosporidium parvum* is common in tropical countries, but the organism is a lumen-dwelling protozoan parasite and usually causes a self-limiting form of enterocolitis.

B (leishmaniasis) and E (trypanosomiasis) are incorrect. Leishmaniasis is caused by numerous *Leishmania* species, including *Leishmania braziliensis, Leishmania donovani,* and *Leishmania tropica* and is usually a cutaneous or mucocutaneous disease. *Trypanosoma brucei* causes African trypanosomiasis (sleeping sickness), while *Trypanosoma cruzi* causes Chagas' disease. The leishmania and trypanosomes are hemoflagellates, so laboratory findings associated with these organisms would differ from laboratory findings associated with plasmodia, which are sporozoans.

D (mucormycosis) is incorrect. Infections with zygomycetes, including *Rhizopus* species and *Mucor* species, cause various forms of mucormycosis, including rhinocerebral, pulmonary, and gastrointestinal mucormycosis. The zygomycetes are fungi, so the laboratory findings associated with these organisms would not be consistent with the case in question.

34. *A* (decreased renal production of 1,25-(OH)2D) is correct. Decreasing renal mass with aging means less production of dihydroxyvitamin D, removing the feedback inhibition of PTH. Increased PTH leads to the degradation of bone matrix.

B (gradually decreasing level of serum PTH) is incorrect. Serum PTH levels increase with aging. Decreased PTH levels slow bone loss and oppose the development of osteoporosis.

C (increased osteoblastic activity) is incorrect. A relative increase in osteoblastic activity strengthens bone.

D (increased renal production of dihydroxyvitamin D) is incorrect. Increased production of dihydroxyvitamin D inhibits PTH secretion.

E (lack of the usual effect of PTH on net renal phosphate secretion) is incorrect. PTH prevents phosphate reabsorption; there is no net secretion of phosphate. If less phosphate is secreted, more is available for bone formation.

35. *A* (coma and respiratory collapse) is correct. Alcohol acts as a central nervous system (CNS) depressant via mechanisms that are still unclear, but possibly by action on GABA receptors. At alcohol levels of 300–400 mg/dL, coma and respiratory collapse are likely. Individuals who chronically abuse the substance will tolerate higher levels.

B   (congestive cardiomyopathy) is incorrect. Long-term, rather than acute, alcohol abuse is strongly associated with congestive cardiomyopathy.

C   (development of acute yellow atrophy of the liver) is incorrect. Although ethanol is a direct hepatic toxin, it would not typically produce such severe damage.

D   (Korsakoff's syndrome) is incorrect. Korsakoff's syndrome, an amnestic syndrome, is a long-term effect of chronic alcoholism due to thiamine deficiency and direct toxicity.

E   (Wernicke's encephalopathy) is incorrect. Wernicke's encephalopathy, which involves confusion, ataxia, and ophthalmoplegia, is a long-term effect of chronic alcoholism due to thiamine deficiency.

36. *C*   (providing written instructions for the patient) is correct. A physician who provides written instructions will enhance compliance with a drug regimen and decrease the possibility that a patient will become confused about a physician's recommendations.

A   (adopting an authoritarian style with the patient) is incorrect. Collaborative relationships facilitate respect. An authoritarian style will likely lead to the patient perceiving the physician as cold, unapproachable, and uncaring.

B   (dividing the dose so the patient takes the drug four times a day) is incorrect. Dividing the dose unnecessarily into multiple dosages complicates instructions and decreases the probability that the patient will take the medication properly.

D   (refusing to serve as the patient's physician if the patient does not comply) is incorrect. Attempting to control the patient's behavior through withdrawal of services will likely lead to poorer compliance. Instead, the physician should attempt to use the ongoing relationship in a more productive manner.

E   (using medical jargon to illustrate the seriousness of the issue) is incorrect. A physician who uses medical jargon will most likely increase the chance that the patient will become confused and be unable to adhere to the recommendations. The diagnosis should be explained to the patient in understandable terms, and the physician should clearly explain how the drug will improve the patient's condition.

37. *A*   (hepatitis A virus) is correct. The virus responsible for the patient's clinical manifestations is hepatitis A virus (HAV), a member of the family *Picornaviridae*. HAV is transmitted by the fecal-oral route, and the incubation period is generally from 2–4 weeks. Manifestations of hepatitis A are due to inflammation-mediated damage to the liver. Although there is no specific treatment for the disease, a vaccine is available to prevent hepatitis A.

B   (hepatitis B virus) and C (hepatitis C virus) are incorrect. Hepatitis B virus (HBV) and hepatitis C virus (HCV) both cause hepatitis. However, HBV is a member of the family *Hepadnaviridae,* and HCV is a member of the family *Flaviviridae.*

D (hepatitis D virus) and E (hepatitis E virus) are incorrect. Hepatitis D virus (HDV) only causes coinfection with HBV. Although hepatitis E virus (HEV) causes a syndrome similar to hepatitis A and is also spread via the fecal-oral route, HEV is a member of the family *Caliciviridae.*

38. *A* (left dorsal and ventral cochlear nuclei) is correct. Information about sound is carried by the cochlear division of the vestibulocochlear nerve (CN VIII) to the ventral and dorsal cochlear nuclei. Beyond this point, the cochlear nuclei project through three pathways to the superior olivary nuclei, each of which must receive fibers from both ears in order to localize sound in space. Thus, lesions that are responsible for total unilateral hearing loss can occur no higher than the level of the cochlear nuclei.

B (left inferior colliculus) is incorrect. Each inferior colliculus contains axons that carry auditory information from both ears. Therefore, damage to the left inferior colliculus would not result in unilateral deafness.

C (left superior colliculus) is incorrect. Most of the fibers in the superior colliculi carry visual information. Some carry auditory and somesthetic information. All of this sensory information is assimilated by the superior colliculus, which then projects caudally to the upper cervical end of the tectospinal tract to facilitate touch and sound, as well as reflex turning of the head to the right. A lesion in the left superior colliculus would not cause unilateral deafness.

D (right medial geniculate nucleus) is incorrect. Most of the neurons in the inferior colliculus carry auditory information and project to the medial geniculate nucleus of the thalamus. However, the colliculi carry auditory information from both ears. Therefore, hearing loss will not occur in only one ear if the right medial geniculate nucleus is damaged.

E (right temporal lobe) is incorrect. The medial geniculate nucleus of the thalamus projects to the auditory cortex in the temporal lobe. This thalamic nucleus receives information from both ears (via the inferior colliculus). Therefore, damage to the right temporal lobe will not cause deafness in only one ear.

39. *E* (recognition of the 5′ splice site) is correct. The patient's clinical and laboratory findings are consistent with the diagnosis of systemic lupus erythematosus (SLE), a chronic immune disorder characterized by multisystem involvement and by clinical exacerbations and remissions. Loss of tolerance to autoantigens is central to the pathogenesis of SLE. Autoantibodies can be formed to DNA-RNA hybrids, ribosomal subunits, and the U1 small nuclear ribonucleoprotein particle (U1 snRNP). U1 snRNP takes part in the splicing of primary transcripts, and it is the snRNP that recognizes the 5′ splice site.

A (assembly of the spliceosome) is incorrect. The spliceosome consists of U4–U6 snRNPs and mRNA.
B (binding to the branch site) is incorrect. U2 snRNP binds to the branch site and polypyrimidine tract.
C (cytoplasmic transport of RNA) is incorrect. U1 snRNP is found in the nucleus, where the splicing takes place, and has no influence on RNA cytoplasmic transport.
D (recognition of the 3′ splice site) is incorrect. U5 snRNP recognizes the 3′ splice site.

40. *D* (prednisone) is correct. Prednisone is frequently used to treat inflammatory bowel disease. The long-term use of glucocorticoids (such as prednisone, prednisolone, and triamcinolone) is associated with various side effects, including muscle weakness, weight gain, redistribution of fat, moon facies, osteoporosis, cataract formation, glaucoma, adrenal insufficiency, and exacerbation of peptic ulcers.

A (azathioprine) is incorrect. Azathioprine is an immunosuppressant agent that has been used for its "steroid-sparing" effect in patients who require long-term treatment to suppress the symptoms of Crohn's disease. The drug is also used to treat rheumatoid arthritis and to prevent organ transplant rejection. Azathioprine is a prodrug that is converted to 6-mercaptopurine (6-MP), the active drug. Since 6-MP is inactivated by xanthine oxidase, the dose of azathioprine would have to be lowered in a patient concomitantly treated with allopurinol.
B (cyclosporine) is incorrect. Cyclosporine is an immunosuppressant agent. Its unlabeled uses include the treatment of inflammatory bowel disease. Its labeled uses include the treatment of rheumatoid arthritis and psoriasis and the prevention of organ rejection in patients receiving allogeneic transplants. Because the metabolism of cyclosporine is inhibited by diltiazem and ketoconazole, either of these drugs can be administered concurrently with cyclosporine to decrease the amount of cyclosporine that is required for treatment and thereby decrease the cost of treatment.
C (olsalazine) is incorrect. Olsalazine is used to maintain the remission of ulcerative colitis in patients who are unable to tolerate sulfasalazine. Olsalazine is a dimer that is converted by bacteria in the distal colon to two molecules of 5-aminosalicylic acid (5-ASA, or mesalamine).
E (sulfasalazine) is incorrect. Sulfasalazine is broken down by bacteria in the distal colon to 5-ASA and sulfapyridine. The 5-ASA is the active moiety in treating inflammatory bowel disease. Since its conversion occurs in the lower bowel, sulfasalazine would not be effective for treating Crohn's disease of the ileum. The sulfapyridine moiety is responsible for the drug's efficacy in the treatment of rheumatoid arthritis and for most of the drug's adverse effects.

41. *D* (partial ptosis of the upper eyelid on the affected side) is correct. The superior cervical ganglion gives rise to all sympathetic nerves to the head. Loss of this function in the head produces a condition known as Horner's syndrome. A symptom of this syndrome is loss of innervation to the superior tarsus muscle, a smooth muscle of the upper eyelid, which causes partial ptosis of the eyelid.

A (dilated pupil on the affected side) is incorrect. Unequal pupil size is another presenting feature of Horner's syndrome, but it is produced by an inability of the pupil to dilate fully on the affected side. Inability to dilate, especially in subdued light, would produce pupils of unequal size.

B (dry eye) is incorrect. Lacrimal secretion is produced by stimulation of parasympathetic nerve fibers, not sympathetic fibers. Parasympathetic fibers to the lacrimal gland arise in the nervus intermedius of the facial nerve (CN VII). Sympathetic innervation to the lacrimal gland is thought to inhibit secretion. Therefore, if anything, the affected side would produce a moist eye.

C (dry mouth) is incorrect. Parasympathetic nerve fibers provide secretomotor stimulation to the salivary glands and the lacrimal gland. These parasympathetics arise in the facial and glossopharyngeal nerves (CN VII and CN IX, respectively). CN VII innervates the submandibular and sublingual salivary glands, and CN IX innervates the parotid salivary gland. Sympathetic stimulation produces the dry mouth that often occurs when a person is nervous or frightened. Thus, absence of sympathetic nerve fibers would not produce dry mouth.

E (persistent sweating from the skin overlying the parotid salivary gland) is incorrect. Loss of sympathetic innervation to the sweat glands of the head on the affected side is a symptom of Horner's syndrome. Sweat glands are innervated only by sympathetic nerve fibers, although these nerve fibers secrete acetylcholine at their effector endings instead of the usual norepinephrine. Loss of sympathetic innervation results in an inability to sweat on the affected side; it occurs as hot, dry, red skin because of loss of sympathetic innervation to sweat glands and to the blood vessels to the head.

42. *C* (DNA analysis of the X chromosome) is correct. This child has fragile X syndrome (FXS). FXS is thought to be a sex-linked recessive syndrome; however, some patients appear to have a sex-linked dominant inheritance pattern, with a fragile site or gap at the end of the long arm of the X chromosome. At this site, there are triplet repeats of three nucleotides (e.g., CGG-CGG-CGG. . .). An interesting phenomenon associated with triplet repeat mutations is that there is progressive worsening of the disease in future generations (called anticipation) and signs of mental retardation or impaired learning in carrier females. The disease is exacerbated because more triplet repeats occur in individuals in each succeeding generation, which explains why female carriers may also express the disease. DNA analysis

of chromosome in lymphocytes identifies the triplet repeats and is considered more sensitive than the fragile X chromosome study.

A (buccal smear) is incorrect. A buccal smear usually is performed to rule out deficient or extra X chromosomes. Normal females have random inactivation of one of the two X chromosomes. Hence, normal females have one Barr body, and normal males have no Barr bodies. The randomly inactivated chromosome becomes an appendage on the nuclear membrane of cells.
B (chromosome study of the father) is incorrect. X-linked conditions are transmitted to males via the carrier female and not by the affected father.
D (serum gonadotropins) is incorrect. The patient shows no clinical evidence of hypogonadism, as in Klinefelter's syndrome, where the testicles are atrophic.
E (testicular biopsy) is incorrect. The patient does not have a testicular neoplasm or signs of Klinefelter's syndrome.

43. C (patient Y has hyperthyroidism) is correct. Patients with hyperthyroidism, or Grave's disease, have hyperthyroidism caused by stimulation of the thyroid TSH receptor by an autoantibody. The resulting rise in serum triiodothyronine (T_3) and thyroxine (T_4) causes a negative feedback response that results in suppression of pituitary TSH production.

A (patient X has a pituitary TSH-secreting tumor) is incorrect. A patient with a pituitary TSH-secreting tumor has elevated TSH levels that do not respond to TRH (escape from normal regulation). TRH normally suppresses TSH secretion from the pituitary, but the tumor is not responsive.
B (patient X has hypothyroidism) is incorrect. TSH secretion is stimulated by TRH, not suppressed by it.
D (patient Y shows a normal response to TRH) is incorrect. Patient Y shows a depressed response to TRH administration, with initial low levels of TSH seen in patients with hyperthyroidism.

44. D (denial) is correct. From extensive interviews with dying patients, research conducted by Elisabeth Kübler-Ross suggests that of the five stages of death, denial is the first stage that many individuals experience when dealing with death. Denial is a primary primitive defense mechanism that allows the patient time to cope with the unexpected and devastating news.

A (acceptance) is incorrect. Acceptance is the final stage associated with death as patients realize their existence is near an end. However, not all patients will fully accept their death prior to its occurrence.
B (anger) is incorrect. Anger often follows denial when a patient is attempting to cope with impending death. This second stage

is characterized by the patient asking questions focused on, "Why me?"

C   (bargaining) is incorrect. Once denial and anger have passed, a patient will commonly enter the bargaining, or third, stage of coping with death. During the bargaining stage, thoughts are focused on a religious or magical intervention that will allow the patient to avoid or postpone death.

E   (depression) is incorrect. The fourth stage of death is depression, which is experienced as the patient begins to fully recognize the finality of death. Depression is a common reaction experienced during the course of terminal illness. An expected grief reaction must be distinguished from clinical depression to avoid additional and/or inappropriate interventions.

45. *A*   (liver) is correct. Oncotic pressure (colloid osmotic pressure) is created by large molecular-weight protein in the blood plasma. About 60%–70% of this protein is albumin, which is synthesized and secreted by the liver. Liver disease could result in a decrease in albumin production and a concomitant decrease in oncotic pressure. When the oncotic pressure is low, the plasma is less able to draw tissue fluid back into capillary beds and to maintain blood volume and blood pressure.

B   (pancreas), C (parotid gland), D (spleen), and E (thyroid gland) are incorrect. A decrease in albumin synthesis or secretion would cause a decrease in oncotic pressure. The liver secretes albumin. The pancreas secretes insulin, glucagon, and pancreatic amylase, lipase, and protease. The parotid gland secretes salivary amylase, and the thyroid gland secretes thyroxine and calcitonin. The primary function of the spleen is to eliminate effete erythrocytes and platelets from the circulatory system and to mount cellular and humoral immune responses against blood-borne antigens.

46. *D*   (directly inhibits protein synthesis) is correct. The patient's clinical and laboratory findings are typical of diphtheria. Although this disease is rare in the United States, numerous outbreaks have occurred in parts of the world where vaccination programs are not maintained. Diphtheria is caused by *Corynebacterium diphtheriae.* The organism is a noninvasive bacterium. It produces diphtheria exotoxin, which causes cell death and systemic manifestations of disease by directly inhibiting protein synthesis.

A   (directly disrupts cell membrane integrity) and E (directly lyses mitochondria) are incorrect. Cell membrane integrity and mitochondrial integrity are not directly affected by *C. diphtheriae* or diphtheria toxin.

B   (directly disrupts microtubules) and C (directly inhibits nucleic acid synthesis) are incorrect. The diphtheria toxin directly inhibits protein synthesis, and any effects on host cell microtubules and nucleic acid synthesis are indirect.

47. **B** (fructose 6-phosphate → fructose 1,6-bisphosphate) is correct. Fructose 6-phosphate is converted to fructose 1,6-bisphosphate by 6-phosphofructokinase (phosphofructokinase 1). This step is the first irreversible reaction specific for glycolysis (a committed step) and is highly regulated. In the liver, the step is inhibited by citrate, glucagon, adenosine triphosphate (ATP), or a low pH. It is stimulated by fructose 2,6-bisphosphate, adenosine monophosphate, adenosine diphosphate, or insulin.

A (1,3-bisphosphoglycerate → 3-phosphoglycerate) is incorrect. 1,3-Bisphosphoglycerate is converted to 3-phosphoglycerate by phosphoglycerate kinase in a reversible reaction.
C (glucose → glucose 6-phosphate) is incorrect. In the liver, glucose is converted to glucose 6-phosphate by glucokinase. This step is irreversible. It is inhibited by fructose 6-phosphate and is activated by fructose 1-phosphate. Note that an extrahepatic glycolytic enzyme, hexokinase, is inhibited by glucose 6-phosphate.
D (glucose 6-phosphate → fructose 6-phosphate) is incorrect. Glucose 6-phosphate is converted to fructose 6-phosphate by glucose-6-phosphate isomerase (phosphohexose isomerase). This is a reversible step.
E (phosphoenolpyruvate → pyruvate) is incorrect. Phosphoenolpyruvate is converted to pyruvate by pyruvate kinase. This is an irreversible step. It is inhibited by a physiologic concentration of ATP and is activated by fructose 1,6-bisphosphate. Pyruvate kinase is also subject to covalent modification. It is active in the dephosphorylated state and inactive in the phosphorylated state.

48. **B** (destruction of the cervical sympathetic plexus by a primary lung cancer) is correct. The patient most likely has a primary squamous cell carcinoma in the left superior pulmonary sulcus. The tumor has invaded and destroyed the cervical sympathetic plexus, producing Horner's syndrome. Horner's syndrome is characterized by ipsilateral lid lag (ptosis), pupil miosis (constriction), and absence of sweating (anhidrosis) on the forehead and face.

A (destruction of the brachial plexus by a primary lung cancer) is incorrect. Tumor invasion of the brachial plexus by superior sulcus tumors usually produces ulnar nerve irritation.
C (extension of a primary lung cancer into the anterior mediastinum) is incorrect. The anterior mediastinum contains the thymus and lymphatic tissue. Tumor invasion of the posterior mediastinum, which contains the sympathetic ganglia and nerves, is responsible for producing Horner's syndrome.
D (uncal herniation secondary to metastatic disease originating in the lung) is incorrect. Uncal herniation refers to herniation of the medial portion of the temporal lobe through the tentorium cerebelli, leading to compression of the midbrain. It is a complication of cerebral edema from any cause, including metastatic dis-

ease to the brain. Uncal herniation commonly is associated with compression of the oculomotor nerve (CN III), which produces lid lag, mydriasis (pupil dilatation), and ophthalmoplegia (eyes deviated downward and outward).

49. **E** (vincristine) is correct. Neurotoxicity is the dose-limiting side effect of vincristine, a vinca alkaloid whose use is associated with various neurologic abnormalities. Suppression of the Achilles tendon reflex is one of the first signs of vincristine-induced neuropathy. Muscle weakness usually affects the lower extremities and can give rise to footdrop. When vincristine treatment is stopped, the muscle weakness may partially or completely resolve, but resolution is slow.

A (asparaginase) is incorrect. Although asparaginase treatment is associated with many side effects (including hypoglycemia, excessive bleeding, and pancreatitis), it is not associated with neurotoxicity.
B (cyclophosphamide) is incorrect. Cyclophosphamide is the most commonly used anticancer drug. Its dose-limiting side effect is bone marrow suppression. Another side effect, hemorrhagic cystitis, can be prevented by concomitant administration of mesna.
C (daunorubicin) is incorrect. Daunorubicin and doxorubicin are anthracycline antibiotics whose dose-limiting side effect is bone marrow suppression. The drugs do not cause neurotoxicity. They are noted for their cumulative cardiomyopathy, which can be minimized by the concomitant use of dexrazoxane.
D (prednisone) is incorrect. Many side effects are associated with prednisone use, but neurotoxicity is not one of them.

50. **B** *(Brucella)* is correct. The clinical and laboratory findings are consistent with the diagnosis of brucellosis, which can be caused by several *Brucella* species. The case described was actually associated with a disease outbreak reported by the Centers for Disease Control and Prevention, and the causative organism was probably *Brucella suis*. This organism infects swine (as well as horses, reindeer, and rodents). It is an intracellular parasite of the reticuloendothelial system, and it typically causes granulomatous lesions in the liver, spleen, bone marrow, and other lymphoid tissues.

A *(Bordetella)* is incorrect. Bordetellae are organisms that are typically associated with infections of the respiratory tract, not the reticuloendothelial system. *Bordetella pertussis,* for example, causes whooping cough.
C *(Francisella)* is incorrect. *Francisella tularensis,* the *Francisella* species that causes infection in humans, is the etiologic agent of several forms of tularemia, including oculoglandular, oropharyngeal, pulmonic, and ulceroglandular tularemia. In the United States, the most common reservoirs of the organism are rabbits and ticks, and transmission usually occurs as a result of handling

infected animals or being bitten by an infected tick. Pigs are not reservoirs of *Francisella.*

D *(Pasteurella)* is incorrect. *Pasteurella* species, such as *Pasteurella multocida,* most commonly cause localized infections in persons who have been scratched or bitten by a dog or cat.

E *(Yersinia)* is incorrect. The yersiniae demonstrate tropism for tissues of the reticuloendothelial tissue. *Yersinia pestis* causes plague, while *Yersinia enterocolitica* and *Yersinia pseudotuberculosis* cause food-borne and water-borne gastrointestinal infections and other diseases. Although *Y. enterocolitica* infects swine, the laboratory findings associated with this organism differ from those described above; *Y. enterocolitica* is facultatively anaerobic, oxidase-negative, and ferments carbohydrates.

Test 2

TEST 2

DIRECTIONS: Each numbered item or incomplete statement is followed by options arranged in alphabetical or logical order. Select the best answer to each question. Some options may be partially correct, but there is only **ONE BEST** answer.

1. A 32-year-old woman has a fever, malaise, and a cough productive of bloody sputum. The sputum is found to contain numerous acid-fast bacilli, which are strict aerobes that grow slowly, are nonmotile, produce niacin, form serpentine cords, and do not form endospores. A chest x-ray shows a cavity containing a dense infiltrate, and an acid-fast stain of a lung biopsy specimen confirms the presence of intracellular and extracellular bacilli. Most of the pathologic manifestations of this patient's disease are attributable to

○ A. disseminated intravascular coagulation
○ B. enzymes produced by the infecting bacilli
○ C. exotoxins produced by the infecting bacilli
○ D. host hypersensitivity
○ E. lipopolysaccharide produced by the infecting bacilli

2. A 55-year-old man complains of weight loss and recurrent episodes of bleeding into the skin. His medical records indicate that 4 months ago he underwent surgery in which the terminal ileum was spared but most of the small intestine was resected. Several months ago, he began treatment with oral antibiotics for a chronic lung infection. He has continued taking antibiotics and says that he has not been taking any vitamin supplements. The patient's current complaints are most likely due to a deficiency of

○ A. intrinsic factor
○ B. vitamin B_{12}
○ C. vitamin C
○ D. vitamin D
○ E. vitamin K

3. A 27-year-old nurse comes to the emergency department because of an apparent bleeding disorder. The physician later discovers that the nurse has taken anticoagulants because she wants to be hospitalized, but she denies this. The most likely diagnosis is

○ A. body dysmorphic disorder
○ B. conversion disorder
○ C. factitious disorder
○ D. hypochondriasis
○ E. malingering

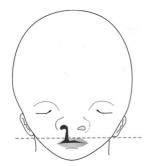

4. Which of the following most likely accounts for the embryologic defect shown in the figure above?

○ A. Exposure to isotretinoin during the last trimester of pregnancy
○ B. Failure of the intermaxillary process to fuse with the right maxillary swelling
○ C. Failure of the nasolacrimal groove to close on the right side
○ D. Failure of the palatine shelves to fuse
○ E. Persistence of the first pharyngeal cleft on the right

5. For the past several weeks, a 39-year-old woman has experienced fatigue, weakness, poor appetite, and weight loss. Physical examination shows hyperpigmentation of the skin and dark patches on the mucous membranes. Laboratory studies show her serum sodium level is 125 mEq/dL, and her serum potassium level is 6.0 mEq/dL. Which of the following is the most likely diagnosis?

○ A. Atrophic adrenals with dense lymphocytic infiltrate
○ B. Carcinoid tumor of the vermiform appendix
○ C. Functional follicular adenoma of the thyroid
○ D. Granulosa cell tumor of the right ovary
○ E. Hyperplasia of all four parathyroid glands

6. A 49-year-old man with temporomandibular joint dysfunction is scheduled to undergo orthognathic surgery. He is given a preanesthetic dose of midazolam, and thiopental is used to induce anesthesia. In addition, he is given a neuromuscular blocking drug (NMBD). Administration of the NMBD produces muscle fasciculations, followed by flaccid paralysis. During the immediate postoperative period, the patient complains of muscle soreness. The NMBD most likely given to the patient was

○ A. atracurium
○ B. mivacurium
○ C. succinylcholine
○ D. tubocurarine
○ E. vecuronium

7. A biopsy of a section of the alveolar septa of the lung of a long-term smoker shows cells containing inhaled tar (carbon) particles. Which of the following cell types is most likely to contain such particles?

○ A. Ciliated cuboidal cells
○ B. Endothelial cells
○ C. Macrophages
○ D. Type I pneumocytes
○ E. Type II pneumocytes

8. A 40-year-old woman who has not menstruated for 3 months complains of a milky discharge from both nipples that began 6 weeks ago. She has also been having frequent retroorbital headaches of increasing severity during this time. An ophthalmologic examination shows bitemporal hemianopia. Which of the following is the most likely cause of these findings?

○ A. Basophilic tumor of the anterior pituitary
○ B. Growth hormone–secreting tumor
○ C. Hashimoto's thyroiditis
○ D. Pinealoma
○ E. Prolactinoma

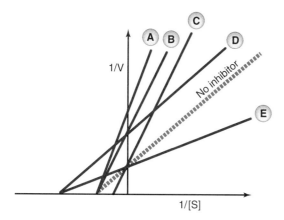

9. A 60-year-old man who has pain in his ankle and knee joints and an elevated level of serum uric acid is prescribed a drug that is a structural analogue of hypoxanthine. The kinetic effect of the drug on xanthine oxidase is best described by which of the plotted lines in the figure above?

○ A. Line A
○ B. Line B
○ C. Line C
○ D. Line D
○ E. Line E

10. About 14 hours after consuming home-canned vegetable soup, a 30-year-old woman develops a headache, weakness, dryness of the mouth, diplopia, dysphagia, dysphonia, and urinary retention. She has no fever, but vomits repeatedly, experiences slight dyspnea, and has dilated pupils. She eventually develops muscle paralysis and dies as a result of respiratory failure. The exotoxin that was responsible for most of the patient's disease manifestations acts by

○ A. blocking the release of postsynaptic inhibitors
○ B. causing the lysis of neurons
○ C. increasing the intracellular level of cyclic adenosine monophosphate (cAMP)
○ D. inhibiting the release of acetylcholine
○ E. inhibiting the synthesis of proteins

11. While undergoing surgery to repair an indirect inguinal hernia, a 13-year-old boy suffers damage to the ilioinguinal nerve. Damage to this nerve would most likely cause which of the following symptoms?

○ A. Infertility
○ B. Numbness of the scrotum and inner side of the thigh
○ C. Numbness over the lateral side of the thigh
○ D. Paralysis of the adductor muscles
○ E. Paralysis of the sartorius muscle

12. A 27-year-old intravenous drug abuser is found dead from an overdose of heroin. Autopsy shows profound pulmonary edema and numerous 3- to 5-mm yellowish white nodules throughout the lungs. Histologic examination shows granulomas with no suggestion of caseous necrosis. Stains for infectious organisms are negative. An examination under polarized light shows small flecks of birefringent material within macrophages. The cause of these granulomas is most likely

○ A. activation of angiotensin-converting enzyme (ACE)
○ B. activation of a previously acquired mycobacterial infection
○ C. concomitant HIV infection
○ D. direct toxicity to alveolar macrophages by heroin
○ E. foreign substance in the injected heroin

13. A 45-year-old woman has a staggering gait and truncal ataxia. Her balance is poor when she walks unaided. She develops nystagmus when she gazes laterally to either side. No other abnormalities are noted. The most likely cause of these findings is a lesion in which of the following areas?

○ A. Basilar pons
○ B. Dentate nucleus
○ C. Medial longitudinal fasciculus
○ D. Midline of the cerebellum
○ E. Midline pontine tegmentum

14. A man finds his 91-year-old mother in a comatose state. While awaiting an ambulance, he discovers an empty bottle that contained a preparation of oxycodone and acetaminophen, which had been prescribed that morning to alleviate his mother's discomfort associated with circulatory insufficiency in her feet. In the emergency department, the patient is found to have markedly depressed respiration, hypotension, and contracted (pinpoint) pupils. The most appropriate therapy aimed at preventing the potential hepatotoxicity associated with her overdose would be

○ A. acetylcysteine
○ B. flumazenil
○ C. lactulose
○ D. naloxone
○ E. sodium bicarbonate

15. A 23-year-old man has moderate urethral discharge for 3 days and occasionally experiences mild dysuria. He has no fever or any visible lesions on his penis. He reports having multiple sex partners. A Gram stain of the urethral discharge specimen is unremarkable, and culture of the specimen on chocolate agar and other bacteriologic media yields negative results. The causative organism is later shown to be a strictly intracellular parasite. Which of the following is the most likely cause of the urethritis?

○ A. *Chlamydia trachomatis*
○ B. *Haemophilus ducreyi*
○ C. *Mycoplasma genitalium*
○ D. *Neisseria gonorrhoeae*
○ E. *Ureaplasma urealyticum*

16. A 69-year-old African-American woman complains of fatigue and pain in her lower back and ribs. She states that she has been having problems with voiding urine for the past few days. Physical examination shows percussion tenderness over the lower vertebrae and rib cage. Renal tubular casts are present in the urine sediment. A radiograph of the chest shows generalized osteopenia in the ribs and thoracic vertebral column and multiple lytic lesions in the ribs. Serum protein electrophoresis (SPE) shows an abnormality in the γ-globulin region. Laboratory studies show:

Rouleaux hemoglobin	7.0 g/dL
Leukocyte count	6500/mm^3
Platelet count	175,000/mm^3
Serum blood urea nitrogen (BUN)	60 mg/dL
Serum creatinine	6 mg/dL
Urine dipstick reaction	Proteinuria 1+ precipitation reaction, sulfosalicylic acid (SSA) 4+

The mechanism responsible for this patient's condition is most closely associated with which of the following?

○ A. Immunoglobulin M–producing lymphoproliferative disorder
○ B. Malignant plasma cell disorder
○ C. Malignant T-cell disorder
○ D. Metastatic disease of undetermined origin
○ E. Renal failure of undetermined origin

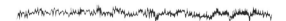

17. A 41-year-old obese woman is referred to a sleep disorders clinic to determine if she has sleep apnea. From 2 AM to 2:30 PM, her electroencephalogram (EEG) consists primarily of the sleep waves shown in the figure above. This patient is most likely

○ A. actively concentrating on a task
○ B. dreaming
○ C. in stage 2 sleep
○ D. in stage 4 sleep
○ E. relaxed but awake

18. A 33-year-old woman is involved in an automobile accident and injured her knee when it was forced against the dashboard. With the knee flexed in a 90-degree position, she now exhibits a positive posterior drawer sign. This positive sign indicates injury to which of the following ligaments?

- ○ A. Anterior cruciate
- ○ B. Lateral collateral
- ○ C. Medial collateral
- ○ D. Patellar
- ○ E. Posterior cruciate

19. A 58-year-old African-American man has a history of type 2 diabetes mellitus that is managed with glyburide therapy. He is taken to the emergency department because of malignant hypertension and is infused with sodium nitroprusside (NP). After 36 hours of high-dose treatment with NP, the patient complains of a headache and lethargy. Hyperventilation is evident, and laboratory studies show lactic acidosis and an increased PO_2 in mixed venous blood. The most likely cause of this patient's reaction and an appropriate treatment would be

- ○ A. cyanide toxicity secondary to decomposition of NP; administer thiosulfate
- ○ B. hypersensitivity reaction to NP; administer epinephrine
- ○ C. hypoglycemia; administer glucose
- ○ D. rare side effect associated with glyburide use; initiate metformin therapy
- ○ E. rhabdomyolysis, a side effect of NP; administer sodium bicarbonate

20. A 33-year-old man with a history of trauma to the right side of the head has a flushed face. He says that his face does not sweat, even on very hot days. A routine physical examination shows right pupillary constriction and ptosis. Which of the following is the most likely cause of these findings?

- ○ A. Horner's syndrome
- ○ B. Infarction in the basilar pons
- ○ C. Infarction in the callosomarginal artery
- ○ D. Inferior alternating hemiplegia
- ○ E. Lesion in the cerebellopontine angle

21. A 20-year-old woman complains of a fever, maculopapular rash, and asymmetric arthritis. She says that she has had the rash for 3 days and that it began on her face and quickly became generalized. Physical examination shows lymphadenopathy affecting the suboccipital and cervical nodes. Bacteriologic and fungal cultures yield negative results, but an enveloped virus with a capsomere-bound protein spike is isolated in cell culture. Which of the following viruses is the most likely cause of the disease?

- ○ A. Adenovirus
- ○ B. Coronavirus
- ○ C. Measles virus
- ○ D. Mumps virus
- ○ E. Rubella virus

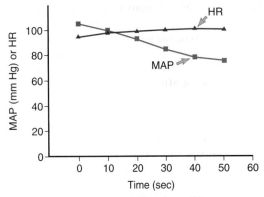

HR = heart rate; MAP = blood pressure

22. The figure above shows the heart rate and blood pressure of a 45-year-old man as he assumes the standing position on first arising in the morning. The first point shows the resting values before arising (*squares* are blood pressure, or MAP = 108 mm Hg; *triangles* are heart rate, or HR = 97/min). Subsequent values show HR and MAP measured every 10 seconds. Which of the following most accurately describes this patient's response?

○ A. He develops tachycardia due to treatment with a cholinergic agonist
○ B. He has a normal baroreflex response to standing up
○ C. He has lost baroreflex function resulting from systemic hypertension
○ D. He is being treated with a sympathetic antagonist
○ E. He recently underwent heart transplantation

23. A 26-year-old man develops uncomplicated watery diarrhea about 48 hours after returning from a trip to Mexico. He does not have a fever. He says he drank tap water in the hotel room before he left for the airport. A stool sample is cultured on MacConkey agar. The causative organism is a gram-negative lactose utilizer, and is facultatively anaerobic and indole-positive. A heat-labile enterotoxin is identified immunologically. This type of enterotoxin exerts its effects by

○ A. increasing intracellular levels of cyclic adenosine monophosphate (cAMP)
○ B. increasing intracellular levels of cyclic guanosine monophosphate (cGMP)
○ C. inducing mucosal inflammation
○ D. inducing the lysis of epithelial cells in the large intestine
○ E. inhibiting protein synthesis and thereby causing cell death

24. During a gynecologic evaluation, a 33-year-old woman mentions that she is concerned because she experiences pain during sexual intercourse. The pain appears to be related to the lack of vaginal lubrication that occurs during foreplay. Vaginal lubrication during sexual activity is a feature of which of the following stages of the normal sexual response for women?

○ A. Desire
○ B. Excitement
○ C. Orgasm
○ D. Plateau
○ E. Resolution

25. In a comatose 80-year-old man, passive movement of the head to the right produces flexion of the left upper extremity, and passive movement of the head to the left produces flexion of the right upper extremity. The man's legs are fixed in extension during all movements. Which of the following is the most likely explanation of these findings?

○ A. Alternating superior hemiplegia
○ B. Brown-Séquard's syndrome
○ C. Decerebrate rigidity
○ D. Decorticate rigidity
○ E. Transection of the spinal cord below T5

26. A 22-year-old medical student volunteers for a hematology research project and is found to be lacking one of four α-globin genes. Previously, he had several hematologic studies that were within normal limits. The significance of this unexpected finding suggests that the student

○ A. has a moderate degree of erythroid hyperplasia in bone marrow
○ B. has an abnormal hemoglobin concentration
○ C. has numerous target cells in the peripheral blood
○ D. is an asymptomatic carrier of α-thalassemia
○ E. may develop severe hemolytic anemia if exposed to oxidant drugs

27. Patients with xeroderma pigmentosum are particularly sensitive to sunlight and prone to developing skin cancer because their skin cells cannot repair damaged DNA. The most common form of this genetic disorder is a result of the absence of which of the following enzymes?

○ A. DNA helicase
○ B. DNA polymerase III
○ C. Endonuclease
○ D. RNA polymerase
○ E. Topoisomerases

28. During several visits to the emergency department, a 46-year-old man has been loud and obnoxious until the physician agrees to see him immediately. To avoid confrontations, the physician always sees this particular patient without delay. Social learning theory predicts that the patient will continue to be loud and obnoxious upon arrival in the emergency department

○ A. if the patient's behavior is routinely ignored
○ B. if the patient is rewarded for pleasant interactions
○ C. if the physician continues to see him immediately
○ D. regardless of any changes the physician attempts
○ E. until the patient is declined medical care

29. A 30-year-old man has explosive diarrhea. He says that 2 weeks before the diarrhea started, he was backpacking in the Rocky Mountains and drank stream water without purifying it. His stool sample is foul-smelling and greasy in appearance. Microscopic examination of the sample shows a stingray-shaped trophozoite with eight flagella, two nuclei, and a sucker. Which of the following organisms is the most likely cause of the diarrhea?

○ A. *Cryptosporidium parvum*
○ B. *Entamoeba histolytica*
○ C. *Giardia lamblia*
○ D. *Toxoplasma gondii*
○ E. *Trypanosoma cruzi*

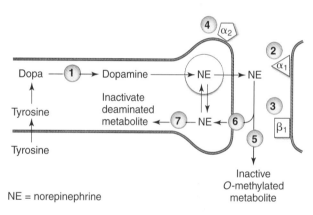

NE = norepinephrine

30. The figure above depicts an adrenergic nerve terminal and postsynaptic adrenergic receptors. The numbers 1 through 7 represent sites of drug action. The antihypertensive effect of methyldopa is best explained by an action at

○ A. site 1
○ B. site 2
○ C. site 3
○ D. site 4
○ E. site 5
○ F. site 6
○ G. site 7

31. A febrile 35-year-old woman complains of a headache, fatigue, and decreased urine output. Physical examination shows bilateral retinal hemorrhages and generalized petechiae and ecchymoses. The peripheral smear shows numerous fragmented red blood cells (RBCs). Laboratory studies show:

Hemoglobin	7.0 g/dL
Leukocyte count	9500/mm^3
Platelet count	30,000/mm^3
Reticulocyte count, corrected	12%
Blood urea nitrogen (BUN), serum	50 mg/dL
Creatinine, serum	5 mg/dL
Partial thromboplastin time (activated, aPTT)	35 seconds
Prothrombin time (PT)	13 seconds
Bleeding time (BT)	>15 minutes
Platelet count	350,000 mm^3
D-dimer assay	Negative

The mechanism most likely responsible for this patient's hematologic disorder is most closely associated with

○ A. circulating anticoagulant
○ B. consumption of coagulation factors
○ C. consumption of platelets
○ D. qualitative platelet disorder
○ E. secondary fibrinolytic disorder

32. A 50-year-old man is taken to the emergency department suffering from abdominal pain, vomiting, and diarrhea. The man is an amateur mushroom hunter and prepared and ate a special mushroom casserole 2 days ago. The patient shows signs of irreversible liver failure. Analysis of leftovers from the mushroom dish shows a high concentration of α-amanitin. Which of the following is the most likely cause of the liver failure in this patient?

○ A. Inability to synthesize proteins because large ribosomal subunit 5.8S RNA is not being produced
○ B. Inability to synthesize proteins because large ribosomal subunit 28S RNA is not being produced
○ C. Inhibition of mitochondrial RNA transcription
○ D. Inhibition of tRNA synthesis
○ E. Lack of mRNA transcription from DNA

33. A 45-year-old man complains of facial paralysis. Physical examination shows a partial ptosis of the left eyelid, weeping from the left eye, drooping of the left corner of the mouth, and failure of that corner of the mouth to respond when the man smiles. Injury to which cranial nerve would produce these symptoms?

○ A. Abducens (CN VI)
○ B. Facial (CN VII)
○ C. Glossopharyngeal (CN IX)
○ D. Trigeminal (CN V)
○ E. Vagus (CN X)

34. A 55-year-old woman with anemia is unknowingly exposed to carbon monoxide (CO) because of a faulty space heater in her home. She appears to be breathing normally, but says she does not feel well. Arterial and venous blood samples are taken. Laboratory studies would most likely show her arterial PaO_2 as

○ A. 120 mm Hg
○ B. 95 mm Hg
○ C. 70 mm Hg
○ D. 50 mm Hg
○ E. 25 mm Hg

35. A 28-year-old man with diabetes mellitus says he has not been monitoring his blood glucose levels regularly because the test strips are expensive. He also mentions that monitoring is a constant reminder of his condition. A medical student in the clinic wants to confront the man about his nonadherence, but an attending physician encourages the student to understand the man's point of view by temporarily "living" in his internal frame of reference. The attending physician is most likely encouraging the student to exercise which of the following skills?

○ A. Assertiveness
○ B. Diagnosis
○ C. Empathy
○ D. Negotiation
○ E. Objective observation

36. A 69-year-old man with a 40-year history of cigarette smoking complains of weight loss, a dragging sensation in his right upper quadrant, and crampy left lower quadrant abdominal pain. He states that he has had alternating bouts of constipation and diarrhea over the past 6 months and has noticed blood coating and mixed with his stools. Physical examination shows an enlarged, nodular liver, external hemorrhoids, and occult blood in the stool. Laboratory studies show:

Hemoglobin	9.0 g/dL
Leukocyte count	6500/mm^3
Platelet count	500,000/mm^3
Mean corpuscular volume	75 μm^3
Ferritin level, serum	3.0 ng/mL

Which of the following disorders best explains the positive stool guaiac in this patient?

○ A. External hemorrhoids
○ B. Hepatocellular carcinoma with metastasis to the colon
○ C. Peptic ulcer disease (PUD)
○ D. Primary colon cancer
○ E. Primary lung cancer with metastasis to the colon

37. Which of the following best explains the change in airway resistance in a patient with interstitial pulmonary edema?

○ A. Decreased because of edema fluid in the interstitial spaces
○ B. Increased because edema fluid interferes with normal lateral traction on the airways
○ C. Increased because of increased work of breathing due to dilution of surfactant
○ D. Increased because zones in the lungs are ventilated but not perfused
○ E. Normal because of little or no fluid in the lumen of the airways

38. A 62-year-old woman has had pain and swelling of her left forearm for 1 day. Examination shows local tenderness and warmth with associated discoloration. Results of Doppler ultrasonography suggest deep venous thrombosis. The patient is treated with an appropriate drug, and the adequacy of the dosage is monitored by measuring the activated partial thromboplastin time (aPTT). The patient is most likely being treated with

○ A. alteplase
○ B. aspirin
○ C. heparin
○ D. streptokinase
○ E. warfarin

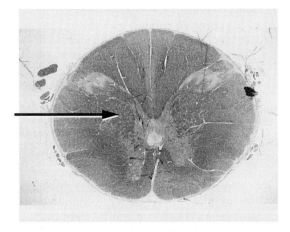

39. Stimulating electrodes have been implanted in a 37-year-old man to test responses to neuronal stimulation. Action potentials in which of the following structures can be detected after axons (at the tip of the arrow in the figure above) have been stimulated?

○ A. Contralateral medial lemniscus
○ B. Contralateral tectum
○ C. Ipsilateral anterior horn
○ D. Ipsilateral red nucleus
○ E. Ipsilateral sympathetic ganglia

40. A 24-year-old man with a history of intravenous drug abuse experiences a sudden onset of fever accompanied by chest pain when he breathes. A chest x-ray shows the presence of numerous small opacities that have black centers and are distributed throughout the upper and lower lobes of both lungs. A Gram stain of aspirated material would most likely show the predominance of

○ A. acid-fast bacilli with a monocytic infiltrate
○ B. gram-positive cocci in clusters with an acute inflammatory infiltrate
○ C. gram-positive filamentous rods with a monocytic infiltrate
○ D. gram-positive lancet-shaped diplocococci with an acute inflammatory infiltrate
○ E. monocytic infiltrate with no visible bacteria

41. A 46-year-old woman with chronic alcoholism wants to abstain from drinking. Her physician recommends a local "12-step" program and prescribes medication that will help her maintain sobriety. One week later, she relapses. Within 15 minutes of ingesting a vodka martini, she experiences nausea, vomiting, flushing of the face and neck, a pulsating headache, dizziness, and hypotension. The medication that was most likely prescribed for this patient was

○ A. chlorpropamide
○ B. disulfiram
○ C. flumazenil
○ D. metronidazole
○ E. naltrexone

42. A physical examination of a 26-year-old man with progressive muscle weakness shows his blood pressure is 152/99 mm Hg. Laboratory studies show his serum pH is 7.6; HCO_3^- is 32 mEq/L; and plasma aldosterone concentration is elevated. The most likely cause of muscle weakness in this patient is

○ A. hyperchloremia
○ B. hyperkalemia
○ C. hypocalcemia
○ D. hypokalemia
○ E. hyponatremia

43. A 30-year-old man develops an acute onset of confusion, ataxia, nystagmus, and ophthalmoplegia shortly after the administration of an intravenous (IV) solution containing 5% glucose and normal saline. The pathogenesis of this patient's neurologic disorder is most closely related to which of the following conditions?

○ A. Central pontine myelinolysis
○ B. Purkinje cell atrophy
○ C. Thiamine deficiency
○ D. Viral encephalitis
○ E. Vitamin B_{12} deficiency

44. A 92-year-old woman complains of hearing loss. Which of the following structures in the organ of Corti would be reduced in size in this patient?

○ A. Diameter of the inner ear tunnel
○ B. Hairs on the surface of inner hair cells
○ C. Thickness of the basilar membrane
○ D. Thickness of the tectorial membrane
○ E. Thickness of the vestibular membrane

45. A 52-year-old long-distance cycler is admitted to the hospital with severe chest pain. He says that the chest pain usually occurs before he gets out of bed in the morning. Cardiac catheterization shows no evidence of coronary artery disease. An ergonovine provocative study shows that the patient experiences severe chest pain associated with ST segment elevation and complete vasospasm of the right anterior descending coronary artery. The medical records indicate that he recently underwent transurethral resection of the prostate and has been taking sildenafil for erectile dysfunction for the past 3 months. The most appropriate therapy for the patient's cardiac condition is

○ A. minoxidil
○ B. nitroglycerin
○ C. prazosin
○ D. propranolol
○ E. verapamil

46. A patient has chronic granulomatous disease. Which of the following would be expected to yield abnormal results?

○ A. Measurement of serum C3 levels
○ B. Measurement of serum IgE and IgA levels
○ C. Testing of the B cell mitogen response
○ D. Use of common skin test antigens
○ E. Use of nitroblue tetrazolium test (NBT)

47. A 7-year-old boy has a neurologic disorder due to a deficiency of a single enzyme. The disorder is characterized by mental retardation, aggressive behavior, and self-mutilation. The cause of the disease is a biochemical defect in the

○ A. catabolism of purine nucleotides
○ B. formation of thymidylate
○ C. pathway of de novo synthesis of purine nucleotides
○ D. production of all pyrimidine nucleotides
○ E. salvage pathway of purines

48. A 33-year-old man has dysuria, meatal erythema and pain, and a purulent urethral discharge. Gram stain of the urethral exudate shows intracellular gram-negative diplococci. The medical records indicate that the patient recently had a severe type I allergic reaction to penicillin. The most appropriate therapy for this patient would be

○ A. ceftriaxone
○ B. ciprofloxacin
○ C. gentamicin
○ D. metronidazole
○ E. vancomycin

49. A 62-year-old woman sees her physician because of "lumps" in her armpits. Physical examination shows small rubbery nodes palpable in the axillae, groin, cervical triangles, and popliteal spaces. Both liver and spleen are palpable. Her leukocyte count is 87,000/mm^3, with 92% small lymphocytes. Biopsy of the lymph nodes shows an infiltrate of small lymphocytes completely effacing the nodal architecture. No suggestion of follicular pattern is apparent. Which of the following is the most likely diagnosis?

○ A. B-cell lymphoma with no involvement of the bone marrow
○ B. High-grade B-cell lymphoma with a rapidly fatal course
○ C. Low-grade B-cell lymphoma with an indolent course
○ D. Lymphoblastic lymphoma originating in the bone marrow
○ E. T-cell lymphoma induced by human T-cell leukemia virus type 1 (HTLV-1)

50. A 24-year-old motorcyclist sustains head trauma after colliding with an automobile and is brought to the emergency department. His breathing is spontaneous, but an abnormal pattern is detected. His chest rises and appears to become "locked" in the inspiratory position, except when interrupted periodically by brief exhalations. This pattern of breathing is most likely the result of

○ A. denervation of central chemoreceptors
○ B. disruption of respiratory circuits in the brainstem
○ C. spinal cord lesion at the first cervical segment
○ D. stroke in the left temporal lobe without brain swelling
○ E. vagotomy and attendant loss of vagal inputs from the lung

ANSWERS AND DISCUSSIONS

1. **D** (host hypersensitivity) is correct. The patient's symptoms, x-ray findings, and laboratory results are consistent with the diagnosis of tuberculosis. The infecting bacillus, *Mycobacterium tuberculosis,* produces no known toxins. The pathologic manifestations of tuberculosis are determined by the patient's hypersensitivity to this organism, particularly hypersensitivity to components of the organism's cell wall, including arabinogalactan and mycosides such as cord factor.

A (disseminated intravascular coagulation) is incorrect. Disseminated intravascular coagulation is not a major factor in the disease described in this patient.
B (enzymes produced by the infecting bacilli) is incorrect. No known enzymes are associated with the pathogenesis of tuberculosis.
C (exotoxins produced by the infecting bacilli) is incorrect. No exotoxins are produced by *M. tuberculosis.*
E (lipopolysaccharide produced by the infecting bacilli) is incorrect. *M. tuberculosis* is cytologically gram-positive and produces no lipopolysaccharide.

2. **E** (vitamin K) is correct. The patient most likely has a vitamin K deficiency resulting from antibiotic treatment, malnutrition, and small intestine resection. Vitamin K is produced by intestinal bacteria and can also be obtained from the diet. Vitamin K is required for the synthesis of blood clotting factors II (prothrombin), VII, IX, and X.

A (intrinsic factor) is incorrect. Gastric parietal cells are responsible for the synthesis of intrinsic factor. The patient did not have a gastrectomy, so he would be unlikely to have a deficiency of intrinsic factor.
B (vitamin B_{12}) is incorrect. Vitamin B_{12} is absorbed in the terminal ileum, which was spared in the patient. Vitamin B_{12} is also stored in the body, and it takes several years to develop a deficiency of this vitamin. Thus, vitamin B_{12} deficiency is unlikely in this patient.
C (vitamin C) is incorrect. Vitamin C deficiency does not cause bleeding into the skin. It causes perifollicular petechiae. In patients who have undergone resection of the small intestine, the absorption of vitamin C is not likely to be impaired.
D (vitamin D) is incorrect. Vitamin D deficiency does not explain the symptoms of the patient. A deficiency of this vitamin can lead to rickets or osteomalacia.

3. **C** (factitious disorder) is correct. Individuals with factitious disorder want to assume a sick role and deliberately produce symptoms to accomplish this goal, such as taking drugs that will necessitate being hospitalized. Additional external incentives do not motivate the behavior.

A   (body dysmorphic disorder) is incorrect. Excessive concern about a self-defined bodily defect and a magnified sense of ugliness characterize body dysmorphic disorder. For example, a woman who is dissatisfied with the size of her nose to the point that she avoids social contact may have body dysmorphic disorder.
B   (conversion disorder) is incorrect. Individuals with conversion disorder develop pseudoneurologic symptoms in response to stress. The process occurs unconsciously, and the prognosis is generally good once the stressor is identified and addressed. For example, a typical conversion reaction might be the sudden onset of blindness secondary to guilt in a man who sees his child hit by an automobile.
D   (hypochondriasis) is incorrect. Hypochondriasis refers to a preoccupation with disease. Individuals with this disorder do not have a medical illness, but they truly believe they do. These individuals focus on any perceived signs of disease. They do not deliberately create symptoms, but they travel from physician to physician seeking a medical diagnosis for their perceived illness.
E   (malingering) is incorrect. Malingering implies a deliberate attempt to produce symptoms because of external incentives (e.g., money, avoidance of responsibilities). Malingering might be suspected when someone is engaged in a lawsuit from a minor motor vehicle accident after developing atypical or excessive physical complaints.

4. **B** (failure of the intermaxillary process to fuse with the right maxillary swelling) is correct. Failure of the maxillary swelling to fuse with the medial nasal prominence of the intermaxillary segment results in a cleft lip. The clefts vary from a small notch in the upper lip to complete clefts of the lip and alveolar part of the palate. Approximately 60%–80% of the affected newborns are males.

A   (exposure to isotretinoin during the last trimester of pregnancy) is incorrect. Isotretinoin and other vitamin A derivatives are well-known teratogens of facial abnormalities. However, the sensitive period for lip and palate formation is 5–10 weeks' gestation. The palate is unaffected because it is formed before the last trimester of pregnancy.
C   (failure of the nasolacrimal groove to close on the right side) is incorrect. The lateral nasal prominences merge with the maxillary swellings by the 5th week of development, forming the nasolacrimal groove, which does not extend to the lip. The nasolacrimal duct develops from the floor of the groove as a solid epithelial cord that canalizes to form the nasolacrimal duct and lacrimal sac.

D   (failure of the palatine shelves to fuse) is incorrect. Failure of the palatine shelves to fuse results in cleft palate, an anomaly that may involve the hard and soft palates. During weeks 8–10 of development, the shelves elevate to a horizontal position and are susceptible to teratogenic agents. Cleft palate may occur simultaneously with cleft lip, but the two defects are induced independently.

E   (persistence of the first pharyngeal cleft on the right) is incorrect. The first pharyngeal cleft, which gives rise to the external auditory meatus, is not involved in formation of the mouth.

5. *A*   (atrophic adrenals with dense lymphocytic infiltrate) is correct. This patient has Addison's disease, as suggested by the fatigue, weakness, poor appetite, and weight loss. Other characteristics include hyperpigmentation of the skin and dark patches on the mucous membranes. In developed countries, the most common cause of Addison's disease is autoimmune destruction of the adrenals, suggested by lymphoid infiltrates in the adrenal glands plus circulating antiadrenal antibodies. In developing countries, tuberculosis would also be a major cause.

B   (carcinoid tumor of the vermiform appendix) is incorrect. A carcinoid tumor limited to the appendix would be clinically silent. In any case, such a tumor does not produce the characteristics associated with Addison's disease.

C   (functional follicular adenoma of the thyroid) is incorrect. This type of thyroid neoplasm would cause typical hyperthyroidism, not Addison's disease.

D   (granulosa cell tumor of the right ovary) is incorrect. A granulosa cell tumor would produce excess estrogen, not Addison's disease.

E   (hyperplasia of all four parathyroid glands) is incorrect. Hyperparathyroidism would cause hypercalcemia, not the electrolyte and pigmentation changes seen in this patient.

6. *C*   (succinylcholine) is correct. Succinylcholine is classified as a depolarizing NMBD. Like acetylcholine, succinylcholine binds to the nicotinic N_M receptor, opens the Na^+,K^+ channel, and causes depolarization of the muscle end plate. When succinylcholine is administered, there is a brief period of uncoordinated muscle activity characterized by muscle fasciculations. Because succinylcholine is not metabolized by acetylcholinesterases at the muscle end plate, the drug then causes persistent depolarization (phase 1 or depolarizing block), which is characterized by flaccid paralysis. The use of cholinesterase inhibitors will augment the depolarizing block. Patients treated with succinylcholine commonly complain of muscle soreness in the postoperative period. Although the relationship of myalgias to fasciculations has

not been established, many anesthesiologists administer a non-depolarizing NMBD prior to administering succinylcholine, and this appears to ameliorate the postoperative soreness.

A (atracurium), B (mivacurium), D (tubocurarine), and E (vecuronium) are incorrect. Atracurium, mivacurium, tubocurarine, and vecuronium are classified as nondepolarizing NMBDs. These drugs act as competitive antagonists at one or both acetylcholine binding sites on the pentameric N_M receptor. This action blocks the depolarizing effect of acetylcholine and results in flaccid paralysis without producing muscle fasciculations. Cholinesterase inhibitors will antagonize the neuromuscular blockade produced by nondepolarizing NMBDs, so these inhibitors can be used to reverse the effects of nondepolarizing NMBDs.

7. *C* (macrophages) is correct. The alveolar macrophage ("dust" cell) wanders over the alveolar surface, phagocytosing bacteria and other inhaled particles, including particles released from inhaled cigarette smoke. These cells digest the phagocytosed bacteria using lysosomal enzymes, which lack carbonase. Carbonase degrades carbon; thus, this lack of carbonase causes the undigested particles of tar to remain in the cells for life.

A (ciliated cuboidal cells) is incorrect. Ciliated cuboidal cells are found in higher (wider) segments of the respiratory tree, not in the alveoli.
B (endothelial cells) is incorrect. Endothelial cells line the alveolar capillaries. Although they reside within the alveolar septum (respiratory membrane), they are not phagocytes. Therefore, they are unlikely to contain lung contaminants (including those introduced by inhaled cigarette smoke).
D (type I pneumocytes) is incorrect. Type I pneumocytes lie within the alveolar septum and face the air in the alveolus. Because they are extremely thin structures, they are able to facilitate the passage of gas between air and blood. They are not phagocytes; therefore, they are unlikely to contain any lung contaminants (including those introduced by inhaled cigarette smoke).
E (type II pneumocytes) is incorrect. Type II pneumocytes reside within the alveolar septum, where they synthesize and release surfactant. These are not phagocytic cells, and are unlikely to contain any lung contaminants (including those introduced by inhaled cigarette smoke).

8. *E* (prolactinoma) is correct. A prolactinoma is a pituitary tumor that secretes prolactin, the hormone responsible for milk production. It also participates in breast development and suppression of ovulation. Excessive amounts of prolactin in the bloodstream can explain all of this patient's symptoms, except the headache and hemianopia. However, the headache may be due

to the mass effect of the tumor on local pain neurons and/or their blood supply, and the hemianopia may be due to the mass effect of the tumor on the optic chiasm.

A   (basophilic tumor of the anterior pituitary) is incorrect. The basophilic cells of the anterior pituitary secrete thyroid-stimulating hormone (TSH), gonadotrophins (which trigger the secretion of follicle-stimulating hormone [FSH], and luteinizing hormone [LH]), and possibly corticotrophins. A tumor originating from gonadotrophs could affect ovulation. Its position within the hypophysis indicates that it could grow into the optic chiasm and cause visual problems. However, it would not cause the milky discharge experienced by this patient.
B   (growth hormone–secreting tumor) is incorrect. Growth hormone is produced by acidophilic cells in the anterior pituitary gland. Excessive growth hormone levels in the blood would cause acromegaly.
C   (Hashimoto's thyroiditis) is incorrect. Hashimoto's thyroiditis is a chronic inflammation of the thyroid gland that is associated with an autoimmune process. Evidence of this condition (e.g., goiter, coexisting autoimmune disorders, or thyroid cancer) was not reported for this patient.
D   (pinealoma) is incorrect. Abnormal milk production points strongly to a pituitary lesion. Since the pituitary gland is near the optic chiasm, a pituitary growth could also cause abnormal vision and headache by means of a mass effect on neighboring structures. A pinealoma can probably be ruled out, however, because of the distance between the pineal gland and the optic chiasm. Also, a pinealoma would not explain the milky discharge from the patient's nipples.

9. *C*   (line C) is correct. The patient's symptoms are consistent with the diagnosis of gout, a disease characterized by frequent attacks of arthritic pain. The hypothetical drug is an inhibitor of xanthine oxidase, the enzyme that converts hypoxanthine and xanthine into uric acid. The kinetic effect of this drug on xanthine oxidase is best described by line C in the figure. Since the drug is structurally similar to the xanthine oxidase substrate, it would be expected to compete for binding at the active site of the enzyme. Competitive inhibition results in a $1/V$ versus $1/[S]$ plot in which the lines of the inhibited and uninhibited reaction intersect on the y-axis. The maximum velocity (V_{max}) is the same in the presence of a competitive inhibitor. However, the Michaelis constant (K_m) is increased in the presence of the competitive inhibitor.

A   (line A) and B (line B) are incorrect. A decrease in V_{max} and no effect on K_m are characteristics of noncompetitive inhibition, in which the inhibitor and substrate bind at different sites on the enzyme.

D (line D) is incorrect. A shift in V_{max} and K_m to yield a plotted line parallel to that of an uninhibited enzyme is characteristic of noncompetitive inhibition.

E (line E) is incorrect. Line E does not follow inhibition kinetics.

10. **D** (inhibiting the release of acetylcholine) is correct. The patient's disease manifestations are consistent with food-borne botulism, a disease caused by *Clostridium botulinum*. This motile, gram-positive, strict anaerobe has subterminally located endospores and is a ubiquitous soil microbe. The organism can be found in home-canned vegetables that have been improperly prepared. The bacterial spores germinate, and the vegetative cells grow and elaborate botulinum toxin. When the toxin is ingested, it causes paralysis by inhibiting the release of acetylcholine from cholinergic synapses. There are seven antigenic types of botulinum toxin.

A (blocking the release of postsynaptic inhibitors) and B (causing the lysis of neurons) are incorrect. Botulinum toxins do not block the release of postsynaptic inhibitors, and they have no direct cytotoxic effect on neurons.

C (increasing the intracellular level of cyclic adenosine monophosphate) and E (inhibiting the synthesis of proteins) are incorrect. Botulinum toxins have no direct effect on cAMP levels or protein synthesis.

11. **B** (numbness of the scrotum and inner side of the thigh) is correct. The ilioinguinal nerve, which travels through the inguinal canal and superficial inguinal ring, innervates the skin of the anterior scrotum and medial thigh. Inguinal incision to repair the hernia may injure the ilioinguinal nerve and/or it may be caught in a suture, causing pain in the L1 dermatome region (anterior scrotum and medial thigh).

A (infertility) is incorrect. Injury to the nerve that travels in the inguinal canal does not cause infertility. Division of the ductus deferens results in sterility on the affected side. Sperm cannot enter the urethra and degenerate in the epididymis and ductus deferens.

C (numbness over the lateral side of the thigh) is incorrect. The lateral femoral cutaneous nerve (L2–L3), which runs under the inguinal ligament lateral to the inguinal canal (not through the inguinal ring), innervates the lateral side of the thigh.

D (paralysis of the adductor muscles) is incorrect. The obturator nerve (L2–L4), which travels along the lateral wall of the lesser pelvis and enters the thigh through the obturator foramen (not the inguinal ring), innervates the thigh adductors.

E (paralysis of the sartorius muscle) is incorrect. The branch of the femoral nerve (L2–L4), which descends through the substance of the psoas major and then behind the inguinal ligament to enter the thigh, innervates the sartorius muscle. It does not travel through the inguinal canal.

12. *E* (foreign substance in the injected heroin) is correct. To increase profits, drug dealers often dilute ("cut") heroin with foreign substances, which is most likely what the patient used. Usually lactose is used, but any white substance is acceptable; the cleanliness of the "lab" is also doubtful. Talc, a common contaminant, is taken up by macrophages, which then form granulomas as a foreign body reaction. Similar granulomas may often be found in the liver, spleen, and lymph nodes. Profound pulmonary edema is often apparent in individuals who die of heroin overdose.

A (activation of angiotensin-converting enzyme) is incorrect. An increased level of ACE is a result of granuloma formation, not a cause of it.
B (activation of a previously acquired mycobacterial infection) is incorrect. Infection directly associated with intravenous heroin use is frequent, but it is typically pyogenic, rather than mycobacterial.
C (concomitant HIV infection) is incorrect. HIV infection frequently accompanies intravenous heroin usage due to needle sharing. Activation of previous tuberculosis at a site now "healed" is possible, as is infection de novo by *Mycobacterium avium-intercellulare*. If this were the case in this patient, the organisms would be readily seen using the appropriate special stains.
D (direct toxicity to alveolar macrophages by heroin) is incorrect. The lung may exhibit hypersensitivity to heroin by developing severe, often fatal, pulmonary edema, but this would not be a direct cause of granuloma formation.

13. *D* (midline of the cerebellum) is correct. The cerebellum coordinates voluntary movement and regulates posture. Postural instability and a broad-based, staggering gait are characteristic findings when a lesion develops along the midline of the cerebellum. A lesion in this area could also result in nystagmus.

A (basilar pons) is incorrect. A lesion in the basilar pons could affect pontocerebellar fibers destined for the neocerebellum, and thus would contribute to the loss of control over voluntary movement. It could also affect upper motor neurons and possibly the abducens nerve (CN VI), which innervates the lateral rectus muscle of the eye. Damage to these structures would not result in nystagmus.
B (dentate nucleus) is incorrect. The dentate nuclei of the cerebellum receive input from the peripheral and central nervous systems (including the cerebellar cortex) and project to motor nuclei in the brain stem and thalamus. Damage to the dentate nuclei would eliminate most of the cerebellar influence on the motor and premotor regions of the cerebral cortex. This would make it difficult to initiate and terminate movement. It would also result in a tremor at the end of each movement, poorly coordinated movement, and the loss of spatial coordination of the hand and

finger muscles. With the exception of the stagger, none of the signs presented by this patient suggest that the dentate nuclei were damaged.

C   (medial longitudinal fasciculus) is incorrect. Upper motor neurons that influence vestibulo-oculomotor reflexes project to the medial longitudinal fasciculus (MLF). These reflexes include the reflex involved when the head is tilted to one side and the eyes rotate toward the opposite side to keep the field of vision on a horizontal plane. An MLF lesion would allow the visual plane to change when the head tilts, but would not induce nystagmus or any of the other signs reported for this patient. A lesion to the MLF results in internuclear ophthalmoplegia.

E   (midline pontine tegmentum) is incorrect. The midline pontine tegmentum includes the abducens nucleus, para-abducens nucleus, and MLF. It does not include structures that, if damaged, could cause the staggering gait and truncal ataxia reported for this patient.

14.   *A*   (acetylcysteine) is correct. When an overdose of acetaminophen is taken, free radicals are formed. These toxic oxidizing metabolites accumulate in excess as they deplete hepatic stores of glutathione, the endogenous reducing agent. The accumulated metabolites cause lipid peroxidation of hepatic membranes, and this leads to hepatic necrosis, coma, and death. In patients who have taken an acetaminophen overdose, treatment with acetylcysteine produces exogenous reducing equivalents to detoxify the oxidizing metabolites. Because acetylcysteine acts as a mucolytic agent, it is also used in the treatment of chronic bronchopulmonary disease.

B   (flumazenil) is incorrect. Flumazenil is a competitive benzodiazepine receptor antagonist and would provide no benefit in an overdose with opioids and acetaminophen.

C   (lactulose) is incorrect. Lactulose is used in the treatment of hepatic encephalopathy. In the colon, bacteria degrade lactulose to form lactate, formate, and acetate. The acidic colonic contents converts ammonia to the ammonium ion, and this traps the ion and prevents its reabsorption. Lactulose acts as an osmotic laxative and removes the trapped ammonium ion from the colon.

D   (naloxone) is incorrect. Naloxone is a pure opioid receptor antagonist. In the patient described, naloxone would reverse oxycodone-induced respiratory depression, but it would not prevent acetaminophen-induced hepatotoxicity.

E   (sodium bicarbonate) is incorrect. Sodium bicarbonate is used to treat severe metabolic acidosis resulting from intoxication with methanol, ethylene glycol, or salicylates. Because sodium bicarbonate alkalinizes the urine, it can also be used to enhance the renal elimination of weak acids or to prevent renal deposition of myoglobulin after severe rhabdomyolysis.

15. *A* *(Chlamydia trachomatis)* is correct. The clinical and laboratory findings are consistent with the diagnosis of urethritis due to *C. trachomatis.* Serovars A, B1, B2, and C of this organism cause trachoma; serovars D through K cause follicular conjunctivitis, neonatal pneumonia, and urogenital infections; and the LGV serotypes (L_1, L_2, and L_3) cause the sexually transmitted disease lymphogranuloma venereum.

B *(Haemophilus ducreyi)* is incorrect. *H. ducreyi* causes a sexually transmitted disease called chancroid. The patient's laboratory findings do not implicate this organism, because *H. ducreyi* is not a strictly intracellular parasite and can be grown on ordinary bacteriologic media.
C *(Mycoplasma genitalium)* is incorrect. *M. genitalium* is an etiologic agent of urethritis. Although it lacks a cell wall, it is not a strictly intracellular parasite and will grow on ordinary laboratory media.
D *(Neisseria gonorrhoeae)* is incorrect. *N. gonorrhoeae* is a major cause of sexually transmitted urethritis. If it had been the etiologic agent in the case described, however, gram-negative diplococci would have been observed in the Gram stain of the urethral discharge, and the organism would have grown on bacteriologic media.
E *(Ureaplasma urealyticum)* is incorrect. *U. urealyticum* is an etiologic agent of urethritis, but is not a strictly intracellular parasite.

16. *B* (malignant plasma cell disorder) is correct. The patient has multiple myeloma (MM) complicated by renal failure due to precipitation of Bence Jones (BJ) protein (light chains) in the renal tubules. MM is the most common primary malignancy of bone, and is more common in African-Americans than in whites. Lytic bone lesions result from secretion of osteoclast-activating factor (interleukin-1) by malignant plasma cells. In >80% of cases, SPE shows a monoclonal spike in the gamma-globulin region. A single clone of malignant plasma cells produces the predominant immunoglobulin (Ig), usually IgG, hence the sharp spike in the gamma-globulin region of SPE. The immunoglobulin's corresponding light chain (kappa or lambda) BJ protein is spilled into the urine. Because urine dipsticks for protein detect only albumin (whereas the SSA detects both albumin and globulins), a disparity between the urine protein dipstick reaction (trace or +1) and SSA (+3 or +4) excludes albumin as the cause of proteinuria and is highly suggestive of BJ protein in the urine. A bone marrow aspirate showing sheets of malignant plasma cells is mandatory to confirm the diagnosis. Serum immunoelectrophoresis identifies the Ig involved. Renal failure is a common cause of death in MM. Note the increase in serum BUN and creatinine levels and renal tubular casts in this patient.

A (immunoglobulin M–producing lymphoproliferative disorder) is incorrect. An IgM–producing lymphoproliferative disorder is called Waldenström's macroglobulinemia. Unlike MM, this malignant disorder is not associated with lytic lesions and acts more like a malignant lymphoma in that it metastasizes to lymph nodes.

C (malignant T-cell disorder) and D (metastatic disease of undetermined origin) are incorrect. Unlike MM, these disorders are not associated with monoclonal spikes or Bence Jones protein.

E (renal failure of undetermined origin) is incorrect. This patient's renal failure is a complication of MM, rather than a cause of her skeletal and hematologic problems.

17. *E* (relaxed but awake) is correct. Alpha waves are present on the EEG of a relaxed individual who is awake.

A (actively concentrating on a task) is incorrect. During active mental concentration, beta waves are most common.

B (dreaming) is incorrect. Dreaming occurs during rapid eye movement (REM) sleep, and the brain waves are of low amplitude but high frequency.

C (in stage 2 sleep) is incorrect. Stage 2 sleep is characterized by sleep spindles and K complexes. During stage 2, peaceful sleep occurs, but the individual is responsive at times to external stimuli.

D (in stage 4 sleep) is incorrect. Delta waves are most prominent during stage 4 sleep, which represents deep sleep.

18. *E* (posterior cruciate) is correct. The integrity of the cruciate ligaments is tested with the knee flexed to a 90-degree position. Rupture of the posterior ligament usually results from a direct blow to the anterior tibia, such as occurs when a knee is forced against the dashboard during an automobile accident. The posterior cruciate ligament limits posterior mobility of the tibia, and rupture of this ligament allows the tibia to assume a position of posterior displacement on the femur when in flexion. A positive drawer sign would be indicated by movement of the tibia backward on the femur.

A (anterior cruciate) is incorrect. The anterior cruciate ligament is tight on extension, and it limits excessive anterior mobility of the tibia on the femur. Rupture of the anterior cruciate ligament allows abnormal anterior displacement of the tibia on the femur in flexion.

B (lateral collateral) is incorrect. The lateral collateral ligament runs from the lateral epicondyle of the femur to the head of the fibula. Together with the medial cruciate ligament, the lateral collateral ligament restrains rotation of the tibia laterally or of the femur medially. Isolated injury to the lateral collateral ligament may have little effect on the stability of the knee. On examination, there is an unnatural mobility toward adduction.

C (medial collateral) is incorrect. The medial collateral ligament, which is critical to the stability of the knee, runs from the medial epicondyle of the femur to the medial surface of the upper end of the tibia. This ligament is most commonly injured by a blow to the lateral side of the knee. Patients with tears of this ligament are unable to extend the knee fully; extension stretches this ligament, causing pain. On examination, there is unnatural mobility toward abduction.

D   (patellar) is incorrect. The patellar ligament is a common tendon of insertion of the four heads of the quadriceps femoris muscle. The main function of the quadriceps is knee extension. If the patellar ligament is ruptured, the patient cannot fully extend the knee. Traumatic disruption of the patellar tendon usually is caused by sudden contraction of the quadratus femoris while running, jumping, or climbing stairs.

19. *A*   (cyanide toxicity secondary to decomposition of NP; administer thiosulfate) is correct. NP is rapidly hydrolyzed and releases free cyanide, which is normally converted to thiocyanate by the mitochondrial rhodanese system in the liver and blood vessels. Prolonged high-dose administration of NP can result in cyanide accumulation, since this enzymatic system exhibits zero-order kinetics. Inhibition of cytochrome oxidase by cyanide causes an increase in anaerobic glycolysis and thereby produces lactic acidosis. It also causes a decrease in O_2 utilization and thereby increases the PO_2 in mixed venous blood. Treatment of NP-induced cyanide toxicity would include administration of thiosulfate.

B   (hypersensitivity reaction to NP; administer epinephrine) is incorrect. The patient's response is not a hypersensitivity reaction to NP. As discussed in A, it is an adverse effect of prolonged high-dose administration of NP.

C   (hypoglycemia; administer glucose) is incorrect. The patient's age, African-American heritage, and medical history may have predisposed him to malignant hypertension, but they would not have increased his risk of NP-induced toxicity. As discussed in A, this toxicity was the result of prolonged high-dose treatment with NP.

D   (rare side effect associated with glyburide use; initiate metformin therapy) is incorrect. Lactic acidosis is not a rare side effect of glyburide use. It is a rare side effect of metformin use and is more likely to occur in patients who have compromised renal function.

E   (rhabdomyolysis, a side effect of NP; administer sodium bicarbonate) is incorrect. Rhabdomyolysis is not a side effect of NP. It is a side effect of the "statin" HMG-CoA reductase inhibitors (such as atorvastatin, fluvastatin, lovastatin, pravastatin, and simvastatin), which are used in the management of hyperlipidemias.

20. *A*   (Horner's syndrome) is correct. This patient exhibits the classic features of Horner's syndrome: ptosis (droopy eyelid) and miosis (constriction of the pupil) on the same side as a lesion that has damaged sympathetic neurons in the hypothalamus or brain stem, ventral spinal roots C8–T2, the superior cervical ganglion,

internal carotid sheath to the iris, or the upper eyelid. The miosis is due to unopposed parasympathetic activity in the pupillary constrictor muscle. The ptosis may be a result of paralysis of the superior tarsal Muller's muscle. The facial flushing and lack of facial sweating may be due to the loss of sympathetic vascular tone.

B (infarction in the basilar pons) is incorrect. An infarction in the basilar pons may disrupt normal activity in the abducens nerve (CN VI), which controls lateral eye movement. The facial nerve (CN VII), which controls muscles of facial expression, and the vestibulocochlear nerve (CN VIII), which transmits signals required for hearing and balance, also exit the brain stem close to this area. No changes in the function of CN VII and VIII were reported for this patient.

C (infarction in the callosomarginal artery) is incorrect. The callosomarginal artery is a branch of the cerebral artery found in the cingulate sulcus. Damage to the cingulum would alter emotional behavior and lead to epilepsy, personality changes, or a lack of inhibition, drive, and initiative. It would not produce the abnormal autonomic findings reported for this patient.

D (inferior alternating hemiplegia) is incorrect. An inferior alternating hemiplegia develops when the lower motor neurons of the hypoglossal nerve (CN XII) are compromised, along with the upper motor neurons in the pyramidal tract. The lesion responsible for this condition occurs in the medulla. It would not cause the findings observed in this patient.

E (lesion in the cerebellopontine angle) is incorrect. A lesion in the cerebellopontine angle would compress afferent fibers within CN VIII, the lower motor neuron of CN VII, and the ipsilateral cerebellar hemisphere. Signs of this lesion would include, respectively, reduction in the sense of hearing and balance; ipsilateral paralysis of the muscles of facial expression below the eyes; and loss of muscle coordination (ataxia) in the ipsilateral limb, intention tremor, or nystagmus.

21. *E* (rubella virus) is correct. The clinical and laboratory findings are consistent with the diagnosis of rubella (German measles). This disease is caused by rubella virus, a member of the genus *Rubivirus* and the family *Togaviridae*. Like other togaviruses, rubella virus is an enveloped, positive-sense, nonsegmented RNA virus with glycoprotein spikes anchored to the capsid. Unlike other togaviruses, which are transmitted by arthropods, rubella virus is transmitted by contact with respiratory tract secretions.

A (adenovirus) is incorrect. Adenoviruses are not enveloped viruses and are not typically associated with a rash. Members of the family *Adenoviridae* are double-stranded, linear DNA viruses.

B (coronavirus) is incorrect. Coronaviruses do not cause a rash. They cause common colds and gastroenteritis. Members of the family *Coronaviridae* are single-stranded, positive-sense, nonsegmented RNA viruses.

C (measles virus) is incorrect. Measles virus is the agent of rubeola. It has glycoprotein spikes, but they are not bound to the capsid. Measles virus is a member of the family *Paramyxoviridae,* which consists of single-stranded, negative-sense, nonsegmented RNA viruses.

D (mumps virus) is incorrect. Mumps virus does not cause rash. It typically causes pain and swelling of the salivary glands. Like measles virus, mumps virus is a member of the family *Paramyxoviridae.*

22. *E* (he recently underwent heart transplantation) is correct. The resting tachycardia (HR = 97/min) and lack of chronotropic response to a decrease in MAP are results of cardiac denervation following heart transplantation.

A (he develops tachycardia due to treatment with a cholinergic agonist) is incorrect. A cholinergic agonist will produce bradycardia. The HR in this patient is virtually unchanged.

B (he has a normal baroreflex response to standing up) is incorrect. The decrease in blood pressure with very little change in HR indicates poor baroreflex function (orthostatic hypotension).

C (he has lost baroreflex function resulting from systemic hypertension) is incorrect. MAP of 108 mm Hg is not in the hypertensive range. The development of hypertension does not eliminate the baroreflex.

D (he is being treated with a sympathetic antagonist) is incorrect. A sympathetic antagonist will not prevent an increase in HR with decreasing blood pressure; the increase in HR is mainly due to decreased parasympathetic activity.

23. *A* (increasing intracellular levels of cyclic adenosine monophosphate) is correct. The clinical and laboratory findings are consistent with the diagnosis of traveler's diarrhea caused by an enterotoxigenic strain of *Escherichia coli.* Enterotoxigenic strains secrete heat-labile enterotoxins and/or heat-stable enterotoxins. The heat-labile type ribosylates the G protein that regulates adenylyl cyclase. This increases intracellular cAMP levels and thereby induces fluid and electrolyte excretion.

B (increasing intracellular levels of cyclic guanosine monophosphate) is incorrect. Unlike the heat-labile type of enterotoxin, the heat-stable type activates guanylyl cyclase and increases intracellular cGMP levels.

C (inducing mucosal inflammation), D (inducing the lysis of epithelial cells in the large intestine), and E (inhibiting protein synthesis and thereby causing cell death) are incorrect. The heat-labile and heat-stable enterotoxins do not mediate mucosal inflammation. They are not known to be cytotoxic, and they do not directly inhibit protein synthesis.

24. ***B*** (excitement) is correct. In their book *Human Sexual Response,* William H. Masters and Virginia E. Johnson described the four phases of the sexual response cycle through their extensive evaluation of sexual functioning. In women, lubrication of the vagina occurs in the first phase, termed excitement. During this phase, men experience penile tumescence and erection.

A (desire) is incorrect. Desire precedes the sexual response cycle and is typically a cognitive process. This phase includes sexual fantasies.
C (orgasm) is incorrect. During the orgasmic phase, both women and men experience contractions, with an increase in pulse rate and blood pressure. This is the phase in which ejaculation occurs. Women may experience multiple orgasms.
D (plateau) is incorrect. In women, the clitoris retracts and vasoconstriction of the outer third of the vagina and the labia minora occurs during the plateau phase. Men display an increase in penile circumference as orgasm is soon approaching.
E (resolution) is incorrect. The clitoris returns to its normal position, and vasoconstriction subsides in females during the resolution phase. Men show a rapid loss of vasoconstriction to the penis and subsequently the size of the penis decreases, the testes descend, and the scrotum relaxes. Men then show a refractory period (typically 10 minutes or more) in which further erection is not possible. Women do not show a refractory period and can respond to additional stimulation.

25. ***D*** (decorticate rigidity) is correct. Decorticate rigidity is characterized by stereotypical arm and leg movements that occur in response to sensory stimulation (e.g., the sensations produced during passive movement of the head). A lesion above the red nucleus (in the cortex or thalamus) could result in flexion in the upper limbs while the lower limbs remain in extension.

A (alternating superior hemiplegia) is incorrect. An alternating superior hemiplegia involves impaired ipsilateral oculomotor (CN III) activity and contralateral hemiparesis. No changes in CN III activity were reported for this patient.
B (Brown-Séquard's syndrome) is incorrect. Brown-Séquard's syndrome is caused by hemisection of the spinal cord and results in ipsilateral paralysis and contralateral loss of pain and temperature sensations. It does not have a bilateral effect on motor activity in the limbs.
C (decerebrate rigidity) is incorrect. Decerebrate rigidity is caused by an intercollicular lesion. It results in all of the limbs being in extension, not just the lower limbs. This effect is due, in part, to the disruption of all descending inhibitory input to the lateral vestibular nucleus.
E (transection of the spinal cord below T5) is incorrect. Motor output to the arm is transmitted through spinal nerves C5–T1. Transection of the spinal cord below T5 would not trigger the responses seen in this patient.

26. *D* (is an asymptomatic carrier of α-thalassemia) is correct. Deletion of one of the four α-globin genes produces a silent carrier state, and no hematologic abnormalities are evident. One of the chromosome 16 genes carries this deficiency. If such an individual has offspring with another carrier, the children could have the α-thalassemia trait. There are four functional α-globin genes; thus, there are four possible degrees of α-thalassemia (based on the loss or one to four genes). This individual has the mildest form; the most severe form is associated with fetal death in utero.

A (has a moderate degree of erythroid hyperplasia in bone marrow), B (has an abnormal hemoglobin concentration), C (has numerous target cells in the peripheral blood), and E (may develop severe hemolytic anemia if exposed to oxidant drugs) are incorrect. Loss of one α-globin allele is silent and results in no hematologic abnormalities, such as hemoglobin Bart's. Sensitivity to oxidant drugs (e.g., antimalarials, sulfonamides, nitrofurantoin, phenacetin, aspirin in large doses, vitamin K derivatives) is associated with glucose-6-phosphate dehydrogenase deficiency, not with α-thalassemia.

27. *C* (endonuclease) is correct. Xeroderma pigmentosum is a rare autosomal recessive disease. In affected patients, the exposure to ultraviolet (UV) light creates severe skin ulcerations and neoplasms. Investigators believe that the removal of pyrimidine dimers in DNA by UV-specific endonuclease is inefficient in these patients, and this causes excisional repair of DNA in skin cells to be defective.

A (DNA helicase) is incorrect. DNA helicase catalyzes adenosine triphosphate–dependent strand separation during DNA replication.
B (DNA polymerase III) is incorrect. DNA polymerase III catalyzes template-dependent DNA chain elongation.
D (RNA polymerase) is incorrect. RNA polymerase catalyzes the formation of RNA in which a strand of DNA or RNA is used as a template.
E (topoisomerases) is incorrect. Topoisomerases regulate the supertwisting of DNA. They create positive or negative supercoils in circular double-stranded DNA.

28. *C* (if the physician continues to see him immediately) is correct. Social learning theory is based on behavioral and cognitive principles of behavior. The theory predicts that individuals act consistently when similar behavior leads to similar consequences. Therefore, altering this patient's behavior would require that the physician alter his own behavior. The physician could reward appropriate behavior (e.g., agree to see the patient only

when he is calm and pleasant) or ignore the inappropriate behavior (e.g., see the patient in the order scheduled or needed regardless of the patient's behavior).

A (if the patient's behavior is routinely ignored) is incorrect. Providing attention for inappropriate behavior is often indirectly reinforcing. Therefore, ignoring the demanding behavior over time will typically lead to a decline in the behavior over time.
B (if the patient is rewarded for pleasant interactions) is incorrect. Positive reinforcement of acceptable behaviors would increase the likelihood that the patient would act appropriately.
D (regardless of any changes the physician attempts) is incorrect. Hopelessness on the part of the physician will not improve the situation. Rather, the physician must learn to remain calm and professional while attempting alternative strategies for dealing with difficult patients.
E (until the patient is declined medical care) is incorrect. Declining health care to an ill patient during an emergency situation is unethical.

29. *C* *(Giardia lamblia)* is correct. The clinical and laboratory findings are consistent with the diagnosis of gastroenteritis caused by the flagellate *G. lamblia*. Infection is acquired by ingesting *G. lamblia* cysts. This patient ingested cysts when he drank contaminated water; however, the cysts can also be transmitted from human to human via the fecal-oral route.

A *(Cryptosporidium parvum)* and B *(Entamoeba histolytica)* are incorrect. *G. lamblia*, *C. parvum*, and *E. histolytica* are all lumen-dwelling protozoan parasites that cause diarrhea. However, *G. lamblia* is a flagellate, *C. parvum* is a sporozoan, and *E. histolytica* is an ameba, so their laboratory findings would differ.
D *(Toxoplasma gondii)* and E *(Trypanosoma cruzi)* are incorrect. *T. gondii* and *T. cruzi* are blood- and tissue-dwelling protozoan parasites. *T. gondii* is a sporozoan parasite capable of causing systemic infection with a wide range of manifestations, but it is not commonly associated with diarrhea. *Toxoplasma* infection is usually acquired via ingestion of improperly cooked meat or via contact with infected cat feces. *T. cruzi* is a hemoflagellate, and would not be found in a stool sample. *T. cruzi* causes Chagas' disease and is transmitted by the bite of the reduviid (kissing) bug.

30. *D* (site 4) is correct. Methyldopa is a prodrug that is decarboxylated by aromatic amino acid decarboxylase (AAAD, or dopa decarboxylase). It is then hydroxylated by dopamine-β-hydroxylase to form the active drug, α-methylnorepinephrine. The active drug acts centrally as an α_2-adrenergic receptor agonist (site 4) and decreases the sympathetic outflow to the vasculature. Cloni-

dine, guanfacine, and guanabenz are other examples of α_2-adrenergic receptor agonists that act centrally to reduce blood pressure.

A (site 1) is incorrect. Site 1 is the site at which carbidopa acts. Carbidopa is a peripheral AAAD inhibitor. By preventing the extracerebral conversion of levodopa to dopamine, it increases the apparent potency of levodopa and decreases some of levodopa's peripheral side effects, such as nausea, vomiting, and arrhythmia.
B (site 2) is incorrect. Site 2 is the site at which α_1-adrenergic receptor antagonists act. These agents, which include prazosin and other "sin" drugs, produce their antihypertensive effect by blocking postsynaptic α_1 receptors.
C (site 3) is incorrect. Site 3 is the site at which β_1-adrenergic receptor antagonists act. These agents, which include propranolol and metoprolol, produce their antihypertensive effect by blocking postsynaptic β_1 receptors.
E (site 5) is incorrect. Site 5 is the site at which tolcapone acts. Tolcapone reversibly inhibits catechol-O-methyltransferase and is used as an adjunct drug in the treatment of Parkinson's disease. When tolcapone is taken concurrently with levodopa, it helps to sustain the levels of levodopa and to minimize the end-of-dose deterioration ("wearing off" effects) associated with levodopa use.
F (site 6) is incorrect. Site 6 is the site at which cocaine acts. Cocaine blocks the neuronal reuptake of norepinephrine and produces somatic side effects via this action. The drug's central reinforcing effects are mediated by the blockade of dopamine reuptake. Its clinical utility as a local anesthetic is attributed to its ability to block Na^+ channels. Other drugs that act at site 6 include tricyclic antidepressants, which block the active transporter for norepinephrine and serotonin.
G (site 7) is incorrect. Site 7 is the site at which monoamine oxidase type A (MAO-A) oxidatively deaminates norepinephrine and serotonin. MAO-A is inhibited by drugs such as phenelzine and tranylcypromine.

31. *C* (consumption of platelets) is correct. The patient has thrombotic thrombocytopenic purpura (TTP), in which a toxin circulating in plasma damages small vessel endothelial cells, resulting in formation of platelet thrombi that occlude the lumen of these vessels throughout the body (e.g., brain, kidneys, heart). Platelets are consumed during this process, which lowers the platelet count and prolongs the BT. The BT primarily evaluates platelet function. Platelet thrombi damage red blood cells, resulting in fragmented cells, called schistocytes, and in an intravascular hemolytic anemia. Renal failure is common, as has occurred in this patient who has a history of oliguria and elevated serum BUN and creatinine levels. Plasmapheresis is the treatment of choice for TTP.

A (circulating anticoagulant) is incorrect. Circulating anticoagulants are antibodies that inhibit specific coagulation factors (e.g., antibodies against factor VIII), hence simulating a coagulation factor deficiency. Normal PTT and PT exclude circulating anticoagulants from the differential diagnosis.

B (consumption of coagulation factors) is incorrect. The thrombi that are formed in the vessel lumen are composed of platelets, not fibrin clots. In other words, TTP is not a variant of disseminated intravascular coagulation (DIC).

D (qualitative platelet disorder) is incorrect. The problem is consumption of platelets in platelet thrombi, and not a disorder involving platelet adhesion or aggregation.

E (secondary fibrinolytic disorder) is incorrect. The D-dimer assay is negative, and the PT and PTT are both normal. Secondary fibrinolysis refers to activation of the fibrinolytic system (plasminogen is converted into plasmin) as a compensatory mechanism to destroy fibrin clots in intravascular coagulation. Plasmin destroys fibrin, fibrinogen, and many of the coagulation factors; therefore, it prolongs the PT and PTT. D-dimers are fibrin monomers in a fibrin clot that have been cross-linked by factor XIII (fibrin-stabilizing factor). Their presence indicates that intravascular coagulation has occurred.

32. *E* (lack of mRNA transcription from DNA) is correct. Eukaryotic RNA polymerase II synthesizes the precursor to messenger RNA (pre-mRNA). It also synthesizes small nuclear RNAs (snRNAs). Forty-eight hours after a toxin is ingested (such as the mushroom toxin α-amanitin) is ingested, important mRNAs will be degraded and no new mRNAs will be produced. This deficiency results in liver failure.

A (inability to synthesize proteins because large ribosomal subunit 5.8S RNA is not being produced) and B (inability to synthesize proteins because large ribosomal subunit 28S RNA is not being produced) are incorrect. Ribosomal RNAs (rRNAs) 5.8S, 18S, and 28S are synthesized by RNA polymerase I, which is insensitive to α-amanitin.

C (inhibition of mitochondrial RNA transcription) is incorrect. Mitochondrial RNA polymerase is a separate polymerase that transcribes all mitochondrial RNAs. It resembles prokaryotic polymerase and is insensitive to α-amanitin, but it can be inhibited by rifampin.

D (inhibition of tRNA synthesis) is incorrect. All transfer RNAs (tRNAs) and the 5S rRNA are produced by RNA polymerase III, an enzyme that is much less sensitive to α-amanitin than is RNA polymerase II. Mushroom poisoning will have a minor effect on RNA polymerase III.

33. *B* (facial) is correct. The facial nerve (CN VII) is one of the more complicated of the cranial nerves. It begins as two roots: a motor root that carries efferent (motor) fibers to the muscles of facial expression, the stylohyoid, posterior digastric, and one of the muscles of the middle ear (stapedius); the nervus intermedius, which carries parasympathetic fibers to the lacrimal gland, nasal

cavity, palate, and submandibular and sublingual salivary glands; and sensory fibers, most of which supply taste to the anterior two thirds of the tongue. CN VII tunnels through the temporal bone, producing a long bony canal, the facial canal.

Paralysis of the facial nerve is termed Bell's palsy. The major presentation is paralysis of the facial (mimetic) muscles, which leads to a slackness of the face on the side of the paralysis and an inability to change the shape of the mouth, as in a smile (or frown); hence, the crooked smile. The other obvious sign is a partial ptosis of the eyelid, a paralysis of the orbicularis oculi muscle, which surrounds and actually closes the eye. This paralysis produces loss of tone of this muscle and slackness of both the upper and lower eyelids, which allows the upper lid to droop and interferes with the lower lid holding the lacrimal secretion in the conjunctival sac. The location of nerve damage determines which functions are lost. Distally, near its exit from the stylomastoid foramen of the skull, the muscles of facial expression are affected, and taste may be involved; in the midpoint (at the second bend), the stapedius is affected; and proximally, near its ganglion (geniculate), the parasympathetic fibers to the lacrimal gland (dry eye) and nasal cavity and palate are affected.

A (abducens) is incorrect. The abducens nerve (CN VI) is a motor nerve to one extraocular muscle of the orbit, the lateral rectus. It has no affect on the muscles of the face.

C (glossopharyngeal) is incorrect. The glossopharyngeal nerve (CN IX) is primarily a sensory nerve to the posterior one third of the tongue for both taste and general sense and to the mucosa of the pharynx, and it provides no innervation to the face. It provides the afferent limb to the gag reflex as well as parasympathetics to the parotid salivary gland. CN IX is a motor nerve to one muscle of the pharynx, the stylopharyngeus muscle.

D (trigeminal) is incorrect. Although the trigeminal nerve (CN V) provides innervation to the face via each of its three divisions (ophthalmic, CN V_1; maxillary, CN V_2; and mandibular, CN V_3), that innervation is only sensory. There are no motor fibers to the face from CN V. One branch, CN V_3, does carry motor fibers, but these are to the four muscles of mastication, one muscle of the palate (tensor palatini), a muscle of the middle ear (tensor tympani), and the suprahyoid muscles.

E (vagus) is incorrect. The vagus nerve (CN X) provides no innervation to the face. In the head and neck, it gives motor innervation to the muscles of the palate (except the tensor palatini), to the muscles of the pharynx (except the stylopharyngeus), and to the intrinsic muscles of the larynx. It also provides sensory innervation to the epiglottis and larynx (above the vocal folds via its internal laryngeal nerve and below the vocal folds via its recurrent laryngeal nerve). CN X is a parasympathetic cranial nerve, with the remainder of its innervations in the thorax and abdomen.

34. *B* (95 mm Hg) is correct. To understand why the patient's PaO_2 is still in the normal range (75–100 mm Hg), it is important to distinguish oxygen-carrying capacity from the oxygen content of blood. The oxygen-carrying capacity is the amount of oxygen the blood can carry when hemoglobin is maximally saturated, whereas the oxygen content of blood is the total amount of oxygen the blood actually contains. In this patient, oxygen content is decreased for two reasons: she has a true anemia due to decreased amount of hemoglobin in her blood; and she has a functional anemia due to CO binding to hemoglobin sites typically reserved for oxygen. However, neither of these problems has any effect on the PaO_2, which depends solely on the amount of oxygen dissolved in plasma. PO_2 is independent of the amount of hemoglobin and the number of sites available to bind oxygen.

A (120 mm Hg) is incorrect. An increase in the PaO_2 indicates an increase in the proportion of oxygen in the plasma compartment of blood. This could result from chemoreceptor stimulation and activation of breathing. CO is not sensed by any physiologic receptor, and breathing is not stimulated, which is why CO is considered dangerous.
C (70 mm Hg), D (50 mm Hg), and E (25 mm Hg) are incorrect. CO reduces the oxygen-carrying capacity of blood, not the oxygen level in plasma, which is indicated by PaO_2. Because the plasma oxygen level is unaffected, the PaO_2 should not fall below normal.

35. *C* (empathy) is correct. A physician develops empathy by placing himself or herself in the position of the patient to facilitate an understanding of how the patient feels. Once empathy is developed for this patient, the student will be better able to assist the patient in resolving the obstacles to monitoring blood glucose levels. An example of an empathic statement would be, "Diabetes is a difficult disease to accept, so I can understand why you might not want to be continually reminded of the fact that you have the disease. Perhaps you could tell me more about how monitoring your blood glucose levels makes you feel."

A (assertiveness) is incorrect. Assertiveness refers to an individual's ability to directly communicate without defensive or accusatory statements and typically is aimed at solving a problem. Sometimes when a physician is assertive with a patient, the patient may feel the interaction is confrontational unless a well-established level of rapport is present. An assertive statement that the medical student might make in this situation could be, "I am concerned that you are not monitoring your blood glucose levels regularly and would like to work with you to problem-solve about how we can get you to do this as suggested."
B (diagnosis) is incorrect. Accurate diagnosis relies on objective data and does not necessarily require an understanding of a patient's subjective point of view regarding an illness.

D   (negotiation) is incorrect. To increase a patient's adherence to treatment recommendations, it is often necessary to negotiate with the patient. When treatment goals are being negotiated, the patient's goals and priorities should be reviewed first. Next, the physician's priorities should be stated and an attempt should be made to establish the order in which issues will be addressed. In this case, the patient's priorities may not revolve around monitoring his blood glucose levels, but he may be willing to monitor them if his priorities are addressed first.

E   (objective observation) is incorrect. Observing a patient's behavior and interactions in an objective manner is critically important to patient care. For example, as part of the clinical interview, a patient's appearance, level of psychomotor activity, gait, speech, affect, and general mannerisms and interactions are all observed and recorded during a mental status examination. These observations are documented to convey a wealth of information about the patient and may provide information that the patient is unaware of about himself.

36. *D*   (primary colon cancer) is correct. The patient has primary colon cancer complicated by iron deficiency anemia (microcytic anemia and low serum ferritin) and metastasis to the liver (nodular, enlarged liver). Key points in the patient's history include weight loss, change in consistency of stools, and blood mixed with stools. Thrombocytosis is common in metastatic cancer and in chronic iron deficiency anemia. The most common cause of iron deficiency in a patient over 50 years of age is colon cancer.

A   (external hemorrhoids) is incorrect. Blood coating stools in the presence of external hemorrhoids always requires further investigation, especially in a patient over 50 years of age. As a rule, external hemorrhoids thrombose; internal hemorrhoids bleed.

B   (hepatocellular carcinoma with metastasis to the colon) is incorrect. Hepatocellular carcinoma (HCC) usually arises from postnecrotic cirrhosis secondary to hepatitis B or hepatitis C. This patient has no history of hepatitis; furthermore, HCC usually metastasizes to the lungs and not to the colon.

C   (peptic ulcer disease) is incorrect. PUD is the most common cause of iron deficiency anemia in men under 50 years of age. Black tarry stools (melena) are more likely to occur than blood coating and mixing with stools. Melena is due to acid conversion of hemoglobin into hematin, a black pigment. PUD alone does not explain the nodular liver in this patient; hence it is not a tenable diagnosis.

E   (primary lung cancer with metastasis to the colon) is incorrect. Metastatic disease to the bowel is more likely to cause signs of obstruction than of bleeding. Although smoking is a risk factor for colon cancer, and primary lung cancer is the most common cause of metastasis to the liver, the overall clinical and laboratory findings do not support lung cancer as the primary diagnosis in this patient.

37. **B** (increased because edema fluid interferes with normal lateral traction on the airways) is correct. Lateral traction exerted by connective tissue helps maintain airway patency. Interstitial edema limits the effects of lateral traction.

A (decreased because of edema fluid in the interstitial spaces) is incorrect. Airway resistance is increased in this case.
C (increased because of the increased work of breathing due to dilution of surfactant) is incorrect. There is no evidence that dilution of surfactant is an important contributor to the pathogenesis of pulmonary edema. Absence of surfactant would not directly affect airway resistance.
D (increased because zones in the lungs are ventilated but not perfused) is incorrect. A major $\dot{V}/\dot{Q}$ abnormality is not likely in interstitial edema; if anything, there would be zones that are perfused but not ventilated.
E (normal because of little or no fluid in the lumen of the airways) is incorrect. Airway resistance is increased in this case.

38. **C** (heparin) is correct. The drug that was administered to the patient was heparin, a drug whose anticoagulant effect must be monitored by measuring the aPTT. The patient's platelet count should also be monitored because heparin is the most frequent cause of drug-induced thrombocytopenia. Heparin acts catalytically to enhance the binding of antithrombin III to activated clotting factors (factors II, IX, X, XI, and XII).

A (alteplase) is incorrect. Alteplase is a recombinant tissue plasminogen activator that preferentially activates fibrin-bound plasminogen. Alteplase is used to lyse thrombi. The adequacy of the dosage of this drug is not monitored by assessing clotting function.
B (aspirin) is incorrect. Aspirin is an antithrombotic drug that inhibits platelet aggregation. It acts by irreversibly inhibiting platelet cyclooxygenase-1 (COX-1) and thereby blocking the production of thromboxane A_2. To prevent thrombosis, patients are usually instructed to take one adult low strength (81 mg) aspirin a day or to take one adult regular strength (325 mg) aspirin every other day. Platelet function can be assessed by monitoring bleeding time.
D (streptokinase) is incorrect. Like alteplase, streptokinase is a "clot buster." Streptokinase acts to catalyze the conversion of plasminogen to plasmin.
E (warfarin) is incorrect. The anticoagulant effect of warfarin is monitored by measuring the patient's prothrombin time (PT). Warfarin inhibits vitamin K epoxide reductase and thereby interferes with the hepatic production of vitamin K–dependent clotting factors (factors II, VII, IX, and X). The patient described would probably begin warfarin therapy while hospitalized and continue this therapy in the outpatient setting.

39. *C* (ipsilateral anterior horn) is correct. The arrow in the figure is pointing to the lateral corticospinal tract below the level of the pyramidal decussation. Most of the fibers in this tract terminate in the ipsilateral anterior horn. Thus, action potentials could be recorded here.

A (contralateral medial lemniscus) is incorrect. The arrow in the figure is pointing to the lateral corticospinal tract, which contains descending motor neurons. Action potentials produced in this tract would not be detected in the medial lemniscus, which carries ascending information about touch and proprioception.

B (contralateral tectum) is incorrect. The arrow in the figure is pointing to the lateral corticospinal tract, which contains descending motor neurons. Specifically, the arrow indicates the area in which the tract has crossed the midline of the central nervous system. Signals produced in this area would be detected caudal to the tectum.

D (ipsilateral red nucleus) is incorrect. The arrow in the figure is pointing to the lateral corticospinal tract just after it has crossed in the pyramidal decussation. The pyramidal decussation lies caudal to the red nucleus and carries descending corticospinal information. Therefore, action potentials would be detected by structures caudal to the pyramids.

E (ipsilateral sympathetic ganglia) is incorrect. The sympathetic ganglia lie adjacent to the spinal cord. The arrow in the figure is pointing to the lateral corticospinal tract just after its decussation.

40. *B* (gram-positive cocci in clusters with an acute inflammatory infiltrate) is correct. In most patients, pneumonia is acquired via aspiration of organisms. In intravenous drug abusers, pneumonia is most commonly acquired via hematogenous spread of *Staphylococcus aureus,* and the x-ray finding of opacities with black centers is indicative of the cavitary type of lesions that result. Based on the patient's history and x-ray findings, the Gram stain would be expected to show a predominance of gram-positive cocci in clusters.

A (acid-fast bacilli with a monocytic infiltrate) is incorrect. The finding of acid-fast bacilli, such as *Mycobacterium tuberculosis,* would be more consistent with chronic pneumonia or an insidious onset of symptoms.

B (gram-positive filamentous rods with a monocytic infiltrate) is incorrect. The finding of gram-positive filamentous rods, such as *Actinomyces israelii,* would be more consistent with an insidious onset of symptoms and with the presence of draining sinus tracts.

C (gram-positive lancet-shaped diplococci with an acute inflammatory infiltrate) is incorrect. The finding of *Streptococcus pneumoniae* would be inconsistent with the x-ray findings, because pneumococcal pneumonia does not result in the loss of lung parenchyma.

E (monocytic infiltrate with no visible bacteria) is incorrect. The finding of a predominantly monocytic infiltrate with no bacteria would be more consistent with a lobar type of pneumonia.

41. **B** (disulfiram) is correct. The patient's response after ingesting ethanol is consistent with a disulfiram reaction. Disulfiram irreversibly inhibits aldehyde dehydrogenase by causing a covalent modification of -SH groups. Aldehyde dehydrogenase is involved in the second step of ethanol oxidation and is the enzyme that catalyzes the conversion of acetaldehyde to acetic acid. When ethanol is ingested, acetaldehyde rapidly accumulates. The acetaldehyde accumulation is responsible for the types of symptoms that were experienced by the patient. Oral disulfiram therapy is prescribed to help "enforce" the state of sobriety in alcoholics who wish to abstain from drinking. It is important to warn these patients that ingesting "disguised" forms of ethanol (such as over-the-counter cough and cold syrups, fermented sauces, and other foods containing ethanol) can cause a disulfiram reaction.

A (chlorpropamide) and D (metronidazole) are incorrect. Chlorpropamide is an oral sulfonylurea drug used in the treatment of diabetes mellitus. Metronidazole is an antibacterial and antiprotozoal agent. Either of these drugs can produce a disulfiram-like reaction when ethanol is ingested, but neither would have been prescribed for this patient.
C (flumazenil) is incorrect. Flumazenil is a benzodiazepine receptor antagonist used to treat benzodiazepine overdoses or to hasten recovery from anesthesia in which benzodiazepines were employed.
E (naltrexone) is incorrect. Naltrexone is a pure opioid receptor antagonist that can be given to alcoholic patients to reduce their craving for ethanol and reduce their rate of relapse to heavy drinking. By blocking the opioid receptors, the drug decreases the reinforcing ("rewarding") effects of ethanol, which are thought to be due in part to the release of opiopetins (endorphins). The concurrent use of ethanol and naltrexone would not have been responsible for the symptoms seen in this patient.

42. **D** (hypokalemia) is correct. Increased aldosterone levels stimulate renal K^+ excretion, thereby producing hypokalemia. Hypokalemia causes muscle weakness by hyperpolarizing the cell membrane, thus moving the membrane potential farther from the threshold.

A (hyperchloremia) is incorrect. An excess of aldosterone induces metabolic alkalosis because aldosterone stimulates renal H^+ secretion, increasing plasma HCO_3^- concentration. The kidney reabsorbs HCO_3^- preferentially, so plasma Cl^- concentration decreases and hypochloremia occurs.
B (hyperkalemia) is incorrect. Increased aldosterone levels lead to hypokalemia, not hyperkalemia.

C   (hypocalcemia) is incorrect. Aldosterone has no direct effects on plasma Ca^{2+} concentration.
E   (hyponatremia) is incorrect. An excess of aldosterone results in Na^+ retention, leading to water retention and extracellular fluid volume expansion. Because water is retained with Na^+, the plasma Na^+ concentration remains normal, but the extracellular fluid volume expansion contributes to the hypertension.

43. *C*   (thiamine deficiency) is correct. The patient has developed acute Wernicke's encephalopathy, which is a clinical syndrome associated with thiamine deficiency. In the United States, alcoholism is the most common cause of thiamine deficiency. Thiamine is a cofactor in the pyruvate dehydrogenase complex, which catalyzes the conversion of pyruvate into acetyl CoA in the mitochondria. In this reaction, NAD^+ is reduced to NADH, which results in the production of 6 ATP in the mitochondria. Decreased levels of acetyl CoA also affect the synthesis of citrate (acetyl CoA + oxaloacetic acid [citrate]); hence the amount of ATP produced by the citric acid cycle is reduced. The reduction in ATP synthesis is primarily responsible for the clinical findings in thiamine deficiency (beriberi). In "wet beriberi," congestive cardiomyopathy leads to left-sided and right-sided heart failure; in "dry beriberi," demyelination results in peripheral neuropathies and the Wernicke-Korsakoff syndrome complex. Administering a glucose-containing solution to a patient with subclinical thiamine deficiency results in the consumption of the remaining thiamine in the pyruvate dehydrogenase complex reaction, which precipitates acute Wernicke's encephalopathy. Clinical features of Wernicke's encephalopathy include confusion, ataxia, nystagmus, and ophthalmoplegia. This underscores the importance of administering thiamine intravenously before infusing glucose-containing solutions.

A   (central pontine myelinolysis) is incorrect. This is a demyelination syndrome associated with a rapid IV administration of saline in a patient who has hyponatremia.
B   (Purkinje cell atrophy) is incorrect. Atrophy of Purkinje cells in the cerebellum is a complication of chronic alcoholism, but does not produce acute Wernicke's encephalopathy.
D   (viral encephalitis) is incorrect. The signs and symptoms of encephalitis are primarily headache and mental status abnormalities.
E   (vitamin B_{12} deficiency) is incorrect. Vitamin B_{12} deficiency is associated with subacute combined degeneration in the spinal cord, with demyelination of the posterior column (lack of proprioception, wide-based gait) and lateral corticospinal tract (spasticity, positive Babinski sign).

44. *B*   (hairs on the surface of inner hair cells) is correct. The term "hairs" refers to stereocilia, which are microvilli, not cilia. The core of the stereocilium contains actin filaments cross-linked with fimbrin near the apical plasmalemma of the hair cell; this

arrangement is responsible for its rigidity. When sound waves move the basilar membrane in the cochlea, the stereocilia are bent, causing the release of the content of the stereocilia into synaptic-like structures. This release excites the afferent nerve fibers that are closely associated with each hair cell. The hairs (stereocilia) on the surface of inner and outer hair cells decrease in number and size during the aging process, thereby reducing the ability to hear.

A   (diameter of the inner ear tunnel) is incorrect. The inner ear tunnel is filled with endolymph. The diameter of this tunnel has nothing to do with the process of hearing.
C   (thickness of the basilar membrane) is incorrect. The basilar membrane supports the organ of Corti in the inner ear. Vibrations in the basilar membrane cause the organ of Corti to move in relation to the overlying tectorial membrane. Hair cells (stereocilia) in the organ of Corti project into the tectorial membrane. The first step in the neurophysiology of hearing is movement of the basilar membrane, which causes the stereocilia to bend. The thickness of the basilar membrane is not as important in the hearing process as a decrease in the number of hairs on hair cells.
D   (thickness of the tectorial membrane) is incorrect. The tectorial membrane overlies the organ of Corti in the inner ear. Hair cells (stereocilia) in the organ of Corti project into the tectorial membrane. The first step in the neurophysiology of hearing occurs when the organ of Corti moves (as occurs when the underlying basilar membrane "vibrates"), causing these cells to bend. The thickness of the tectorial membrane is not as important in the hearing process as a decrease in the number of hairs on hair cells.
E   (thickness of the vestibular membrane) is incorrect. The vestibular membrane is the part of the cochlear duct that faces the scala vestibuli. It does not play a role in the process of hearing. Furthermore, this membrane is two cells thick throughout life.

45. *E* (verapamil) is correct. The patient's clinical and ECG findings are consistent with the diagnosis of Prinzmetal's angina (also called variant angina or vasospastic angina). Verapamil and other calcium channel blockers are effective for the management of Prinzmetal's angina and for the management of classic angina (also called typical angina, exertional angina, or angina of effort).

A   (minoxidil) and C (prazosin) are incorrect. Minoxidil and prazosin have no role in the management of Prinzmetal's angina or classic angina.
B   (nitroglycerin) is incorrect. Nitroglycerin and other nitrates are indicated for the management of Prinzmetal's angina and classic angina. However, they are contraindicated in patients who are taking sildenafil for erectile dysfunction. The concurrent use of a nitrate and sildenafil can cause a profound fall in blood pressure and result in death.

D (propranolol) is incorrect. Propranolol and other β-adrenergic receptor antagonists may worsen Prinzmetal's angina and are indicated only for the management of classic angina. If propranolol were used in Prinzmetal's angina, the β_2 receptors (which normally mediate vasodilation) would be blocked, and the α_1 receptors (which normally mediate vasoconstriction) would be unopposed.

46. *E* (use of nitroblue tetrazolium test) is correct. Patients with chronic granulomatous disease typically suffer from recurrent fungal and bacterial infections characterized by the formation of granulomas, rather than pustules. The NBT test is used to assay neutrophil microbicidal function. Because the cells of patients with chronic granulomatous disease lack NADPH oxidase, NBT reduction fails to occur.

A (measurement of serum C3 levels) is incorrect. Changes in C3 and other complement levels are not associated with granulomatous disease and the inability to produce pus.
B (measurement of serum IgE and IgA levels) is incorrect. The ability to form IgE and IgA is not impaired in patients with chronic granulomatous disease.
C (testing of the B cell mitogen response) is incorrect. The ability to obtain an antibody response is not impaired in patients with chronic granulomatous disease. Therefore, testing of the B cell mitogen response would not be helpful.
D (use of common skin test antigens) is incorrect. When a common skin test antigen (such as *Candida* antigen) is used in skin tests, the lack of a delayed-type hypersensitivity (DTH) reaction indicates a possible problem with T helper activity. DTH reactions are not impaired in patients with chronic granulomatous disease.

47. *E* (salvage pathway of purines) is correct. The patient's clinical findings are consistent with the diagnosis of Lesch-Nyhan syndrome, an X-linked recessive disorder affecting only males. This syndrome is caused by a deficiency of hypoxanthine-guanine phosphoribosyltransferase (HGPRT), an enzyme found in the salvage pathway of purines. Nucleotides are synthesized by two types of pathways: de novo synthesis pathways and salvage pathways. Salvage pathways recycle bases and nucleosides to nucleotides.

A (catabolism of purine nucleotides) is incorrect. Catabolism of purine nucleotides leads to uric acid. A defect in this pathway results in gout.
B (formation of thymidylate) is incorrect. Thymidylate is a pyrimidine nucleotide. The deficient enzyme is in the purine salvage pathway.
C (pathway of de novo synthesis of purine nucleotides) is incorrect. The de novo synthesis of purines is a synthesis of nucleotides from precursors such as ribose 5-phosphate, carbon dioxide, glycine, glutamine, aspartate, and derivatives of tetrahy-

drofolate. Free bases are not intermediates in the de novo pathway.

D (production of all pyrimidine nucleotides) is incorrect. The deficient enzyme is in the purine salvage pathway.

48. **B** (ciprofloxacin) is correct. The patient has gonorrhea. Ciprofloxacin, given as a single oral dose, is effective for the treatment of *Neisseria gonorrhoeae* infections and is considered the drug of choice in penicillin-allergic patients. Presumptive therapy for *Chlamydia trachomatis* in patients with gonorrhea would include concomitant administration of doxycycline in men and non-pregnant women or concomitant administration of a macrolide (erythromycin) in pregnant women.

A (ceftriaxone) is incorrect. Ceftriaxone, given as a single intramuscular injection, is considered the drug of choice for uncomplicated urethral gonococcal infections. However, cross-sensitivity to cephalosporins is seen in 5%–15% of patients who are allergic to penicillins. Because ceftriaxone is a cephalosporin, it would not have been used to treat the penicillin-allergic patient described.

C (gentamicin) and D (metronidazole) are incorrect. Aminoglycosides (such as gentamicin) and metronidazole are ineffective in the treatment of *N. gonorrhoeae* infections.

E (vancomycin) is incorrect. Vancomycin is effective only against gram-positive bacteria. Its use is reserved for treatment of the following: methicillin-resistant *Staphylococcus aureus* infections, *Clostridium difficile* infections that are not amenable to therapy with metronidazole, and bacterial endocarditis in penicillin-allergic patients.

49. **C** (low-grade lymphoma with an indolent course) is correct. Small lymphocytic lymphoma, which makes up about 4% of all non-Hodgkin's lymphomas (NHL), is a member of the low-grade group of the Working Formulation Classification. Of the low-grade lymphomas, only small lymphocytic lymphoma does not have a follicular (nodular) architecture.

A (B-cell lymphoma with no involvement of the bone marrow) is incorrect. Although almost all (>95% of cases) small lymphocytic lymphomas are of a B cell immunophenotype, about 60% of affected patients have involvement of the bone marrow.

B (high-grade B-cell lymphoma with a rapidly fatal course) is incorrect. Small lymphocytic lymphoma is an incurable but generally indolent tumor. Prolonged survival is expected.

D (lymphoblastic lymphoma originating in the bone marrow) is incorrect. Lymphoblastic lymphoma is a disease of the young population and would be formed of large lymphoid cells with prominent nuclei.

E (T-cell lymphoma induced by human T-cell leukemia virus type 1) is incorrect. HTLV-1 causes a T-cell lymphoma that is characterized by skin involvement, generalized lymphadenopathy, hepatosplenomegaly, hypercalcemia, and circulating multilobed T lymphocytes.

50. *B* (disruption of respiratory circuits in the brainstem) is correct. The first suspicion a physician may have when faced with a patient with an abnormal breathing pattern is central nervous system involvement. The neurons involved in automatic control of respiration extend from the medullary to pontine regions of the brainstem. Space-occupying lesions, increased intracranial pressure, a ruptured aneurysm, or a stroke within the brainstem can disturb normal breathing. The breathing pattern described for this patient is apneustic (i.e., the patient tends to hold his breath during the inspiratory phase and has very short periods of expiration).

A (denervation of central chemoreceptors) is incorrect. If there were total denervation of the central chemoreceptors, automatic breathing could not be sustained due to loss of central drive. This patient is breathing, although abnormally.
C (spinal cord lesion at the first cervical segment) is incorrect. If central neurons passing through the upper cervical spinal cord were damaged, respiratory movements would be faint, or possibly nonexistent.
D (stroke in the left temporal lobe without brain swelling) is incorrect. A stroke in higher regions of the brain will have little effect on spontaneous breathing. A patient could be in a persistent vegetative state (coma) and have absolutely normal spontaneous breathing (as if sleeping).
E (vagotomy and attendant loss of vagal inputs from the lung) is incorrect. Vagotomy has little effect on human breathing.

Test 3

TEST 3

DIRECTIONS: Each numbered item or incomplete statement is followed by options arranged in alphabetical or logical order. Select the best answer to each question. Some options may be partially correct, but there is only **ONE BEST** answer.

1. A 43-year-old woman has a 16-year history of a psychiatric disorder characterized by disorganized thinking (including looseness of associations), poverty of speech (alogia), blunted affect, anhedonia, and social withdrawal. Since her original diagnosis, she has been hospitalized 18 times and has failed to respond to various drugs considered appropriate for the management of her disorder. Three months after her physician begins treating her with a new drug, she complains of a sore throat, fever, malaise, weakness, and chills. Her white blood cell count (WBC) is 4100/mm³, with a differential of 31% neutrophils. The medical records indicate that 1 week earlier her WBC was 6300/mm³ and her differential was 57%. Treatment with which drug is the most likely cause of the patient's current clinical manifestations and laboratory results?

○ A. Carbamazepine
○ B. Clozapine
○ C. Fluphenazine
○ D. Flurazepam
○ E. Risperidone

2. A neonate born at 34 weeks' gestation is of appropriate weight and appears to be healthy. About 1 hour after birth, the infant displays retraction of the ribs, and grunting sounds are heard during each respiratory cycle. Over the next several hours, the infant has breathing difficulties and subsequently develops cyanosis. Rales over both lung fields are heard on auscultation. Blood gases show increased $PaCO_2$ and decreased PaO_2. The neonate's respiratory difficulty is primarily caused by

○ A. aspiration of meconium
○ B. lack of pulmonary surfactant
○ C. in utero infection with cytomegalovirus
○ D. in utero infection with parvovirus
○ E. in utero infection with *Toxoplasma gondii*

3. Several hours after eating chicken fried rice, a 33-year-old man develops nausea, vomiting, and cramps but does not have a fever. His symptoms persist for 18 hours. A gram-positive, penicillin-resistant, spore-forming, facultatively anaerobic rod is isolated from samples of the implicated food and the patient's stool. Which of the following organisms is the most likely cause of the gastroenteritis?

○ A. *Bacillus cereus*
○ B. *Bacillus subtilis*
○ C. *Clostridium difficile*
○ D. *Clostridium perfringens*
○ E. *Staphylococcus aureus*

4. A 75-year-old man is diagnosed with multiple myeloma. He has had numerous infections and currently has anemia, a high monoclonal paraprotein level, hypercalcemia, bone pain, and evidence of malignant myeloma cells in the bone marrow. Both before and after they are transformed, myeloma cells have

○ A. many apical secretory granules
○ B. many secondary lysosomes
○ C. numerous polysomes
○ D. numerous profiles of smooth endoplasmic reticulum (SER)
○ E. prominent Golgi complex

5. The mother of an 8-month-old boy takes her son to a pediatric clinic because of fever and irritability, and he has been tugging at his right earlobe. Pneumatic otoscopic examination shows an opaque, bulging tympanic membrane with limited mobility. Empiric therapy with amoxicillin is initiated. Three days later, the mother reports that her son's condition has not improved. Since examination shows little change, the pediatrician decides to treat the patient with amoxicillin plus clavulanic acid. The rationale for the change in therapy is because clavulanic acid

○ A. inhibits beta-lactamases and potentiates the activity of amoxicillin
○ B. inhibits carboxypeptidases and potentiates the activity of amoxicillin
○ C. inhibits DNA gyrase and extends the spectrum of amoxicillin to cover *Pseudomonas* species
○ D. inhibits protein synthesis and has a synergistic effect with amoxicillin
○ E. inhibits transpeptidases and has an additive effect with amoxicillin

6. A 30-year-old woman with a fractured proximal radius is unable to extend the metacarpophalangeal (MCP) and proximal interphalangeal (PIP) joints of the ring and little fingers. On examination, there is flexion attitude of the joints of the ring and little fingers at the MCP and PIP joints. The nerve involved in this injury

○ A. derives from the medial cord
○ B. lies deep to the flexor retinaculum
○ C. runs superficial to the flexor retinaculum
○ D. supplies the skin over the hypothenar eminence
○ E. travels through the supinator muscle

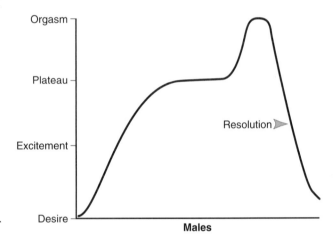

7. To appropriately treat a 42-year-old man diagnosed with premature ejaculation disorder, the physician must determine the phase of the sexual response cycle when premature ejaculation occurs. This disorder most likely occurs during which of the following phases (see the figure above)?

○ A. Desire
○ B. Excitement
○ C. Orgasm
○ D. Plateau
○ E. Resolution

8. A 46-year-old moderately obese woman is suffering from heartburn and regurgitation of acid saliva that is worse after eating a large meal. She is treated with cimetidine. During the course of therapy, her serum creatinine concentration increases by 11%, with no other changes in serum electrolytes. The most likely explanation for the increase in serum creatinine is that cimetidine is

○ A. being reabsorbed by the nephron in exchange for creatinine
○ B. blocking synthesis of creatinine by skeletal muscle
○ C. causing acute renal failure
○ D. competing with creatinine for renal tubular secretion
○ E. inhibiting uptake of creatinine ingested with food

9. A 14-year-old boy has a history of prolonged bleeding from minor cuts and trauma. Hematologic studies show normal prothrombin time and normal partial thromboplastin time. An earlobe bleeding time is 14 minutes. Platelet aggregation tests with adenosine diphosphate (ADP), epinephrine, and collagen are normal. Platelets fail to aggregate with ristocetin, even with the addition of normal von Willebrand factor (vWF). A diagnosis of Bernard-Soulier syndrome is confirmed. In a patient with this condition, platelets fail to

○ A. aggregate
○ B. bind vWF
○ C. degranulate
○ D. form thromboxane A_2
○ E. release ADP

10. A 53-year-old man with a 30-year history of alcoholism develops painful lesions on the mucous membranes of his mouth and tongue and has pigmented keratotic scaling lesions on his face and hands. He complains of weakness, forgetfulness, burning sensations in various parts of the body, and diarrhea. A deficiency of which of the following is most likely to account for these findings?

○ A. Biotin
○ B. Folic acid
○ C. Niacin
○ D. Riboflavin
○ E. Vitamin C

11. A 9-month-old girl has symptoms of acute febrile pharyngitis, including fever, sore throat, and a cough. Physical examination shows an erythematous pharyngeal mucosa without vesicles or ulcerations. She has no rash or other abnormal physical findings. Routine bacteriologic cultures yield negative results. Viral cultures grow a nonenveloped DNA virus with icosahedral symmetry and distinctive pentons. The virus completely agglutinates monkey erythrocytes. The virus that is the etiologic agent of this patient's pharyngitis is also associated with

○ A. gastroenteritis
○ B. hemorrhagic fever
○ C. meningitis
○ D. mononucleosis
○ E. paralytic encephalitis

12. A 49-year-old woman decides to have her cholesterol levels checked during her company's "Wellness Fair," since she has a family history of "bad lipids." Her findings include a nonfasting high-density lipoprotein (HDL) cholesterol concentration of 58 mg/dL, total cholesterol concentration of 310 mg/dL, and tendinous xanthomas. Results of a fasting lipoprotein profile indicate no elevation in the triglyceride concentration but an elevation in the low-density lipoprotein (LDL) cholesterol concentration. The woman is counseled about appropriate dietary modifications and is instructed to begin therapy with a drug that blocks the synthesis of cholesterol. This drug is most likely

○ A. colestipol
○ B. gemfibrozil
○ C. lovastatin
○ D. nicotinamide
○ E. nicotinic acid

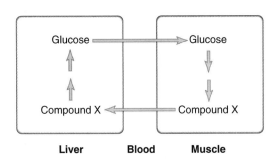

Liver   Blood   Muscle

13. In the figure above, which depicts the Cori cycle, compound X is

○ A. citrate
○ B. glucose
○ C. α-ketoglutarate
○ D. lactate
○ E. malate

14. A 19-year-old man suffering from a gunshot wound is brought to the emergency department with rapidly developing profound hypovolemic shock from acute hemorrhaging. The bleeding is controlled, and he is admitted to the intensive care unit. One day after surgery, he appears to be in distress. Arterial blood gas analysis shows a pH of 7.28, $PaCO_2$ of 60 mm Hg, and PaO_2 of 70 mm Hg. Moist rales are heard over both lung fields on auscultation. He is using accessory muscles of respiration to aid in breathing and is subsequently diagnosed with adult respiratory distress syndrome (ARDS). In the pathogenesis of ARDS, the final common pathway primarily involves defective or damaged

○ A. alveolar capillary endothelium
○ B. Clara cells
○ C. pulmonary surfactant
○ D. type I pneumocytes
○ E. type II pneumocytes

15. An 84-year-old woman began to demonstrate deficits in recent and remote memory 10 years ago. Over time, these deficits worsened, and she developed wandering behavior and confusion. Laboratory tests conducted before her death showed decreased choline acetyltransferase activity. A postmortem brain biopsy showed neurofibrillary tangles and senile plaques with amyloid-dense cores. No other significant causes of memory loss were identified. This woman most likely had

○ A. acute limbic encephalitis
○ B. Alzheimer's disease
○ C. Parkinson's disease
○ D. Pick's disease
○ E. transient global amnesia

16. During a routine physical examination of a newborn infant, meconium is found at the umbilicus. The appearance of this material is a sign of which of the following?

- ○ A. Fistula of the ascending colon with the umbilical cord
- ○ B. Herniation of the transverse colon at the umbilicus
- ○ C. Normal presentation as part of severing the umbilical cord
- ○ D. Persistence of a remnant of the vitelline duct
- ○ E. Persistence of the allantois

17. A previously healthy 26-year-old woman is involved in an automobile accident and sustains injuries that cause severe hemorrhaging. On arrival at the emergency department, she is conscious and oriented to time, place, and person. Her blood pressure is 95/65 mm Hg, pulse is 115/min, and respirations are rapid. The hemodynamic response to hemorrhage would most likely include which of the following?

- ○ A. Decreased coronary blood flow
- ○ B. Decreased sympathetic tone to the venous system
- ○ C. Increased blood flow to the skin, intestines, and kidneys
- ○ D. Increased cholinergic vasoconstrictor tone of skeletal muscle arterioles
- ○ E. Normal cerebral blood flow

18. A 19-year-old man is suspicious and tangential, uses peculiar words and odd sentence structure, and displays magical thinking and eccentric ideas. Hallucinations and delusions are absent. He appears to have functioned at a similar level throughout his life. The most likely diagnosis of this patient is

- ○ A. borderline personality disorder
- ○ B. organic delusional syndrome
- ○ C. paranoid schizophrenia
- ○ D. schizotypal personality disorder
- ○ E. undifferentiated schizophrenia

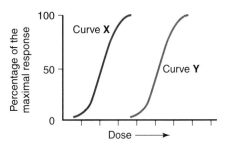

19. The figure above shows dose-response curves for a particular drug when the drug is given in the absence *(curve X)* or presence *(curve Y)* of another pharmacologic agent. The figure most accurately reflects

- ○ A. the chronotropic effect of acetylcholine in the absence *(curve X)* or presence *(curve Y)* of neostigmine
- ○ B. the hypertensive effect of norepinephrine in the absence *(curve X)* or presence *(curve Y)* of phenoxybenzamine
- ○ C. the inotropic effect of isoproterenol in the absence *(curve X)* or presence *(curve Y)* of propranolol
- ○ D. the inotropic effect of pindolol in the absence *(curve X)* or presence *(curve Y)* of a maximal inotropic dose of isoproterenol
- ○ E. the therapeutic effect of levodopa in the absence *(curve X)* or presence *(curve Y)* of carbidopa

20. A 42-year-old man has a deep laceration in his right thigh but does not seek medical attention until there is considerable pain, edema, and discoloration of the tissue at the site of the original trauma. Physical examination shows necrosis of the biceps femoris and evidence of toxemia (including fever, tachycardia, and hypotension) without signs of muscle spasms. Gram-stained exudate from the lesion shows gram-positive rods without endospores. Exudate is inoculated on sheep blood agar plates and aerobic cultures show no growth. Anaerobic cultures grow gram-positive rods, some of which have central endospores, and produce target hemolysis on the blood agar. The rods are nonmotile and aerotolerant. Which of the following *Clostridium* species is the most likely cause of the disease?

○ A. *Clostridium butyricum*
○ B. *Clostridium difficile*
○ C. *Clostridium histolyticum*
○ D. *Clostridium perfringens*
○ E. *Clostridium septicum*

21. A 16-year-old girl has stiff joints, skeletal abnormalities, and clouding of the cornea. Biochemical tests show the presence of dermatan sulfate in the urine. The findings are most likely attributable to which of the following?

○ A. Ehlers-Danlos syndrome
○ B. Glycogen storage disease
○ C. Marfan syndrome
○ D. Mucopolysaccharidosis
○ E. Sphingolipidosis

22. An autopsy performed on a 40-year-old man with dementia shows atrophy of the frontal and temporoparietal lobes of the brain. Histologic examination shows senile plaques. The pathogenesis of the dementia in this patient is most closely related to which of the following?

○ A. β-Amyloid protein
○ B. Decreased dopamine levels
○ C. Slow virus disease
○ D. Triplet repeat mutation

23. A 74-year-old woman is brought to the emergency department lethargic and in obvious heat stress. Her blood pressure is 100/65 mm Hg, her body temperature is 38.4° C (101.3° F), and her breathing is rapid and shallow. A urinalysis shows a very dark and concentrated urine free of blood, proteins, glucose, and bicarbonate. Plasma Na^+ concentration is 159 mEq/L. She is suffering from severe dehydration and is started on an intravenous infusion of 500 mL physiologic saline solution. Which of the following is the most appropriate hydration therapy for this patient?

○ A. Hyperosmotic volume expansion with hydration of both intracellular and extracellular compartments
○ B. Hyperosmotic volume expansion with intracellular hydration and extracellular dehydration
○ C. Hyposmotic volume expansion with hydration of both intracellular and extracellular compartments
○ D. Hyposmotic volume expansion with intracellular hydration and extracellular dehydration
○ E. Isosmotic volume expansion with no change in intracellular or extracellular osmolalities

24. A 37-year-old man who reports to a dermatology clinic to have a melanoma removed indicates that he is not routinely taking any medications. During the surgical procedure, the patient experiences excessive bleeding. When questioned again about taking medications, he indicates that he had a headache 4 days ago and took an analgesic at that time. The analgesic that this patient most likely took was

○ A. acetaminophen
○ B. aspirin
○ C. ibuprofen
○ D. salsalate
○ E. warfarin

25. A 50-year-old woman has difficulty moving her thumb toward the palmar surface of the digiti minimi. She also experiences pain over the palmar surface of the thumb and index and middle fingers. Pressure and tapping over the lateral portion of the flexor retinaculum cause tingling of the thumb and third and fourth digits, indicating nerve damage. This compressed nerve travels

○ A. between the flexor digitorum superficialis and flexor digitorum profundus
○ B. between the two heads of the flexor carpi ulnaris
○ C. superficial to the flexor retinaculum
○ D. through the coracobrachialis muscle
○ E. through the supinator muscle

26. A 14-year-old boy is rushed to the emergency department by his parents, who were frightened by his loss of consciousness. The previous day, the boy had complained of a stiff neck and headache. The physician suspects bacterial meningitis and orders a cerebrospinal fluid (CSF) culture. CSF will be obtained from which of the following structures?

○ A. Cerebellomedullary cistern (cisterna magna)
○ B. Fourth ventricle
○ C. Lateral ventricles
○ D. Lumbar cistern
○ E. Pontine cistern

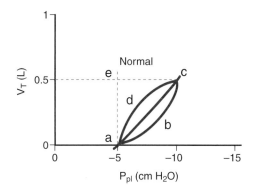

27. The region of inspiratory airflow resistance (R) shown in the figure above is

○ A. R ~ a-b-c-a
○ B. R ~ a-c-d-a
○ C. R ~ a-c-e-a
○ D. R ~ a-b-c-d-a
○ E. R ~ a-b-c-e-a

28. A 35-year-old woman has multiorgan failure resulting from toxic shock syndrome. Laboratory findings in this patient would include

○ A. fulminant septicemia
○ B. high levels of T cell cytokines
○ C. high ratio of CD8+ cells to CD4+ cells
○ D. hypergammaglobulinemia
○ E. positive results in the limulus test

29. A 26-year-old man is scheduled to begin cisplatin treatment for bladder cancer that is no longer amenable to surgery or radiotherapy. To minimize or prevent cisplatin-induced nausea and vomiting, he is first given prochlorperazine. One hour later, he complains of severe pain in the eyes and neck and is found to have a fixed upward gaze and twisting upward torsion of the head. This dystonic reaction to prochlorperazine is caused by blockade of

○ A. α_1-adrenergic receptors
○ B. dopamine D_2 receptors
○ C. histamine H_1 receptors
○ D. muscarinic receptors
○ E. serotonin receptors

30. A 55-year-old woman has a 10-year history of episodes of confusion and fainting that occur either on first arising in the morning or after exercising. The episodes are preceded or accompanied by shaking, sweating, and palpitations. The woman's husband has noticed that when his wife faints, she shows no signs of seizures and that eating prevents the symptoms. Her history and physical examination are otherwise unremarkable. Which of the following is the most likely cause of this patient's symptoms?

○ A. Autonomic insufficiency leading to orthostatic hypotension
○ B. Benign insulin-secreting tumor causing periodic hypoglycemia
○ C. Glucagon-secreting tumor causing periodic hypoglycemia
○ D. Meningioma in the region of the frontal cortex
○ E. Norepinephrine-secreting tumor causing periodic hyperglycemia

31. An afebrile 50-year-old man with a 30-year history of cigarette smoking complains of flushing in his face, watery diarrhea, and weight loss over the past 6 months. Physical examination shows an enlarged, nodular liver and a grade 3 pansystolic murmur heard best along the left parasternal border. S_3 and S_4 heart sounds are present, and the heart sounds and murmur increase in intensity on inspiration. The patient's neck veins are distended, and the jugular venous pulse shows a giant *c-v* wave. Which of the following laboratory studies would be most useful in confirming the diagnosis of this patient's clinical disorder?

○ A. Blood cultures
○ B. Complete blood cell count
○ C. Liver function tests
○ D. Serum electrolytes
○ E. Urine test for 5-hydroxyindoleacetic acid (5-HIAA)

32. A 43-year-old man is found to have hypermobility of the joints and hyperextensibility of the skin while undergoing a routine physical examination. The patient's medical history includes a corneal rupture. Recent laboratory studies show a deficiency of lysyl hydroxylase. Which of the following is the most likely diagnosis?

○ A. Cystic fibrosis
○ B. Ehlers-Danlos syndrome
○ C. Familial hypercholesterolemia
○ D. Fragile X syndrome
○ E. Marfan syndrome

33. For the past 2 months, a 28-year-old man says he has experienced fatigue, is sleeping more, and has feelings of worthlessness and guilt. He is otherwise physically healthy and denies previous psychiatric problems. He and his wife divorced 4 months ago. The most likely diagnosis is

○ A. acute stress disorder
○ B. adjustment disorder with depressed mood
○ C. dysthymia
○ D. major depressive disorder
○ E. posttraumatic stress disorder

34. A 24-year-old woman in her first trimester of pregnancy complains of heat intolerance. Physical examination shows a slightly enlarged, nontender thyroid gland. Thyroid function studies show a serum thyroxine (T_4) level of 14 μg/dL and a serum thyroid-stimulating hormone (TSH) level of 3.0 μU/mL. Which of the following best explains the results of these studies?

○ A. Decreased thyroid-binding globulin
○ B. Increased synthesis of T_4
○ C. Increased synthesis of triiodothyronine (T_3)
○ D. Thyroiditis-induced release of T_4
○ E. Normal finding in pregnancy

35. Pharmacologic strategies to enhance motor function in patients with Parkinson's disease include which of the following?

○ A. Decreasing release of presynaptic dopamine
○ B. Decreasing synthesis of dopamine
○ C. Increasing dopamine synaptic reuptake
○ D. Increasing levels of acetylcholine in the putamen
○ E. Stimulating postsynaptic dopamine receptors

36. A healthy man and woman have two healthy daughters; they had two sons who died in early infancy of a genetic defect that only affects male offspring. The mode of inheritance for this defect is

○ A. autosomal dominant
○ B. autosomal recessive
○ C. multifactorial
○ D. X-linked dominant
○ E. X-linked recessive

37. A 30-year-old man from Arizona experiences a sudden onset of fever and myalgia. He is admitted to the hospital with tachycardia and tachypnea. His condition quickly worsens, and he dies of respiratory failure. Bacterial and fungal cultures of blood and sputum samples yield negative results, but an enveloped virus with a helical nucleocapsid is isolated in cell culture. Which of the following viruses is the most likely cause of the disease?

○ A. California encephalitis virus
○ B. Coltivirus
○ C. Dengue virus
○ D. Hantavirus
○ E. Lassa virus

38. A 62-year-old man has right-sided ptosis and cannot adduct his right eye. This patient most likely has a small lesion involving which structure shown in the figure below?

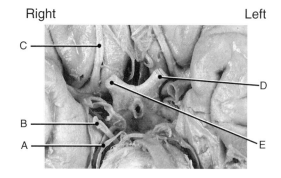

A. Structure A
B. Structure B
C. Structure C
D. Structure D
E. Structure E

39. A 17-year-old girl has lost about 10 kg (22 lb) within a 10-week period and is now 20% below her expected body weight. Further examination shows that she has an intense fear of becoming fat and has a distorted body image, uses vigorous exercise to avoid weight gain, and has missed her last five consecutive menstrual cycles. The most likely diagnosis is

○ A. anorexia nervosa
○ B. body dysmorphic disorder
○ C. bulimia nervosa
○ D. pica
○ E. rumination disorder

40. A 61-year-old man who has been treated with a "heart drug" for 3 years now has hypertension and begins concurrent treatment with furosemide. Six days later, he develops anorexia, nausea, vomiting, fatigue, xanthopsia (yellow vision), and photophobia. An ECG shows atrial tachycardia with pronounced slowing of the atrioventricular (AV) node conduction velocity. The patient's "heart drug" is most likely

○ A. digoxin
○ B. milrinone
○ C. propranolol
○ D. quinidine
○ E. verapamil

41. A 14-year-old boy with a sore throat, dyspnea, and fever is examined in the physician's office and given a prescription for oral amoxicillin. The following day, the boy's mother notes changes in the boy's behavior. He appears to alter between hyperactivity and withdrawal and has developed a fear of drinking fluids. Later that day he has a seizure and is taken to the hospital. On admission, he is found to be hyperventilating, incoherent, and suffering from hallucinations. Physical examination shows tachycardia and hypotension. No rash is present. A virus that reacts with specific anti–G protein antibody is isolated from a sample of cerebrospinal fluid. Which of the following viruses is the most likely cause of the disease?

○ A. Eastern equine encephalitis virus
○ B. Ebola virus
○ C. Echovirus
○ D. Hantavirus
○ E. Rabies virus

42. A 30-year-old woman with emphysema and bronchitis has been living in a highly polluted industrial area for the past 20 years. She says that one of her brothers died of lung disease. The serum protein electrophoresis pattern shows a decrease in the α_1 electrophoretic peak. The defective protein can be best characterized as

○ A. a cysteine protease inhibitor
○ B. primarily an inhibitor of elastase released by macrophages and neutrophils
○ C. showing specificity for trypsin
○ D. synthesized in the lungs and inhibits surfactant production
○ E. thought to be inherited in an X-linked manner

43. A 53-year-old man complains of weakness in his right leg. He has hyperactive muscle stretch reflexes, a positive Babinski sign, and diffuse areas of weakness in the right leg. He can accurately distinguish sharp and dull pain in the right leg but not in the left. The most likely cause of these findings is a lesion in the

○ A. cerebellum
○ B. internal capsule, left anterior limb
○ C. left lateral funiculus
○ D. reticular formation
○ E. right frontal lobe

44. While skiing, a 23-year-old woman falls forward over her skis, hyperextending her knees. Which of the following ligaments is most likely to be injured?

○ A. Anterior cruciate
○ B. Fibular collateral
○ C. Posterior cruciate
○ D. Posterior meniscofemoral
○ E. Tibial collateral

45. A 50-year-old man who works as a gardener seeks medical help for an indurated, inflamed, erupting ulcer on his right hand. Examination shows regional lymphadenopathy and multiple subcutaneous nodules that appear to follow lymphatic channels away from the primary lesion. He is afebrile, and the remainder of the physical examination is unremarkable, except for manifestations related to his history of alcoholism. A dimorphic fungus is cultured from exudate obtained from the primary lesion. Which of the following organisms is the most likely cause of the disease?

○ A. *Blastomyces dermatitidis*
○ B. *Candida albicans*
○ C. *Coccidioides immitis*
○ D. *Histoplasma capsulatum*
○ E. *Sporothrix schenckii*

46. A 68-year-old woman who begins taking a drug to prevent influenza A develops mild pitting edema of the ankles and a purplish red mottling of the skin on her lower leg. The mottled region does not itch or cause pain, but its color intensifies when she stands up or goes outdoors in the cold weather. Treatment with which drug is most likely to have caused these adverse effects?

○ A. Acyclovir
○ B. Amantadine
○ C. Foscarnet
○ D. Oseltamivir
○ E. Ribavirin
○ F. Zidovudine

47. A tall, obese 13-year-old boy has bilateral gynecomastia, decreased testicular volume for his age, and sparse axillary and pubic hair. He had the usual childhood infections, except for mumps. A CT scan of the pituitary gland is normal. A buccal smear preparation shows a single Barr body extending off the nuclear membrane of many squamous cells. The results of a chromosome study are pending. Which of the following sets of laboratory studies would be expected in this patient?

	Serum FSH	Serum LH	Serum Testosterone
○ A.	High	High	Low
○ B.	High	Normal	Normal
○ C.	Low	Low	Low
○ D.	Normal	High	Low

FSH, Follicle-stimulating hormone; *LH,* luteinizing hormone.

48. An 8-year-old girl who plays outdoors in the spring and early summer sneezes and suffers from acute conjunctivitis and inflammation of the nasal membranes. Her eyes and nose are continuously itchy. Her condition is an example of which of the following types of hypersensitivity reaction?

○ A. Type I
○ B. Type II
○ C. Type III
○ D. Type IV

49. A psychiatrist has referred a patient diagnosed with narcissistic personality disorder to a cardiologist because of a cardiovascular condition. Prior to the evaluation, the cardiologist should remember that this patient is most likely to exhibit which of the following traits?

○ A. Be guarded and have difficulty disclosing personal information
○ B. Demonstrate an excessive need for order and control and ask many questions
○ C. Demonstrate a need for lavish personal attention and have a grandiose sense of self-importance
○ D. Have difficulty making decisions and be overly reliant on the physician
○ E. Interact in a flirtatious manner and display seductive behavior

50. A 28-year-old man who was hit by a car while crossing the street is immediately taken by ambulance to a nearby hospital. Physical examination shows diminished pulse, cold, clammy skin, and blood pressure of 60/40 mm Hg. Additional findings include an open right femoral fracture and tenderness over the left lower rib cage. The patient is infused with 3 L of 0.9% normal saline and a blood sample is drawn. Which of the following results would be expected from this sample?

○ A. Low hemoglobin (Hgb) and low hematocrit (Hct)
○ B. Low mean corpuscular volume (MCV)
○ C. Low serum glucose concentration
○ D. Low serum sodium concentration
○ E. Low white blood cell (WBC) count

ANSWERS AND DISCUSSIONS

1. **B** (clozapine) is correct. The patient has a history of schizophrenia, and her current symptoms and laboratory results are consistent with clozapine-induced agranulocytosis. Because patients who take clozapine are at risk for agranulocytosis, they must have their blood tested every week during the first 6 months of therapy and every other week thereafter in order to obtain the next supply of medicine. Clozapine, an atypical antipsychotic drug, was most likely prescribed for this patient because she has treatment-resistant schizophrenia with predominantly negative symptoms (including affective flattening, anhedonia, alogia, and withdrawal), rather than positive symptoms (such as delusions and hallucinations). In contrast to typical antipsychotic drugs, the atypical antipsychotic drugs have greater efficacy against the negative symptoms of schizophrenia. They also have a lower incidence of extrapyramidal side effects, including acute effects (such as dystonia, akathisia, and parkinsonism) and chronic effects (such as tardive dyskinesia).

A (carbamazepine) is incorrect. While the use of carbamazepine has been associated with the development of agranulocytosis, the drug would not have been appropriate for management of this patient's treatment-resistant schizophrenia.
C (fluphenazine) and D (flurazepam) are incorrect. Fluphenazine is a typical antipsychotic drug, and flurazepam is a benzodiazepine hypnotic. Neither drug would have been employed for the management of this patient's treatment-resistant schizophrenia. Neither drug has been associated with the development of agranulocytosis.
E (risperidone) is incorrect. Because risperidone is an atypical antipsychotic drug, it would have been appropriate for management of this patient's treatment-resistant schizophrenia. However, its use is not associated with the development of agranulocytosis.

2. **B** (lack of pulmonary surfactant) is correct. This is a classic presentation of idiopathic respiratory distress syndrome (RDS) due to lack of formation of pulmonary surfactant by type II pneumocytes. Histologic examination of the lungs at this time would show hyaline membranes lining the alveolar ducts. The increased work of respiration causes exhaustion of the infant, resulting in decreased ventilation and increased $PaCO_2$. Multiple foci of atelectasis produce ventilation/perfusion ($\dot{V}/\dot{Q}$) ratios near 0, which causes venous dilution of oxygenated blood, producing a decline in PaO_2.

107

A (aspiration of meconium) is incorrect. Meconium aspiration is associated with fetal distress. It may cause immediate difficulties with respiration after birth, but it is not expected to cause the usual progression of idiopathic RDS.

C (in utero infection with cytomegalovirus) and E (in utero infection with *Toxoplasma gondii*) are incorrect. Although pneumonitis is frequently seen with TORCH infections (toxoplasmosis, rubella, cytomegalovirus, herpes simplex), it would not be expected to produce RDS.

D (in utero infection with parvovirus) is incorrect. Parvovirus infection causes hydrops fetalis and spontaneous abortion.

3. ***A*** *(Bacillus cereus)* is correct. The patient's clinical and laboratory findings are consistent with self-limited gastroenteritis caused by *B. cereus*. This organism produces emetic and diarrheal enterotoxins and is often found in rice dishes that are improperly refrigerated and then reheated.

B *(Bacillus subtilis)* is incorrect. Although *B. subtilis* has occasionally been reported to cause gastroenteritis, it is a strict aerobe.

C *(Clostridium difficile)* and D *(Clostridium perfringens)* are incorrect. Although both *C. difficile* and *C. perfringens* cause gastroenteritis, they are strict anaerobes.

E *(Staphylococcus aureus)* is incorrect. Although *S. aureus* causes gastroenteritis, it is a gram-positive coccus.

4. ***E*** (prominent Golgi complex) is correct. Myeloma cells are transformed plasma cells. Before and after transformation, they have a prominent Golgi apparatus. They also have a well-developed rough endoplasmic reticulum (RER).

A (many apical secretory granules) and B (many secondary lysosomes) are incorrect. Secretory granules are a cytoplasmic characteristic of a regulated secretory pathway, and secondary lysosomes are a cytoplasmic characteristic of phagocytic cells. Myeloma cells are transformed plasma cells. They lack secretory granules and secondary lysosomes. Plasma cells secrete antibody, have a well-developed RER, and are found in lymphoid tissues with activated lymphoid nodules. Plasma cells secrete via a constitutive secretory pathway, a pathway in which the product is transported to the cell surface by small vesicles that are undetected by a light microscope.

C (numerous polysomes) and D (numerous profiles of smooth endoplasmic reticulum) are incorrect. The presence of many polysomes is a cytoplasmic characteristic of cells that synthesize but do not secrete protein. The presence of numerous profiles of SER is a characteristic of steroid-secreting cells. Myeloma cells are plasma cells. They do not have numerous polysomes or profiles of SER. They secrete protein (antibody), have a well-developed RER, and are found in lymphoid tissues with activated lymphoid nodules.

5. *A* (inhibits beta-lactamases and potentiates the activity of amoxicillin) is correct. The patient has acute otitis media due to viral or bacterial pathogens. Empiric therapy directed against the most common bacterial pathogens (*Streptococcus pneumoniae,* *Haemophilus influenzae,* and *Moraxella catarrhalis*) most likely failed because of bacterial resistance from production of plasmid-encoded beta-lactamases. Although clavulanic acid is not an antibiotic, it effectively inhibits both plasmid-encoded and non-inducible chromosomal beta-lactamases. Thus, clavulanic acid potentiates the activity of amoxicillin.

B (inhibits carboxypeptidases and potentiates the activity of amoxicillin) is incorrect. Clavulanic acid does not inhibit carboxy-peptidase activity. It inhibits beta-lactamase activity.
C (inhibits DNA gyrase and extends the spectrum of amoxicillin to cover *Pseudomonas* species) is incorrect. Clavulanic acid does not inhibit DNA gyrase. The fluoroquinolone antimicrobials act by this mechanism and are active against *Pseudomonas.*
D (inhibits protein synthesis and has a synergistic effect with amoxicillin) is incorrect. Clavulanic acid does not inhibit protein synthesis. Antimicrobials that do inhibit protein synthesis include chloramphenicol, clindamycin, aminoglycosides, tetracyclines, and macrolides.
E (inhibits transpeptidases and has an additive effect with amoxicillin) is incorrect. Clavulanic acid does not inhibit transpeptidase activity. All of the beta-lactam antimicrobials (including amoxicillin) inhibit transpeptidases and thereby prevent cross-linking of the bacterial cell wall.

6. *E* (travels through the supinator muscle) is correct. The nerve involved in this patient's injury is the deep branch of the radial nerve, which travels through the supinator muscle and then becomes the posterior interosseous nerve. Injury to the posterior interosseous nerve when the ring and little fingers are initially involved is described as a "pseudoulnar clawhand." There is no hyperextension at the MCP joints of the ring and little fingers, usually seen with a lower ulnar nerve lesion as in "clawhand."

A (derives from the medial cord) is incorrect. The radial nerve is derived from the posterior cord, not the medial cord.
B (lies deep to the flexor retinaculum) is incorrect. The median nerve travels deep to the flexor retinaculum. In the hand, this nerve innervates the muscles of the hypothenar eminence (flexor pollicis brevis, abductor pollicis brevis, and opponens pollicis) and only the first and second lumbricals.
C (runs superficial to the flexor retinaculum) is incorrect. The ulnar nerve travels superficial to the flexor retinaculum. Injury to the ulnar nerve may cause a condition known as "clawhand," which is characterized by the hyperextension at the metacarpophalangeal joints and flexion at the proximal interphalangeal joints of the ring and little fingers.

D (supplies the skin over the hypothenar eminence) is incorrect. The ulnar nerve, not the radial nerve, supplies the skin over the hypothenar eminence.

7. *C* (orgasm) is correct. Premature ejaculation, as discussed in the *Diagnostic and Statistical Manual of Mental Disorders,* 4th ed. (DSM-IV), occurs during the orgasmic phase and refers to a pervasive pattern of orgasm and ejaculation with minimal sexual stimulation. In this disorder, the man ejaculates before, on, or shortly after penetration. Male orgasmic disorder (i.e., inability to achieve orgasm following a phase of normal sexual excitement) is an example of another disorder in men that occurs in the orgasmic phase.

A (desire) is incorrect. Hypoactive sexual desire disorder, sexual aversion disorder, or disorders of desire secondary to general medical conditions or substance use are examples of dysfunctions of men in the desire phase.

B (excitement) and D (plateau) are incorrect. The DSM-IV consolidates the two phases (excitement and plateau) into a single excitement phase. Male erectile disorder (i.e., impotence) occurs in the excitement phase. In their book *Human Sexual Response,* William H. Masters and Virginia E. Johnson delineated the excitement and plateau phases.

E (resolution) is incorrect. During the resolution phase, men exhibit a refractory period (typically 10–45 minutes) in which orgasm is not possible. Postcoital dysphoria or headache after sexual activity can occur in this phase.

8. *D* (competing with creatinine for renal tubular secretion) is correct. Cimetidine and creatinine are both organic cations that compete for the same renal tubular secretion mechanism. Inhibiting creatinine secretion will lead to an increase in its serum concentration.

A (being reabsorbed by the nephron in exchange for creatinine) is incorrect. If cimetidine is being reabsorbed in exchange for creatinine, creatinine excretion will increase and its serum concentration will decrease.

B (blocking synthesis of creatinine by skeletal muscle) is incorrect. Blocking synthesis of creatinine lowers its serum concentration.

C (causing acute renal failure) is incorrect. Although acute renal failure leads to an increase in serum creatinine concentration, it also elevates serum K^+ and BUN (blood urea nitrogen). Because the other serum electrolyte values have not changed, acute renal failure is unlikely.

E (inhibiting uptake of creatinine ingested with food) is incorrect. Inhibiting uptake of creatinine from the intestine lowers its serum concentration.

9. *B*   (bind vWF) is correct. Bernard-Soulier syndrome is an autoso-
    mal recessive disorder characterized by giant platelets with mem-
    branes lacking glycoprotein Ib, the locus of the vWF receptor.
    This prevents the platelets from binding to the subendothelium
    and interferes with their ability to form a hemostatic plug in a
    focus of vascular injury.

    A   (aggregate) is incorrect. Platelets with an inability to aggre-
    gate are characteristic of thrombasthenia. The symptoms of Glanz-
    mann's thrombasthenia, a rare autosomal recessive disorder,
    include mucosal and postoperative bleeding.
    C   (degranulate) is incorrect. Platelets with an inability to degran-
    ulate are characteristic of storage pool disease, a group of mild
    bleeding disorders with defective secretion of platelet granule con-
    tents that stimulate platelet aggregation.
    D   (form thromboxane A_2) is incorrect. Cyclooxygenase inhibi-
    tors such as aspirin block the formation of thromboxane A_2, a po-
    tent platelet-aggregating agent.
    E   (release ADP) is incorrect. Platelets with an inability to release
    ADP are characteristic of storage pool disease, a group of mild
    bleeding disorders with defective secretion of platelet granule con-
    tents (especially ADP) that stimulate platelet aggregation.

10. *C*   (niacin) is correct. The patient's clinical manifestations are
    consistent with the diagnosis of pellagra. This life-threatening
    disease is characterized by dermatitis, diarrhea, and dementia
    (the "three d's") and is caused by a deficiency of niacin. Niacin
    absorption from the stomach and small intestine may be im-
    paired as a result of chronic alcoholism.

    A   (biotin) is incorrect. Biotin deficiency associated with poor
    dietary intake is rare. A large percentage of the biotin in humans
    is supplied by intestinal bacteria. Experimental biotin deficiency is
    characterized by dermatitis, hair loss, muscle pain, paresthesias,
    and hypercholesterolemia. Some of these signs and symptoms
    have been observed in persons consuming large amounts of
    raw eggs, in patients receiving long-term high-dose antibiotic
    treatment, and in patients receiving long-term parenteral
    nutrition.
    B   (folic acid) is incorrect. A deficiency of folic acid results in
    megaloblastic anemia. It is rarely associated with neurologic
    abnormalities.
    D   (riboflavin) is incorrect. The signs and symptoms of riboflavin
    deficiency include cheilosis, glossitis, angular stomatitis, burn-
    ing of the eyes, and anemia.
    E   (vitamin C) is incorrect. Vitamin C deficiency results in im-
    paired collagen synthesis. It is not associated with neurologic
    symptoms.

11. **A** (gastroenteritis) is correct. The clinical and laboratory findings are consistent with the diagnosis of acute febrile pharyngitis caused by an adenovirus. Adenoviruses cause many types of infections, including gastroenteritis, pneumonia, conjunctivitis, hemorrhagic cystitis, and pharyngoconjunctival fever.

B (hemorrhagic fever) is incorrect. Adenoviruses are not known to be etiologic agents of hemorrhagic fever. Agents of hemorrhagic fever include filoviruses (such as Ebola virus and Marburg virus), yellow fever virus, and dengue virus.
C (meningitis) is incorrect. Adenoviruses are not significant causes of meningitis. Major viral causes of meningitis include enteroviruses, herpesviruses (such as herpes simplex viruses 1 and 2, cytomegalovirus, and Epstein-Barr virus), and mumps virus.
D (mononucleosis) is incorrect. Adenoviruses do not cause mononucleosis. Epstein-Barr virus and cytomegalovirus are the major causes of mononucleosis.
E (paralytic encephalitis) is incorrect. Adenoviruses are not major causes of paralytic encephalitis. Major causes of this disease include poliovirus, enterovirus types 70 and 71, and coxsackievirus type A7.

12. **C** (lovastatin) is correct. The patient's clinical and laboratory findings are consistent with a diagnosis of type IIa familial hypercholesterolemia, a form of hyperlipoproteinemia that is frequently treated with lovastatin. Lovastatin and other "statin" drugs act by inhibiting HMG-CoA reductase and blocking the rate-limiting step in the synthesis of cholesterol. Inhibition of HMG-CoA leads to an increase in the number of high-affinity LDL receptors and an increase in the liver's extraction of LDL and LDL precursors (VLDL remnants). This in turn reduces the serum level of LDL cholesterol. The adverse effects of "statin" drugs include myalgia and rhabdomyolysis.

A (colestipol) is incorrect. Colestipol and cholestyramine are bile acid–binding resins indicated for the management of primary hypercholesterolemia. The drugs enhance the elimination of bile acids, triggering an increase in bile acid synthesis. The synthesis of bile acids requires the liver to take up more cholesterol, thereby lowering the LDL cholesterol concentration in the serum. The adverse effects of bile acid–binding resins are primarily gastrointestinal and include constipation, flatulence, and fecal impaction. The drugs may increase VLDL and triglyceride concentrations and should not be used to treat patients with hypertriglyceridemia.
B (gemfibrozil) is incorrect. Gemfibrozil, a fibric acid derivative, is used primarily for the treatment of hypertriglyceridemia. The drug acts by stimulating lipoprotein lipase activity. This results in an increase in the catabolism of VLDL and intermediate-density lipoprotein (IDL). The adverse effects of gemfibrozil include gallstones and myopathy; incidence of myopathy is increased when gemfibrozil is given concomitantly with a "statin" drug.

D (nicotinamide) is incorrect. Nicotinamide is used to correct niacin deficiency and to prevent pellagra. The drug is referred to as the "nonflushing" form of niacin because it lacks vasodilative activity. Nicotinamide also lacks hypolipidemic activity and therefore would have no value in treating patients with hyperlipidemia.

E (nicotinic acid) is incorrect. Nicotinic acid (also called niacin or vitamin B_3) is useful for the management of all types of hyperlipidemia. It acts by inhibiting hepatic VLDL secretion. Its adverse effects include flushing and abdominal itching (both of which can be prevented by taking aspirin) and hepatotoxicity.

13. **D** (lactate) is correct. Lactate is released into the blood by cells that lack mitochondria (such as red blood cells) and by exercising skeletal muscle. Lactate diffuses out of active skeletal muscle and into the blood and is then carried to the liver. The lactate that enters the liver is oxidized to pyruvate, which is then converted to glucose. Glucose enters the blood and is transported to skeletal muscle. Contracting skeletal muscle derives adenosine triphosphate from the glycolytic conversion of glucose to lactate. These reactions constitute the Cori cycle.

A (citrate), C (α-ketoglutarate), and E (malate) are incorrect. Citrate, α-ketoglutarate, and malate do not enter the Cori cycle.

B (glucose) is incorrect. Glucose is not transported to the liver from active skeletal muscle in the Cori cycle.

14. **A** (alveolar capillary endothelium) is correct. The pathologic equivalent of ARDS is termed diffuse alveolar damage, which is primarily associated with endothelial injury. When the endothelium is injured, protein-rich fluid leaks into the extravascular space, which produces interstitial and intra-alveolar pulmonary edema. Hyaline-like membranes form, and organization of the exudate eventually occurs.

B (Clara cells) is incorrect. Clara cells are unciliated cells found in the epithelium of the respiratory and terminal bronchioles. These cells do not play a significant role in a patient with ARDS.

C (pulmonary surfactant) is incorrect. Lack of surfactant in the newborn causes respiratory distress syndrome (RDS). Although RDS shares some histologic similarities with the acute phase of ARDS, its origin is entirely different, and it does not progress to pulmonary fibrosis.

D (type I pneumocytes) is incorrect. Toxic gases may damage type I cells and lead to denudation of the alveolar surface. However, this does not account for the leakage of fluid into the extravascular space. Proliferation of type II cells eventually replaces the lost type I cells, resulting in the characteristic "cobblestone" appearance of the alveoli.

E (type II pneumocytes) is incorrect. Type II cells seem remarkably resistant to injury and account for much of the repair that occurs in the resolution of ARDS.

15. *B* (Alzheimer's disease) is correct. Alzheimer's disease is characterized by a progressive loss of cognitive function, which is associated with the presence of senile plaque and neurofibrillary tangles in cortical and subcortical gray matter. It usually begins with the loss of recent memory and loss of the ability to learn new information. Patients often exhibit behavioral disorganization and are unable to perform activities of daily living.

A (acute limbic encephalitis) is incorrect. Limbic encephalitis is one of several sensory neuronopathies that may accompany small cell lung carcinoma. Patients first exhibit anxiety and depression and eventually memory loss, confusion, and abnormal behaviors. As an acute condition, however, its onset is abrupt, as opposed to the progressive development of dementia described for this patient. In addition, it would probably be resolved through cancer therapy, but no mention of cancer was made in the autopsy report.

C (Parkinson's disease) is incorrect. Parkinson's disease is characterized by a "poverty of movement"—a subtle resting tremor in one limb and slow, reduced voluntary movements that are difficult to initiate. Memory loss is not a characteristic of Parkinson's disease.

D (Pick's disease) is incorrect. Pick's disease is a form of dementia characterized by the progressive deterioration and eventual death of neurons in the frontal and temporal lobes and, in some cases, the striatum. Patients often have Pick bodies (inclusions), which consist of a loose aggregation of abnormal filaments. These inclusions react to the same types of antibodies that are used to identify the neurofibrillary tangles of Alzheimer's disease, but they are structurally distinct.

E (transient global amnesia) is incorrect. Transient global amnesia is short-term loss of memory of all past events and sensory information. It can be ruled out in this patient because of its fleeting nature.

16. *D* (persistence of a remnant of the vitelline duct) is correct. The vitelline duct, a remnant of the yolk sac of early development, is attached to the midgut and extends into the umbilical cord. Normally, as the gut undergoes physiologic herniation and returns to the abdominal cavity, the vitelline duct disappears. However, it may persist as a diverticulum of the distal ileum, which sometimes extends into the umbilical cord. If the vitelline duct is present within the umbilical cord, it will be cut with the rest of the cord, creating an opening to the surface.

Consequently, meconium (fecal material) may appear at the umbilicus and is diagnostic of a persistent vitelline duct, termed Meckel's diverticulum. Remember the "rule of 2's" when thinking of Meckel's diverticulum: it arises from the ileum; it is located approximately 2 feet from the ileocecal junction; it is generally about 2 inches long; it occurs in about 2% of the population; and it involves 2 types of ectopic tissue (gastric or pancreatic). It is often asymptomatic, but can contain gastric mucosa in its lining. It does not always extend into the umbilical cord. Gastric mucosa and associated hydrochloric acid secretion is harmful when located in the small intestine, which has a very basic pH. Like the appendix of the cecum, a Meckel's diverticulum can become infected and inflamed.

A   (fistula of the ascending colon with the umbilical cord) is incorrect. Although a fistula between the ascending colon and the umbilicus might result in the appearance of fecal material at the umbilicus, it is highly unlikely this would occur. The ascending colon courses up the right side of the abdomen against the posterior body wall. As such, it would not be readily available to the umbilicus, which is situated in the midline on the anterior abdominal wall.
B   (herniation of the transverse colon at the umbilicus) is incorrect. Because the transverse colon crosses the upper anterior abdomen, it could theoretically become positioned relative to the umbilicus. It might even be involved in an umbilical hernia. However, a better explanation for fecal material at the umbilicus, especially in a newborn, is an abnormality involving the midgut region of the small intestine.
C   (normal presentation as part of severing the umbilical cord) is incorrect. Fecal material is not normally present at the umbilical cord in newborns.
E   (persistence of the allantois) is incorrect. Persistence of the allantois, related to the developing bladder, does occur. The allantois, a blind pouch continuous with the urinary bladder (urogenital sinus) developmentally, extends into the umbilical cord. However, the allantois supposedly regresses and persists only as a fold of connective tissue in the midline of the anterior abdominal wall between the anterosuperior aspect of the bladder (apex) and the umbilicus (median umbilical fold or ligament). If the lumen of the allantois does persist, severing of the umbilical cord would also sever the remnant of the allantois. As a result, urine (not fecal material) would appear at the umbilicus, a sign of a patent urachus or persistent allantois.

17. E   (normal cerebral blood flow) is correct. Cerebral blood flow is autoregulated to maintain neural function. This patient's state of consciousness and orientation support this conclusion.

A   (decreased coronary blood flow) is incorrect. The coronary circulation is also effectively autoregulated, primarily by a metabolic mechanism. Cardiac muscle hypoxia causes the release of adenosine from the cardiac myocytes, and adenosine vasodilates the coronary resistance vessels.
B   (decreased sympathetic tone to the venous system) is incorrect. Hemorrhage results in widespread increased sympathetic tone, including tone to the veins.

C (increased blood flow to the skin, intestines, and kidneys) is incorrect. The widespread stimulation of sympathetic nerve activity that occurs in hemorrhage causes vasoconstriction and decreased blood flow in these vascular beds.

D (increased cholinergic vasoconstrictor tone of skeletal muscle arterioles) is incorrect. Skeletal muscle vasoconstriction is adrenergic, not cholinergic.

18. **D** (schizotypal personality disorder) is correct. This description is consistent with schizotypal personality disorder. Individuals with schizotypal personality disorder exhibit magical thinking, eccentric beliefs, ideas of reference, oddities in thought and speech, and inappropriate affect, but they do not display psychosis.

A (borderline personality disorder) is incorrect. Instability in affect, behavior, relationships, and self-image combined with impulsivity typifies borderline personality disorder.

B (organic delusional syndrome) is incorrect. Organic delusional disorder applies when delusions or other schizophrenic-like symptoms develop secondary to a general medical condition (e.g., head trauma). The nonspecific neuroanatomic findings seen in schizophrenia do not qualify as evidence of cerebral disease or damage.

C (paranoid schizophrenia) is incorrect. Schizophrenia must be present before the subtype paranoid can be applied. In this subtype, hallucinations and delusions are prominent, while affect, speech, and motor functioning are only mildly impacted.

E (undifferentiated schizophrenia) is incorrect. The diagnosis of undifferentiated schizophrenia is assigned when there is impaired functioning and at least some symptoms of schizophrenia are evident for a minimum of 6 months. Two or more active-phase symptoms (e.g., delusions, hallucinations, disorganized speech, grossly disorganized or catatonic behavior, and negative symptoms) also must be present for at least 1 month. The subtype undifferentiated schizophrenia is assigned when other subtypes are not evident or multiple subtypes occur concurrently.

19. **C** (the inotropic effect of isoproterenol in the absence *[curve X]* or presence *[curve Y]* of propranolol) is correct. In this figure, isoproterenol is the agonist, and propranolol is a competitive antagonist at all β-adrenergic receptor subtypes. The dose-response curves of any agonist in the absence or presence of a competitive antagonist would be expected to look like the curves in the figure. The competitive antagonist causes a parallel shift to the right in the agonist's dose-response curve, reflecting a decrease in apparent potency.

A (the chronotropic effect of acetylcholine in the absence *[curve X]* or presence *[curve Y]* of neostigmine) is incorrect. Neostigmine is a cholinesterase inhibitor. Its presence would cause a parallel shift to the left in the curve for acetylcholine, reflecting an increase in apparent potency. A shift to the left is the classic shift of an agent that acts to potentiate a response.

B   (the hypertensive effect of norepinephrine in the absence *[curve X]* or presence *[curve Y]* of phenoxybenzamine) is incorrect. Phenoxybenzamine is a noncompetitive α-adrenergic receptor antagonist. Like all antagonists, a noncompetitive antagonist will shift the curve to the right (reflecting a decrease in apparent potency). Unlike other antagonists, a noncompetitive antagonist will also cause a diminished maximal response (reflecting a decrease in efficacy), since its presence causes a reduction in available receptors with which the agonist may interact. The curves in this case would look as follows:

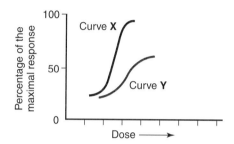

D   (the inotropic effect of pindolol in the absence *[curve X]* or presence *[curve Y]* of a maximal inotropic dose of isoproterenol) is incorrect. Pindolol is a partial agonist, and isoproterenol is a full agonist. When given alone, pindolol would never reach 100% response, as a full agonist would. In the presence of a maximal concentration of a full agonist, such as isoproterenol, pindolol would act as an antagonist. Thus, the response of isoproterenol would decrease as the dose of pindolol is increased until the maximal response to pindolol alone is reached. The curves in this case would look as follows:

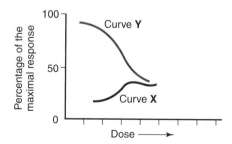

E   (the therapeutic effect of levodopa in the absence *[curve X]* of or presence *[curve Y]* of carbidopa) is incorrect. Carbidopa potentiates the response to levodopa by inhibiting aromatic amino acid decarboxylase (dopa decarboxylase) and preventing its peripheral conversion to dopamine. Thus, the presence of carbidopa would result in a parallel shift to the left in the curve for levodopa.

20. **D** *(Clostridium perfringens)* is correct. The clinical and laboratory findings are consistent with the diagnosis of clostridial myonecrosis (gas gangrene), a disease caused most frequently by *C. perfringens*. This organism is commonly found in soil and water and is also a resident of the gastrointestinal tract. Target hemolysis on blood agar is a finding characteristic of this species. The zone of complete hemolysis is caused by the theta toxin, and the zone of incomplete hemolysis is caused by the alpha toxin.

    A *(Clostridium butyricum)* is incorrect. *C. butyricum* rarely causes disease in humans, but it does produce botulinum toxin.
    B *(Clostridium difficile)* is incorrect. *C. difficile* does not cause myonecrosis. It causes antibiotic-associated gastroenteritis.
    C *(Clostridium histolyticum)* and E *(Clostridium septicum)* are incorrect. Both *C. histolyticum* and *C. septicum* cause clostridial myonecrosis, but these species do not produce the theta toxin, so they would not cause target hemolysis.

21. **D** (mucopolysaccharidosis) is correct. Mucopolysaccharidoses are rare disorders in which the deficiency of a specific lysosomal enzyme causes one or more partly degraded glycosaminoglycans (such as heparan sulfate, dermatan sulfate, or keratan sulfate) to accumulate in the lysosomes of many tissues. Most mucopolysaccharidoses are inherited in an autosomal recessive manner.

    A (Ehlers-Danlos syndrome) is incorrect. Ehlers-Danlos syndrome refers to a heterogeneous group of disorders of connective tissue. Some of the disorders result from genetic defects of collagen chain structure, while others result from deficiencies of enzymes needed for collagen processing. Common signs are weakness, hypermobility of the joints, and hyperextensibility of the skin. Patients may have significant amounts of procollagen in extracts of their skin and tendons.
    B (glycogen storage disease) is incorrect. Glycogen storage diseases result in abnormal glycogen metabolism and accumulation of glycogen in cells. The most affected organs are the liver (hepatomegaly and cirrhosis) and muscles.
    C (Marfan syndrome) is incorrect. Marfan syndrome results from a genetic defect in the structure of elastin.
    E (sphingolipidosis) is incorrect. Sphingolipidoses are storage diseases of glycosphingolipids, such as sphingomyelin, ceramide, and globoside. They are caused by a deficiency of lysosomal enzymes that degrade glycosphingolipids.

22. *A* (β-Amyloid protein) is correct. Senile plaques are characteristic of Alzheimer's disease (AD), which is the most common cause of dementia in patients over 65 years of age. Senile plaques contain a core of A-β amyloid surrounded by neurites. The explanation for the age disparity in this case is that the patient has Down syndrome with three functioning chromosome number 21 (e.g., trisomy 21). Chromosome 21 codes for an Alzheimer precursor protein (APP), part of which is amyloid-β (A-β) protein. This protein is toxic to neurons; hence the extra chromosome 21 codes for more of the protein, which results in AD at an early age.

B (decreased dopamine levels) is incorrect. This describes Parkinson's disease, where there is degeneration and depigmentation of neurons in the substantia nigra and locus ceruleus and a corresponding decrease in the synthesis of the neurotransmitter dopamine. Patients have extrapyramidal signs and symptoms and occasionally develop dementia.

C (slow virus disease) is incorrect. Slow virus diseases include subacute sclerosing panencephalitis (associated with measles), progressive multifocal leukoencephalopathy (associated with papovavirus), and Creutzfeldt-Jakob disease (associated with prions). Although all of these diseases produce dementia, senile plaques are not present in the brain tissue.

D (triplet repeat mutation) is incorrect. A triplet repeat mutation associated with dementia is Huntington's disease, which is an autosomal dominant disease with triplet repeats of CAG on the short arm of chromosome 4. Atrophy and loss of striatal neurons occur in the caudate nucleus, putamen, and frontal cortex; however, there are no senile plaques in the tissue. Furthermore, patients have chorea and extrapyramidal signs, which are not seen in AD.

23. *C* (hyposmotic volume expansion with hydration of both intracellular and extracellular compartments) is correct. Dehydration is suggested in this patient by the elevated plasma Na^+ concentration and body temperature; body fluids will be expected to be hypertonic (>300 mOsm/L). The 500 mL of physiologic saline solution will correct this by replacing both Na^+ and water. Physiologic saline (~300 mOsm/L) is given to expand the extracellular space (plasma and interstitial compartments). Since this exogenous solution is hypotonic to body fluids, the tonicity of the intracellular regions continues to exceed extracellular tonicity. As a result, some of the extracellular water also moves across cell membranes by osmosis, thereby hydrating intracellular spaces as well. Normally, a reduced fluid volume or a more highly concentrated fluid triggers the thirst mechanism. This mechanism is regulated by hypothalamic osmoreceptors. This thirst mechanism is diminished and dehydration occurs more easily in elderly individuals, making it especially important to keep them hydrated on hot summer days.

A (hyperosmotic volume expansion with hydration of both intracellular and extracellular compartments) and B (hyperosmotic volume expansion with intracellular hydration and extracellular dehydration) are incorrect. A hyperosmotic solution (i.e., a solution that is hypertonic to body fluids) would add solute to an already solute-rich extracellular environment. The resulting osmosis would draw fluid from the intracellular space, resulting in crenation. Thus, each of these approaches would lead to extracellular hydration and intracellular dehydration.

D (hyposmotic volume expansion with intracellular hydration and extracellular dehydration) is incorrect. Adding a solution that is hyposmotic to extracellular fluid would reduce the concentration of extracellular solute and push water into cells. After osmotic balance is achieved, both intracellular and extracellular regions will be hydrated.

E (isosmotic volume expansion with no changes in intracellular or extracellular osmolalities) is incorrect. Adding a solution with the same concentration as the existing extracellular fluid would not result in osmosis. Thus, neither solute nor fluid moves from one compartment to the other in a significant amount, and the state of intracellular dehydration remains virtually unchanged.

24. **B** (aspirin) is correct. Unlike other nonsteroidal anti-inflammatory drugs (NSAIDs), aspirin irreversibly inhibits platelet cyclooxygenase (COX). Inhibition of COX prevents the formation of thromboxane A_2. This inhibits platelet hemostasis and causes an increase in bleeding time. Since platelets are enucleated "end cells," the restoration of normal platelet function requires the synthesis of new platelets, a process that takes 7–10 days. If the patient took aspirin (acetylsalicylic acid) 4 days before surgery, he would be expected to experience excessive bleeding during surgery. To avoid this problem, patients should be instructed to stop taking aspirin 1 week before elective surgery and to stop taking other NSAIDs 2 days before elective surgery.

A (acetaminophen) is incorrect. Acetaminophen is a centrally acting inhibitor of COX. Because acetaminophen does not affect platelet function, it would not have caused increased bleeding in the patient described.

C (ibuprofen) is incorrect. Aspirin and ibuprofen are both NSAIDs that inhibit platelet COX. However, aspirin causes irreversible inhibition, whereas ibuprofen causes reversible inhibition. Normal platelet function in the patient would have returned 4 days after taking ibuprofen.

D (salsalate) is incorrect. Salsalate, a nonacetylated salicylate, does not significantly affect platelet function and is considered the NSAID of choice in patients who have an iatrogenic or idiopathic bleeding diathesis.

E (warfarin) is incorrect. Warfarin is an orally administered anticoagulant that increases bleeding. However, warfarin would not have been taken by the patient, because it has no efficacy in the management of headaches.

25. *A* (between the flexor digitorum superficialis and flexor digitorum profundus) is correct. To confirm the diagnosis of carpal tunnel syndrome, the physician may tap over the palmar carpal ligament. Tingling in the distribution of the median nerve (i.e., over the thumb, index, and middle fingers) will confirm the diagnosis.

   The median nerve, which passes into the forearm between the two heads of the pronator teres, between the two heads of the flexor digitorum superficialis, and then between the flexor digitorum superficialis and flexor digitorum profundus, passes into the hand through the carpal tunnel by deep or antebrachial fascia.

   The flexor retinaculum, a ligament that stretches across the wrist from scaphoid and trapezium laterally to the pisiform and hook of the hamate, medially converts the carpal groove formed by carpal bones into the osteofibrous canal known as the carpal tunnel. The tendons of the flexor digitorum superficialis, flexor digitorum profundus, and flexor pollicis longus, as well as the median nerve, travel through the carpal tunnel, making it a very "crowded" area. Therefore, any increase in bulk caused by local factors and/or systemic diseases compresses the median nerve, causing the condition known as "carpal tunnel syndrome."

   B (between the two heads of the flexor carpi ulnaris) is incorrect. The ulnar nerve, not the median nerve, travels between the two heads of the flexor carpi ulnaris.
   C (superficial to the flexor retinaculum) is incorrect. At the wrist, the median nerve travels deep to the flexor retinaculum, and the ulnar nerve is superficial to it.
   D (through the coracobrachialis muscle) is incorrect. The musculocutaneous nerve travels through the coracobrachialis muscle.
   E (through the supinator muscle) is incorrect. The radial nerve travels through the supinator muscle.

26. *D* (lumbar cistern) is correct. The lumbar cistern contains the largest and most accessible pool of CSF. It is located between the end of the spinal cord (L1 or L2) and the end of the dural sheath (S2). Because the only neural tissue in this region is the cauda equina, there is little chance of damaging the central nervous system when withdrawing CSF from this compartment.

   A (cerebellomedullary cistern) is incorrect. Theoretically, CSF can be drawn from the cerebellomedullary cistern (cisterna magna) in infants. However, even though the lumbar cistern has not reached adult size by that time, it is preferred for most patients, including infants.

B (fourth ventricle) is incorrect. The fourth ventricle is not appropriate because it contains only approximately 1 mL of CSF. To withdraw CSF from this ventricle, the physician would have to penetrate the cerebellum or brain stem, which could result in brain damage.

C (lateral ventricles) is incorrect. The lateral ventricles are not appropriate CSF sources, because their CSF volume is limited (approximately 9 mL each). To withdraw CSF from the ventricles, the physician would have to penetrate the cerebral cortex, which may result in brain damage.

E (pontine cistern) is incorrect. The pontine cistern is a small cistern located between the base of the pons and the clivus (a bony surface extending posterorostrally from the foramen magnum toward the occipital bone), and is quite inaccessible.

27. *A* (R ~ a-b-c-a) is correct. This figure is a compliance plot. Compliance is defined as the change in volume per change in pressure (indicated by the slope of the lines). The straight line (a-c) represents static compliance, when no air is flowing. The bowed curves (a-b-c- and c-d-a) represent dynamic compliance, which occurs when air is flowing against resistance. If airflow resistance were negligible, the dynamic and static compliance lines would overlap each other. During inspiration, the intrapleural pressure (P_{pl}) becomes more negative and allows the alveolar pressure to drop to a subatmospheric level; this results in a gradient that promotes the flow of air into the lungs. Because of airflow resistance, however, the change in lung volume always lags behind the change in alveolar pressure; the recording of these changes results in a bowed curve. Thus, the area inscribed a-b-c-a represents inspiratory airflow resistance.

B (R ~ a-c-d-a) is incorrect. This area represents expiratory airflow resistance.

C (R ~ a-c-e-a) is incorrect. This area is proportional to the elastic properties of the lungs and compliance.

D (R ~ a-b-c-d-a) is incorrect. This area is a combination of inspiratory and expiratory airflow resistance.

E (R ~ a-b-c-e-a) is incorrect. This area represents a combination of compliance and airflow resistance, and is related to the total work of breathing.

28. *B* (high levels of T cell cytokines) is correct. Patients with toxic shock syndrome (TSS) have high levels of T cell cytokines, because staphylococcal enterotoxins act as superantigens that nonspecifically bind to and activate T cells.

A (fulminant septicemia) is incorrect. In nearly all cases of TSS, the infection is localized, rather than systemic. The toxin is systemic.

C (high ratio of CD8+ cells to CD4+ cells) is incorrect. A high ratio of CD8+ cells to CD4+ cells is not a finding associated with TSS. It is a finding associated with Epstein-Barr virus infections and with other diseases in which there may be polyclonal activation of B cells.

D (hypergammaglobulinemia) is incorrect. Hypergammaglobulinemia is indicative of nonspecific activation of B cells, so it would not be a finding in TSS.

E (positive results in the limulus test) is incorrect. Positive results in the limulus test indicate the presence of an endotoxin from a gram-negative organism. TSS is caused by *Staphylococcus aureus,* and toxic shock–like syndrome is caused by *Streptococcus pyogenes.* Both organisms are gram-positive.

29. *B* (dopamine D_2 receptors) is correct. Dystonic reactions can occur during the first few hours or days after the administration of a phenothiazine drug, such as prochlorperazine. In this case, the patient's dystonia is characterized by oculogyric crisis and torticollis. Dystonias and other acute extrapyramidal side effects (such as parkinsonism and akathisia) are thought to arise when the blockade of postsynaptic D_2 receptors causes a decrease in the dopamine and acetylcholine input to the striatum (nigrostriatal dopaminergic pathway). Treatment with an antimuscarinic agent, such as benztropine or diphenhydramine, can effectively alleviate dystonic reactions.

A (α_1-adrenergic receptors) is incorrect. The α_1-adrenergic receptor blockade by prochlorperazine is responsible for side effects such as nasal stuffiness, orthostatic hypotension, and miosis.

C (histamine H_1 receptors) is incorrect. The H_1 receptor blockade by prochlorperazine is responsible for the sedative side effect of the drug.

D (muscarinic receptors) is incorrect. Muscarinic receptor blockade by prochlorperazine is responsible for side effects such as dry mouth, urinary retention, constipation, and blurred vision.

E (serotonin receptors) is incorrect. Prochlorperazine does not block serotonin receptors.

30. *B* (benign insulin-secreting tumor causing periodic hypoglycemia) is correct. Confusion or fainting that occurs when blood glucose levels are low (e.g., when fasting or exercising) and is relieved or prevented by eating suggests hypoglycemia. A benign insulin-secreting tumor, also known as an insulinoma, will induce symptomatic hypoglycemia when blood glucose levels are low.

A (autonomic insufficiency leading to orthostatic hypotension) is incorrect. Symptoms of autonomic insufficiency are not relieved by eating and are not likely to be episodic.

C (glucagon-secreting tumor causing periodic hypoglycemia) is incorrect. Glucagon stimulates hepatic glucose release and produces hyperglycemia, not hypoglycemia.

D (meningioma in the region of the frontal cortex) is incorrect. Seizures and headaches are the primary presenting symptoms of meningiomas.

E (norepinephrine-secreting tumor causing periodic hyperglycemia) is incorrect. Norepinephrine-secreting tumors, also known as pheochromocytomas, cause hypertension and headaches; they do not cause fainting.

31. *E* (urine test for 5-hydroxyindoleacetic acid) is correct. The patient has the clinical findings of a carcinoid syndrome complicated by tricuspid insufficiency. To develop a carcinoid syndrome, a carcinoid tumor secreting serotonin must metastasize to the liver. In the liver, the tumor nodules secrete serotonin directly into hepatic vein tributaries and gain access to the systemic circulation, where the tumor produces flushing (due to vasodilatation), diarrhea, and right-sided valvular lesions. All carcinoid tumors are malignant; however, their ability to metastasize to the liver occurs when they are >2 cm. This explains why carcinoid tumors of the appendix (usually <2 cm) rarely metastasize to the liver, whereas those in the terminal ileum have the potential to metastasize; hence their notoriety as the most common primary site for tumors associated with carcinoid syndrome. The classic laboratory finding in carcinoid syndrome is an increase in urine levels of 5-HIAA, which is the liver-derived metabolic end product of serotonin.

Serotonin elicits a fibrogenic response in the valvular tissue that may result in tricuspid insufficiency or pulmonic stenosis. This patient has tricuspid insufficiency with the classic pansystolic murmur, giant *c-v* wave (due to blood entering the right atrium during systole), and S_3 and S_4 heart sounds (due to volume overload in the right ventricle). Because inspiration increases negative intrathoracic pressures, more blood enters the right side of the heart than is present in the left side. Hence, all abnormal heart sounds and murmurs increase in intensity on inspiration in lesions on the right-side, as opposed to left-sided lesions, which increase in intensity on expiration.

Smoking has no relationship with carcinoid tumors or carcinoid syndrome. Bronchial carcinoids rarely produce carcinoid syndrome and are not associated with smoking. Furthermore, it is not necessary for bronchial carcinoids to metastasize to the liver to produce the syndrome, because serotonin has direct access to the systemic circulation.

A (blood cultures) is incorrect. The patient does not have infective endocarditis (IE) of the tricuspid valve; IE does not explain the nodular liver, flushing, and diarrhea. IE involving the tricuspid valve is most often associated with intravenous drug abuse.
B (complete blood cell count) is incorrect. There are no distinct hematologic features that characterize carcinoid syndrome.
C (liver function tests) is incorrect. Liver function tests are usually normal in patients with liver metastasis due to the focal, rather than diffuse, involvement of the liver parenchyma.
D (serum electrolytes) is incorrect. Serum electrolytes have no distinct diagnostic profile for carcinoid syndrome.

32. **B** (Ehlers-Danlos syndrome) is correct. Ehlers-Danlos syndrome is a multitude of disorders caused by a defect in an autosomal recessive gene involved in the synthesis of collagen or collagen cross-linking events. At least 10 varieties of this disorder are known. This patient may have variant VI, which is characterized by decreased hydroxylation of lysyl residues in type I and type III collagen.

A (cystic fibrosis) is incorrect. Cystic fibrosis is the most common lethal genetic disease affecting white children. It is caused by a defect in the function of all exocrine glands. The organs most likely to be seriously affected are the lungs and pancreas, because this disorder results in abnormally viscous secretions blocking the airways and the pancreatic ducts.
C (familial hypercholesterolemia) is incorrect. Familial hypercholesterolemia is a genetic disease caused by mutations in the gene for receptor proteins. It results in defective catabolism and excessive biosynthesis of cholesterol. This patient's symptoms suggest abnormal collagen formation; familial hypercholesterolemia does not play a role in collagen formation.
D (fragile X syndrome) is incorrect. Fragile X syndrome occurs in males and is characterized by mental retardation and macroorchidism. It is identified by an abnormal banding pattern on the affected X chromosome, which represents the amplification of sets of three nucleotides and which disrupts the normal function of the gene.
E (Marfan syndrome) is incorrect. Marfan syndrome is an autosomal dominant disorder that results in a defect in the production of fibril, a structural glycoprotein secreted by fibroblasts that forms microfibrillar aggregates in the extracellular matrix. These aggregates serve as scaffolds for normal elastic fibers. The most serious clinical sign of Marfan syndrome is loss of elasticity in the tunica media of the aorta. This defect is the pathologic basis for aortic aneurysm, which can result in aortic dissection or rupture.

33. **B** (adjustment disorder with depressed mood) is correct. When an individual develops clinically significant emotional and behavioral symptoms within 3 months of a psychosocial stressor, the diagnosis of adjustment disorder is appropriate. The patient experienced decreased energy, increased sleep, and feelings of worthlessness and guilt for 2 months after a major stressor, his divorce.

A (acute stress disorder) is incorrect. In acute stress disorder, symptoms similar to posttraumatic stress disorder occur, but they begin within 4 weeks of the traumatic event and only last from 2 days to 4 weeks. This patient has been experiencing symptoms for 2 months.
C (dysthymia) is incorrect. Dysthymia refers to a chronic low level of depression that persists for at least 2 years in adulthood. This patient's symptoms are of much shorter duration.

D (major depressive disorder) is incorrect. This patient is not reporting enough symptoms suggestive of depression to meet the diagnostic criteria to warrant a diagnosis of major depression. Major depressive disorder applies only when a seriously depressed mood or anhedonia is present for at least 2 weeks in conjunction with three or four additional symptoms of depression, also displayed with functional impairment.

E (posttraumatic stress disorder) is incorrect. Posttraumatic stress disorder is diagnosed when a person has difficulty coping with exposure to a life-threatening traumatic event. Following the trauma, maladaptive patterns of reexperiencing the trauma and avoidance of stimuli related to the event occur. These criteria do not apply to this patient.

34. *E* (normal finding in pregnancy) is correct. The total serum T_4 level reflects free T_4 (unbound and metabolically active) and T_4 bound to thyroid-binding globulin (TBG, metabolically inactive). The increase in estrogen that normally occurs during pregnancy stimulates liver synthesis of TBG. Because T_4 normally occupies one third of the binding sites on TBG, the additional TBG with its bound fraction increases the total level of T_4. The amount of T_4 synthesized by the thyroid gland is in balance with the levels of free T_4 in the serum; hence the free T_4 levels remain the same and the patient is clinically euthyroid. Because free T_4 has a negative feedback relationship with TSH, the serum TSH level also remains normal. Thus, an increase in serum T_4 in the presence of a normal TSH level indicates that the patient has an increase in TBG, most likely secondary to an increase in estrogen. An enlarged thyroid gland and heat intolerance are normal findings in a pregnant patient.

A (decreased thyroid-binding globulin) is incorrect. Estrogen increases liver synthesis of TBG.

B (increased synthesis of T_4) and C (increased synthesis of T_3) are incorrect. The patient's TSH level is normal, indicating that free hormone levels must be normal.

D (thyroiditis-induced release of thyroxine) is incorrect. The TSH level is normal, indicating that the patient is euthyroid. Patients with hyperthyroidism have increased free T_4 levels and corresponding TSH suppression.

35. *E* (stimulating postsynaptic dopamine receptors) is correct. Parkinson's disease is characterized by the degeneration of several dopaminergic pathways, including the nigrostriatal pathway, which projects from the substantia nigra pars compacta to the striatum. The loss of this excitatory input modifies basal ganglia output and results in resting tremor, increased muscle tone, and difficulty in initiating movement, which is characteristic of this disease. Pharmacologic strategies would include drugs that can stimulate dopaminergic fibers.

A (decreasing release of presynaptic dopamine) is incorrect. Blocking the release of dopamine from presynaptic fibers reduces the amount of dopamine available to bind with postsynaptic receptors and excite postsynaptic fibers. Because patients with Parkinson's disease have already lost dopaminergic fibers, factors that would decrease dopamine levels even further would worsen their condition.
B (decreasing synthesis of dopamine) is incorrect. Reducing the production of dopamine in patients whose condition is caused by a lack of dopaminergic fibers would only worsen their condition.
C (increasing dopamine synaptic reuptake) is incorrect. Reuptake by presynaptic fibers reduces the amount of dopamine available in the synaptic cleft to bind with postsynaptic receptors.
D (increasing levels of acetylcholine in the putamen) is incorrect. One of the treatments for patients with Parkinson's disease involves decreasing, rather than increasing, the level of acetylcholine.

36. *E* (X-linked recessive) is correct. An X-linked recessive disorder is transmitted from mother to son. The mutant gene is on chromosome X. The mother is heterozygous for that gene, but she is not affected by the disorder. Her son will have only one X chromosome, so he will display the disorder. Hemophilia A is an example of an X-linked disorder.

A (autosomal dominant) is incorrect. Autosomal dominant diseases result from the mutation of one gene of a pair coding for a structural protein. An individual with an autosomal dominant disorder is affected by a disease. Each child of the affected individual has a 50% chance of being affected. An example of an autosomal dominant disorder is von Willebrand's disease.
B (autosomal recessive) is incorrect. Autosomal recessive disorders occur when both maternal and paternal genes of a gene pair have a mutation. Heterozygous individuals do not have symptoms of the disease. If both parents are heterozygous for a gene, each child has a 25% chance of being affected. Many enzyme deficiencies, including phenylketonuria (PKU) and homocystinuria, are inherited in this manner.
C (multifactorial) is incorrect. Multifactorial disorders affect both sexes and are believed to be caused by a combination of genetic and environmental factors. An example of a multifactorial disorder is cleft lip.
D (X-linked dominant) is incorrect. The term X-linked dominant refers only to expression in females. In an X-linked dominant disorder, the affected female transmits the disorder to 50% of her sons and 50% of her daughters. An example of an X-linked dominant disorder is vitamin D–resistant rickets.

37. *D* (hantavirus) is correct. The clinical, epidemiologic, and laboratory findings are consistent with the diagnosis of hantavirus pulmonary syndrome, an emerging infectious disease in the United States. The deer mouse is the primary reservoir, and

transmission to humans occurs via the inhalation of aerosolized virions from mouse excrement. Hantaviruses are members of the family *Bunyaviridae,* a family consisting of enveloped RNA viruses that have a helical nucleocapsid.

A (California encephalitis virus) is incorrect. California encephalitis virus is also a member of the family *Bunyaviridae,* but it predominantly infects the central nervous system.
B (coltivirus) is incorrect. Coltiviruses include the virus responsible for Colorado tick fever and are members of the family *Reoviridae.* This family consists of nonenveloped RNA viruses that have an icosahedral nucleocapsid.
C (dengue virus) is incorrect. Dengue virus is the agent of dengue fever, a disease characterized by fever, arthritis, myalgia, and rash. It is also an agent of hemorrhagic fever. Dengue virus is a member of the family *Flaviviridae,* which consists of enveloped RNA viruses that have an icosahedral nucleocapsid.
E (Lassa virus) is incorrect. Lassa virus is an agent of hemorrhagic fever, so its clinical manifestations differ from those in the patient described. Lassa virus is a member of the family *Arenaviridae.* This family, like the family *Bunyaviridae,* consists of enveloped RNA viruses that have a helical nucleocapsid.

38. ***B*** (structure B) is correct. The oculomotor nerve (CN III) innervates all of the muscles of the eye, except the superior oblique and lateral rectus muscles. It also innervates the striated muscle in the eyelid. Damage to oculomotor fibers serving the right eye results in right-sided ptosis and the inability to adduct the right eye.

A (structure A) is incorrect. The superior cerebellar artery serves the superior surface of the cerebellum, which receives much of its input from the cerebral cortex via pontine nuclei. Damage to this artery interferes with cerebellar functions, including the ability to maintain equilibrium and posture and plan voluntary movement. It does not play a role in eye movement.
C (structure C) is incorrect. The olfactory tract extends from the olfactory bulb directly to the olfactory cortex in the cerebrum. The olfactory bulb receives bundles of unmyelinated fibers (fila) that have passed through the ethmoid bone. It contains sensory neurons that transmit information about odor. It does not contain motor neurons and therefore cannot control muscle activity in the eye.
D (structures D) and E (right optic nerve) are incorrect. The left and right optic nerves consist of the axons of retinal ganglion cells, which project to the optic disc. These are sensory nerves that transmit information about vision. They do not contain motor neurons and therefore do not regulate muscle activity in the eye.

39. *A* (anorexia nervosa) is correct. The cardinal characteristic of anorexia nervosa is emaciation, which is achieved through rigorous exercise and drastic restriction of food intake. To assign a diagnosis of anorexia nervosa, patients must be 15% or more below expected body weight, and amenorrhea (an absence of the menstrual cycle) must be present for at least 3 consecutive menstrual cycles in female patients. Body image disturbances, conflicts about sexuality, and excessive need for control and perfection also are often present.

B (body dysmorphic disorder) is incorrect. Excessive concern about a self-defined bodily defect and a magnified sense of ugliness characterize body dysmorphic disorder.
C (bulimia nervosa) is incorrect. Binge eating followed by purgative behaviors, such as self-induced vomiting; use of laxatives, diuretics, and enema abuse; or excessive fasting and exercise constitutes a diagnosis of bulimia nervosa.
D (pica) is incorrect. The ingestion of nonnutritive substances (e.g., dirt, cigarette butts, paint chips) is termed pica.
E (rumination disorder) is incorrect. Rumination disorder is typically seen in infancy and involves the ingestion of regurgitated food. The technique is sometimes used by adults with eating disorders to minimize weight gain.

40. *A* (digoxin) is correct. The patient's clinical and ECG findings are consistent with digoxin intoxication precipitated by the concurrent use of furosemide. Furosemide-induced hypokalemia increases the likelihood of digoxin cardiotoxicity by increasing the binding of digoxin to Na^+,K^+-ATPase. Atrial tachycardia that is evoked by delayed after-depolarizations and occurs in the presence of AV slowing or AV block is a classic rhythm disturbance seen in patients with digoxin intoxication.

B (milrinone) is incorrect. Milrinone is administered intravenously and is indicated only for the short-term management of congestive heart failure. It does not interact with furosemide and does not have the side effect profile that is described.
C (propranolol) and E (verapamil) are incorrect. Propranolol and verapamil do not interact with furosemide and do not have the side effect profile that is described.
D (quinidine) is incorrect. The extracardiac toxic effects of quinidine would include the classic signs of cinchonism (tinnitus, headache, blurred vision, and vertigo). The cardiac toxic effects of quinidine are not consistent with those described for the patient and would show a marked widening of the QRS complex, prolongation of the QT interval, and torsade de pointes.

41. *E* (rabies virus) is correct. The clinical and laboratory findings are consistent with the diagnosis of rabies encephalitis. In the United States, this disease occurs sporadically and can be transmitted by contact with saliva from an infected animal or by inhalation of the aerosolized rabies virus. Like other members of

the family *Rhabdoviridae,* rabies virus is a single-stranded, negative-sense, nonsegmented RNA virus. The G proteins are glycoproteins found in the envelope of the virus.

A (eastern equine encephalitis virus) and C (echovirus) are incorrect. Eastern equine encephalitis virus and echoviruses are etiologic agents of encephalitis. However, they do not cause the types of behavioral changes described in this case, and they lack G proteins. Eastern equine encephalitis virus is a member of the family *Togaviridae,* and echoviruses are members of the family *Picornaviridae.* These two families consist of single-stranded, positive-sense, nonsegmented RNA viruses.
B (Ebola virus) is incorrect. Although Ebola virus can cause encephalitis, it is more commonly associated with hemorrhagic fever. The virus lacks G protein but is a member of the family *Filoviridae,* a family whose genome has the same characteristics as the family *Rhabdoviridae.*
D (hantavirus) is incorrect. Hantaviruses are not associated with encephalitis. They are members of the family *Bunyaviridae,* which consists of single-stranded, negative-sense, segmented RNA viruses.

42. *B* (primarily an inhibitor of elastase released by macrophages and neutrophils) is correct. The patient's clinical and laboratory findings are consistent with the diagnosis of α_1-antitrypsin deficiency. The main physiologic function of α_1-antitrypsin is to protect the lungs from elastase released by neutrophils. It can also protect lung tissue from proteases released by dying cells during inflammation. In α_1-antitrypsin deficiency, elastase degrades lung tissue. Cigarette smoking or air pollution can contribute to the disease by oxidizing any α_1-antitrypsin that is present.

A (a cysteine protease inhibitor) is incorrect. α_1-Antitrypsin is not a cysteine protease inhibitor; it is a serine protease inhibitor.
C (showing specificity for trypsin) is incorrect. α_1-Antitrypsin has in vitro activity against many serine proteases, including trypsin, plasmin, thrombin, chymotrypsin, and neutrophil elastase.
D (synthesized in the lungs and inhibits surfactant production) is incorrect. α_1-Antitrypsin is synthesized in the liver, not in the lungs.
E (thought to be inherited in an X-linked manner) is incorrect. α_1-Antitrypsin deficiency is inherited as an autosomal codominant trait. Both alleles contribute to the disease, and neither is dominant over the other.

43. *C* (left lateral funiculus) is correct. The lateral funiculus (also known as the lateral column) is a column of white matter that lies lateral to the dorsal and ventral horns in the spinal cord and carries pain signals to the brain and motor and autonomic signals from the brain. A lesion in the left lateral funiculus could block signals descending from upper motor neurons to spinal in-

terneurons and alpha motor neurons to control local reflexes. Loss of such control would result in hyperactive stretch reflexes, a positive Babinski's sign, and diffuse areas of weakness in the right leg. Since pain fibers usually do not cross the midline of the spinal cord until they have risen a few levels above the level of entry, a lesion on the left at the point of entry for pain fibers traveling from the left leg would block pain sensations from the left leg.

A (cerebellum) is incorrect. A lesion in the cerebellum would result in abnormal voluntary movement and poor balance. It would not affect sensory function or pain pathways.
B (internal capsule, left anterior limb) is incorrect. The anterior limb of the internal capsule contains fibers projecting from the frontal lobe to the pons. These fibers do not descend to the spinal interneurons. Therefore, they would not affect reflexes that involve the limbs.
D (reticular formation) is incorrect. Some pain signals are transmitted by the spinoreticular tract to the reticular formation and from there to the thalamus. Thus, a lesion in the reticular formation would block some pain signals. However, it would not account for the complete absence of pain sensation in the left leg, nor for the abnormal motor and reflex activity reported for this patient.
E (right frontal lobe) is incorrect. The frontal lobe contains the primary motor and premotor cortices. A lesion in the right frontal lobe would block motor signals destined for alpha motor neurons governing the right side of the body. These are motor fibers; therefore, the lesion would not affect pain sensations from the leg.

44. A (anterior cruciate) is correct. The anterior cruciate ligament (ACL), together with the posterior cruciate ligament, is important in providing stability to the knee during extension and flexion of the joint. These intracapsular ligaments, which lie within the joint cavity (but outside the synovial cavity), are so-named because they form an "X" inside the knee joint. Their names also derive from their sites of attachment to the tibia. The ACL attaches anteriorly to the intercondylar eminence of the tibia and posteriorly into the lateral condyle of the femur. The femur tends to glide anteriorly on the tibia during flexion of the knee and posteriorly on the tibia during extension of the joint. The ACL tightens during leg extension, limits extension, and prevents hyperextension of the knee. In addition, the ligament prevents anterior dislocation of the tibia on the femur during extension of the leg. The ACL is commonly damaged in two ways: in hyperextension, as in a headlong fall, as in this case; and by a blow from the posterior leg, which forces the tibia anteriorly, as in a "clip" in football (a hit from the side, below the knee).

B (fibular collateral) is incorrect. The fibular (lateral) collateral ligament spans the knee joint between the lateral condyle of the femur and the head of the fibula and protects against forced adduction of the leg at the knee. In addition, it acts with the tibial collateral ligament to prevent lateral rotation of the tibia in an extended knee. The origin of this ropelike ligament, which splits the tendon of insertion of the biceps femoris, is adjacent to the origin of the popliteus muscle from the lateral femoral condyle. The fibular collateral ligament is seldom damaged, partly because it is strong, but primarily because blows to the medial side of the knee to adduct the leg are uncommon.

C (posterior cruciate) is incorrect. The posterior cruciate ligament, in addition to the ACL, is important in providing stability to the knee during flexion of the joint. These two intracapsular ligaments that lie within the joint cavity (but outside the synovial cavity) are so-named because they form an "X" inside the knee joint. Their names also derive from their sites of attachment to the tibia. The posterior cruciate ligament attaches posteriorly on the tibia and anteriorly into the medial condyle of the femur, and provides stability to the knee, particularly during flexion. It is relatively loose in an extended knee. In addition, the posterior cruciate ligament prevents anterior dislocation of the femur (posterior dislocation of the tibia) during flexion of the knee.

D (posterior meniscofemoral) is incorrect. The posterior meniscofemoral ligament, which extends from the posterior aspect of the lateral meniscus to the medial condyle of the femur, plays no role in knee-joint stability beyond anchoring the lateral meniscus to the femur. One of the most common football injuries is the so-called "unhappy triad," which results from a blow to the posterolateral aspect of the knee. The blow forcibly adducts the leg, tearing the tibial collateral ligament and the medial meniscus, and drives the tibia anteriorly, tearing the ACL—hence, the term "unhappy triad."

E (tibial collateral) is incorrect. All ligaments of the knee provide for increased stability during movement. The major function of the tibial (medial) collateral ligament is to prevent abduction of the knee. This ligament is most taut when the leg is extended and relatively loose when the leg is in flexion. It prevents lateral rotation of the tibia related to the femur in an extended knee. The tibial collateral ligament is most commonly injured by a blow to the lateral aspect of the knee, forcing abduction of the leg. It is less susceptible to involvement in a hyperextension injury. Morphologically, the tibial collateral ligament is a broad flat band attached to the medial condyle of the femur and the medial condyle and upper body of the tibia. An important feature of the tibial collateral ligament is that it attaches to the medial meniscus. As a result, when the tibial collateral ligament is torn, the medial meniscus is also often damaged.

45. *E* *(Sporothrix schenckii)* is correct. The patient described has a classic case of lymphocutaneous sporotrichosis, a disease that is also known as alcoholic rose gardener's syndrome and is caused by *S. schenckii.* The dimorphic fungus is ubiquitous in the environment and is often found in vegetation. Individuals at increased risk for sporotrichosis include those who are constantly exposed to potential sources of inoculation and those who have underlying diseases.

A *(Blastomyces dermatitidis),* B *(Candida albicans),* C *(Coccidioides immitis),* and D *(Histoplasma capsulatum)* are incorrect. All of these fungi are dimorphic and can cause skin lesions. However, they rarely cause multiple lesions that follow lymphatic channels.

46. *B* (amantadine) is correct. The patient has classic manifestations of amantadine-induced livedo reticularis. This adverse effect, which occurs in up to 80% of patients treated with amantadine, is benign and reversible. It is thought to be due to amantadine-stimulated local release of norepinephrine, which causes vasoconstriction and changes in the permeability of cutaneous blood vessels.

A (acyclovir), C (foscarnet), and F (zidovudine) are incorrect. Acyclovir, foscarnet, and zidovudine are not effective against influenzavirus A, and their use is not associated with the development of livedo reticularis. Acyclovir is used to treat herpes simplex virus (HSV) and varicella-zoster virus (VZV) infections. Foscarnet is used to treat retinitis caused by cytomegalovirus (CMV) and to treat acyclovir-resistant HSV infections in immunocompromised patients. Zidovudine is a nucleoside reverse transcriptase inhibitor that is used in combination with other drugs for the treatment of HIV infection.
D (oseltamivir) is incorrect. Oseltamivir is indicated for the treatment of acute influenza A or B in patients who have had symptoms for a short period (≤ 2 days). The drug acts to inhibit viral neuraminidase, an enzyme required for the release of the virus from infected cells.
E (ribavirin) is incorrect. Ribavirin is sometimes used in the management of influenza A and B, although it is not labeled for this use. Ribavirin treatment has not been associated with the development of livedo reticularis.

47. *A* (high FSH; high LH; low testosterone) is correct. The patient has Klinefelter's syndrome, which is a sex-chromosome disorder with 47 chromosomes (XXY). These patients have one Barr body, because one of the two X chromosomes is randomly inactivated. Abnormal numbers of chromosomes are usually due to nondisjunction in the first step of meiosis. Most patients are diagnosed in adolescence, when males fail to show appropriate secondary sex characteristics of puberty. Physical examination shows disproportionately long arms and legs (eunuchoid proportions), decreased testicular volume for age, sparse axillary and pubic hair, and gynecomastia; the last two findings are related to hyperestrinism. Both testicles are atrophic, with atrophy and fibrosis of the seminiferous tubules and no evidence of spermatogenesis (azoospermia). There is hyperplasia of the Leydig cells. The absence of Sertoli cells in the fibrosed seminiferous tubules results in decreased synthesis of the hormone inhibin, which normally has a negative feedback relationship with FSH. Hence, FSH levels in Klinefelter's syndrome are markedly elevated. Because FSH normally increases the synthesis of aromatase in Leydig cells, hyperplasia of the Leydig cells causes an even greater conversion of testosterone into estradiol than normal. Therefore, the patient develops signs of hyperestrinism and hypogonadism, due to low testosterone levels. Decreased synthesis of testosterone, which normally has a negative feedback on LH, leads to an increase in LH.

B (high FSH; normal LH; normal testosterone) is incorrect. These findings are consistent with pure seminiferous tubule failure. Loss of inhibin leads to an increase in FSH. Because Leydig cells are functional, serum LH and testosterone are normal.
C (low FSH; low LH; and low testosterone) is incorrect. These findings are consistent with hypopituitarism, where FSH and LH are decreased, with low LH leading to decreased testosterone synthesis.
D (normal FSH; high LH; low testosterone) is incorrect. These findings are consistent with a pure Leydig cell failure, where a decrease in testosterone leads to an increase in LH. FSH is normal, because the seminiferous tubules are normal.

48. *A* (type I) is correct. The patient's clinical manifestations are consistent with the diagnosis of hay fever. In this form of allergic rhinitis, attacks occur seasonally in response to exposure to pollens and other antigens. Allergic rhinitis is an example of type I hypersensitivity, which is IgE-mediated. Type I hypersensitivity reactions are also called immediate or anaphylactic reactions.

B (type II) is incorrect. Type II hypersensitivity is antibody-mediated cytotoxic hypersensitivity. Type II reactions are also called antibody-dependent reactions.
C (type III) is incorrect. Type III hypersensitivity is immune complex-mediated hypersensitivity.
D (type IV) is incorrect. Type IV hypersensitivity is delayed-type hypersensitivity. Type IV reactions are also called cell-mediated reactions.

49. *C* (demonstrate a need for lavish personal attention and have a grandiose sense of self-importance) is correct. Individuals with narcissistic personality disorder show a pervasive pattern of grandiosity, an excessive need for admiration, and lack empathy for others. These individuals believe they are "special" and expect others (including their physicians) to treat them as special.

A (be guarded and have difficulty disclosing personal information) is incorrect. Excessive suspiciousness is a trait most commonly associated with paranoid personality disorder or psychotic disorder.
B (demonstrate an excessive need for order and control and ask many questions) is incorrect. Preoccupation with orderliness, perfection, and control is typically a sign of an obsessive-compulsive personality disorder.
D (have difficulty making decisions and be overly reliant on the physician) is incorrect. Patients with dependent personality disorder are more likely to be submissive and overly reliant on the physician.
E (interact in a flirtatious manner and display seductive behavior) is incorrect. Inappropriate seductive behavior is often associated with histrionic or borderline personality disorder. Affected individuals need excessive attention and are highly emotional.

50. *A* (low hemoglobin and low hematocrit) is correct. The patient is in hypovolemic shock secondary to blood loss from the open femoral fracture and a possible ruptured spleen. Initially, loss of whole blood does not alter the Hgb and Hct concentrations because equal amounts of red blood cells (RBCs) and plasma are lost. Within a few hours, however, sodium-containing fluid reabsorbed by the kidneys, along with fluid from the interstitial space, is added to the vascular compartment to restore volume. This uncovers the RBC deficit, leading to a decrease in the Hgb and Hct. If the patient is not transfused with packed RBCs, over the next few weeks to months, the bone marrow replaces the RBC deficit until the Hgb and Hct return to the normal range. However, if a patient with massive blood loss is infused with 0.9% normal saline to increase the blood pressure, the RBC deficit is uncovered immediately and the expected decrease in Hgb and Hct is noted in a complete blood cell count.

B (low mean corpuscular volume) is incorrect. The size of the RBCs is not altered by the immediate loss of RBCs.
C (low serum glucose concentration) is incorrect. The patient received 0.9% normal saline without glucose.
D (low serum sodium concentration) is incorrect. The concentration of sodium remains the same because 0.9% normal saline is isotonic with plasma.
E (low white blood cell count) is incorrect. Trauma causes the release of catecholamines, which decrease adhesion molecule synthesis, causing release of the marginating neutrophil pool in the peripheral blood into the circulating pool. This results in an absolute neutrophilic leukocytosis.

Test 4

TEST 4

DIRECTIONS: Each numbered item or incomplete statement is followed by options arranged in alphabetical or logical order. Select the best answer to each question. Some options may be partially correct, but there is only **ONE BEST** answer.

1. A 25-year-old woman has not had her menstrual period for the past 8 months. She is 62 inches tall and weighs 41 kg (90 lb), and she says that she has been trying to lose weight for her upcoming wedding. A urine pregnancy test is negative. The patient is given an intramuscular injection of progesterone. Ten days later she reports that she has had no withdrawal bleeding. Laboratory studies show the following serum levels:

Prolactin	10 ng/mL
Follicle-stimulating hormone (FSH)	3 mIU/mL
Luteinizing hormone (LH)	2 mIU/mL
Thyroid-stimulating hormone (TSH)	4.1 µU/mL
Estradiol	Low
Cortisol (AM)	35 µg/dL
Growth hormone	10 ng/mL

Which of the following is the most likely diagnosis?

- ○ A. Acromegaly
- ○ B. Cushing's syndrome
- ○ C. Hypopituitarism
- ○ D. Primary ovarian disease
- ○ E. Weight loss syndrome

2. A 34-year-old man with a history of several sexually transmitted diseases visits an outpatient clinic and is found to have fever, pharyngitis, lymphadenopathy, leukopenia, splenomegaly, and a maculopapular rash. Laboratory studies to determine the cause of his manifestations show nothing definitive and are remarkable only for an increased antibody titer to cytomegalovirus (CMV). Two months later, he is admitted to the hospital with shortness of breath and a spiking fever. Bronchoscopy is diagnostic of *Pneumocystis carinii* pneumonia. Laboratory studies show a CD4+ cell count of 300/mm^3, and antibodies to another virus (not CMV) are identified by enzyme-linked immunosorbent assay (ELISA) and the Western blot test. The virus causing the underlying disease replicates its genome

- ○ A. after enclosure in a new viral capsid
- ○ B. after integration into the host chromosome
- ○ C. freely within the host nucleus
- ○ D. in the cytoplasm of host cells
- ○ E. in the endoplasmic reticulum of host cells

3. A 58-year-old woman has diminished sensations in her left forehead and eyelid. She feels no pain in her left cornea and has no tearing in that eye. A lesion in which of the following areas is most likely to cause these findings?

○ A. Left frontal lobe
○ B. Left motor nucleus of the trigeminal nerve (CN V)
○ C. Left ventral posterolateral (VPL) nucleus of the thalamus
○ D. Ophthalmic division of the left trigeminal nerve
○ E. Right nucleus of CN V

4. While undergoing a routine physical examination, an asymptomatic 65-year-old man has a blood pressure reading of 165/110 mm Hg in both arms and legs. An abdominal bruit is heard on auscultation. His serum electrolytes are normal. Six months ago, he was normotensive. The most likely cause of hypertension in this patient is

○ A. arteriosclerotic narrowing of a renal artery
○ B. benign aldosterone-secreting tumor
○ C. coarctation of the aorta
○ D. essential hypertension
○ E. increased aortic compliance due to normal aging

5. A 4-year-old girl is brought to the pediatrician for evaluation because her father is concerned that the child's language skills are not at the same level his other children displayed at the same age. The girl responds to simple directions, follows simple commands, and understands pronouns. She also uses utterances, imitates sounds, refers to herself by name, and appears to know about 100 words. She does not exhibit other higher order language skills. Of the following language-related statements, the most appropriate conclusion is that the child's

○ A. expressive skills are intact but receptive language is impaired
○ B. receptive language is intact but expressive skills are impaired
○ C. language is progressing as expected
○ D. language is within 1 year of her expected level
○ E. language is seriously impaired and warrants further evaluation

6. A febrile 23-year-old woman complains of fatigue, right upper quadrant pain, and difficulty swallowing. Physical examination shows exudative tonsillitis, palatal petechiae, tender cervical lymphadenopathy, splenomegaly, and tender hepatomegaly. A complete blood cell count shows mild microcytic anemia, lymphocytic leukocytosis with ~20% of the lymphocytes having atypical features, and a mild thrombocytopenia. Which of the following laboratory findings is expected in this patient?

○ A. Low total iron-binding capacity
○ B. Normal serum ferritin
○ C. Normal serum transaminases
○ D. Positive hepatitis B surface antigen
○ E. Positive heterophile antibody test

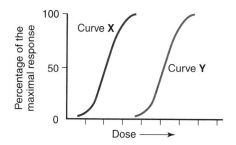

7. In the figure above, *curve X* and *curve Y* represent the dose-response curves when a drug is given under two different conditions. The figure most accurately reflects

○ A. analgesic effect of morphine given concurrently with naltrexone *(curve X)* or morphine given alone *(curve Y)*
○ B. antiparkinsonian effect of levodopa given concurrently with carbidopa *(curve X)* or levodopa given alone *(curve Y)*
○ C. chronotropic effect of isoproterenol given concurrently with metoprolol *(curve X)* or isoproterenol given alone *(curve Y)*
○ D. hypnotic effect of lorazepam given concurrently with flumazenil *(curve X)* or lorazepam given alone *(curve Y)*
○ E. sedative effect of diazepam given to an individual who is physically dependent on ethanol but is sober and drug-free at the time of taking the diazepam *(curve X)* or diazepam given to an individual who is not physically dependent on ethanol and is sober and drug-free at the time of taking the diazepam *(curve Y)*

8. A 45-year-old man complains of chronic back pain that radiates down into the leg. A CT scan shows a posterolateral rupture of the intervertebral disk between L3 and L4.

The pain and discomfort, particularly in the thigh, is caused by the hernial sac exerting pressure on which of the following spinal nerves?

○ A. Second lumbar (L2)
○ B. Third lumbar (L3)
○ C. Fourth lumbar (L4)
○ D. Fifth lumbar (L5)
○ E. First sacral (S1)

9. An otherwise healthy 85-year-old white woman has suffered from numerous ophthalmologic disorders, including macular degeneration, retinitis pigmentosa, glaucoma, cataracts, and corneal ulcers. Which cell type is affected in macular degeneration?

○ A. Cones
○ B. Endothelial cells (trabecular meshwork)
○ C. Keratocytes
○ D. Lens fibers
○ E. Rods

10. A 21-year-old woman begins suffering from chills, nausea, diarrhea, abdominal cramps, and intermittent emesis about 4 hours after eating a cheese sandwich that had been left at room temperature all morning. The manifestations resolve in about 24 hours without complications. The agent is presumed to be a gram-positive coccus that grows in clusters and produces numerous toxins. Which of the following toxins is most likely responsible for the disease manifestations?

○ A. Alpha toxin
○ B. Heat-labile enterotoxin
○ C. Heat-stable enterotoxin
○ D. Pyrogenic exotoxin
○ E. Toxic shock syndrome toxin 1 (TSST-1)

11. A 34-year-old man has polydipsia and polyuria. A 24-hour urine sample shows a volume of 7.8 L and osmolality of 135 mOsm/kg. His urine is negative for red blood cells, leukocytes, protein, and glucose. His blood pressure and heart rate are both normal. Which of the following is a likely cause of polyuria in this patient?

○ A. Acute attack of diabetes mellitus without glucosuria
○ B. Acute renal failure with a severe decrease in glomerular filtration rate (GFR)
○ C. Cerebrovascular accident damaging the anterior pituitary gland
○ D. Renal supersensitivity to the effects of antidiuretic hormone (ADH)
○ E. Suppression of ADH secretion due to polydipsia

12. A 72-year-old man complains of sudden onset of left flank pain and dizziness when he stands up quickly. When he is lying down, his blood pressure is 100/80 mm Hg, and his pulse is 110/min. When he is moved to a sitting position, his blood pressure is 80/60 mm Hg, and his pulse is 160/min. A pulsatile mass is palpated in the abdomen. The pathogenesis of the patient's flank pain and hypotension is most closely attributed to structural weakness of the aorta due to

○ A. genetic defect in collagen
○ B. genetic defect in fibrillin
○ C. immunocomplex-mediated disease
○ D. normal changes associated with aging
○ E. severe atherosclerosis

13. A 28-year-old woman is suffering from depression and is having trouble sleeping. The physician refers her to a sleep disorders clinic for evaluation. Which polysomnogram finding is most likely to be found on this patient's sleep electroencephalogram (EEG)?

○ A. Decreased awakenings
○ B. Decreased length of first period of rapid eye movement (REM) sleep
○ C. Increased period of REM latency
○ D. REM sleep onset
○ E. Reduced slow wave sleep of stages 3 and 4

14. An 8-year-old boy touches a hot stove and burns his hand. Blisters form when edema causes the separation of which of the following structures?

○ A. Epidermis and dermis
○ B. Hypodermis and deep fascia
○ C. Hypodermis and dermis
○ D. Papillary layer and reticular layer of the dermis
○ E. Stratum corneum and stratum granulosum

15. A 26-year-old woman was thrown into the windshield during an automobile accident and sustained a deep gash to her face, just lateral to her upper lip. The facial artery is severed, resulting in substantial arterial bleeding. At which point, apart from at the wound itself, might pressure be placed to stop the bleeding?

○ A. Internal carotid artery just inferior to the mandible
○ B. Medial angle of the eye
○ C. Midpoint of the neck just posterior to the sternocleidomastoid muscle
○ D. Skin overlying the mandible just anterior to the insertion of the masseter muscle
○ E. Temporal region just anterior and superior to the ear

16. A 55-year-old man experienced a headache, sore throat, and vomiting for 3 days before developing a stiff neck. He is admitted to the hospital and found to have a persistent fever and progressive paralysis of the lower limbs. Examination of a cerebrospinal fluid sample shows pleocytosis with normal glucose and protein levels. Bacterial and fungal cultures yield negative results, but a member of the family *Picornaviridae* is grown in cell culture. The patient says that 1 week before being admitted to the hospital, he had held his 2-month-old grandson and that the grandson had received his first round of childhood immunizations the day before. Which of the following viruses is the most likely cause of the patient's disease?

○ A. Mumps virus
○ B. Poliovirus
○ C. Rubella virus
○ D. Rubeola virus
○ E. Varicella-zoster virus

17. A 22-year-old woman who is about to undergo debridement of a large purulent decubitus ulcer receives local injections of a lidocaine formulation that contains epinephrine. The time to onset of the anesthetic effect is markedly prolonged, and the formulation is less effective than usual. These responses could best be explained by

○ A. decrease in hepatic cytochrome P450 metabolism of lidocaine
○ B. decrease in lipid solubility of lidocaine
○ C. increased fraction of lidocaine in the ionized form
○ D. rapid diffusion of lidocaine from the site of action
○ E. rapid hydrolysis of lidocaine by pseudocholinesterases

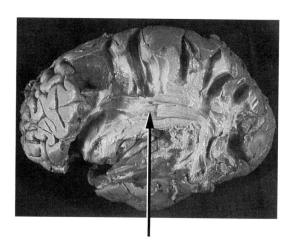

18. An 82-year-old man who is right-handed has a lesion in the area of the brain highlighted in the figure above. Which of the following findings is most likely to be reported in this patient's history?

○ A. Akinetopsia
○ B. Bitemporal hemianopia
○ C. Impaired repetition
○ D. Ipsilateral deafness
○ E. Nystagmus

19. A new test to detect breast cancer is administered to 500 patients. The results of the test are as follows:

Test Results	Patients with Breast Cancer	Patients without Breast Cancer
Positive	80	40
Negative	20	360

The specificity of the test is

○ A. 20%
○ B. 66.67%
○ C. 80%
○ D. 90%
○ E. 94.7%

20. A 69-year-old terminally ill man with liver failure receives a baboon liver transplant. After 1 week, he shows signs of rejection. This patient's rejection is most likely mediated by

- ○ A. action of complement and other serum mediators
- ○ B. action of neutrophils
- ○ C. combination of T lymphocytes and antibody-mediated mechanisms
- ○ D. preformed antibodies
- ○ E. T lymphocytes

21. Complete renal failure would most likely occur in which of the following conditions?

- ○ A. Arterial pressure is too low to produce renal blood flow
- ○ B. Circulating levels of antidiuretic hormone (ADH) are suppressed
- ○ C. Filtration fraction falls to 0%
- ○ D. Tubuloglomerular feedback is maximally stimulated
- ○ E. Water clearance is 0 mL/min

22. A 2-week-old girl is brought to the emergency department in a state of shock. Physical examination shows ambiguous genitalia and severe dehydration due to vomiting and diarrhea. Laboratory studies show hyperkalemia, hyponatremia, hypoglycemia, and acidosis. The most likely cause of these findings is a deficiency of

- ○ A. 11β-hydroxylase
- ○ B. 16α-hydroxylase
- ○ C. 17α-hydroxylase
- ○ D. 21α-hydroxylase
- ○ E. 3β-hydroxysteroid dehydrogenase

23. A 65-year-old man with symptoms of congestive heart failure (CHF) is taken to the emergency department. Appropriate therapy with a drug whose activity is increased with hypokalemia is initiated. The clinical efficacy of this drug in the management of CHF is attributed to

- ○ A. inhibition of Ca^{2+} reuptake into the sarcoplasmic reticulum
- ○ B. inhibition of cyclic adenosine monophosphate (cAMP) phosphodiesterases
- ○ C. inhibition of Na^+,K^+-ATPase
- ○ D. stimulation of β_1-adrenergic receptors
- ○ E. stimulation of phospholipase C

24. A 29-year-old Greek medical missionary, who recently returned to the United States after spending 3 months in Africa, is diagnosed with malaria due to *Plasmodium vivax*. After 4 days of therapy with primaquine, he develops a fever, chills, low back pain, and dark urine. A complete blood cell count shows his hemoglobin is 6 g/dL, leukocyte count is 15,000/mm^3, and platelet count is 450,000/mm^3. A corrected reticulocyte count is 12%. The peripheral smear shows polychromasia and numerous red blood cells (RBCs) that are missing parts of their membrane. Urine dipstick is positive for blood. Urine sediment is normal. Which of the following additional laboratory studies would most likely be reported for this patient?

- ○ A. Abnormal hemoglobin electrophoresis
- ○ B. Low mean corpuscular hemoglobin concentration (MCHC)
- ○ C. Low serum ferritin concentration
- ○ D. Positive direct Coombs' test
- ○ E. Positive Heinz body preparation

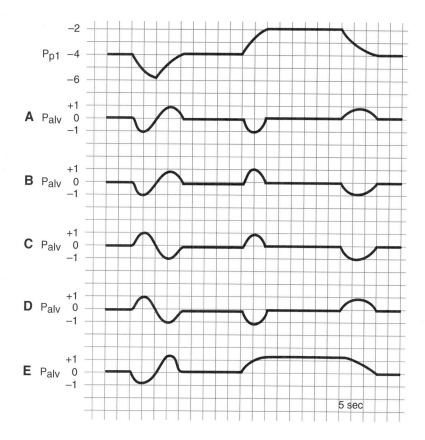

25. A 24-year-old woman with breathing difficulties is asked to swallow a balloon-tipped catheter to measure lung compliance. The catheter comes to a resting position within the thoracic esophagus, allowing the physician to estimate her intrapleural pressure. Which alveolar pressure tracing (P_{alv}) shown in the figure above properly matches the fluctuations in intrapleural pressure (P_{pl}) that were recorded in this patient? (All pressures are expressed in units of cm H_2O.)

○ A. Tracing A
○ B. Tracing B
○ C. Tracing C
○ D. Tracing D
○ E. Tracing E

26. A 65-year-old man who is right handed has had a stroke. Although his speech is fluid and melodic and he articulates well, he makes little sense and uses few meaningful words. He is unable to name common objects and does not seem to understand the physician's questions. He has diminished sensation in his right arm and hand. This patient's stroke has most likely affected which of the following arteries?

○ A. Anterior cerebral
○ B. Callosomarginal
○ C. Lenticulostriate
○ D. Middle cerebral
○ E. Posterior cerebral

27. While conducting a physical examination, a male physician has difficulty keeping an elderly female patient focused. The patient is talkative, discusses issues unrelated to the reason for the visit, and expresses her pleasure at having someone listen to her. The physician is ordinarily more assertive and redirects patients, but listens passively to her. Later, he recognizes that he behaved differently because this patient reminded him of his deceased grandmother. The physician's behavior is best explained by which of the following terms?

○ A. Codependency
○ B. Countertransference
○ C. Projection
○ D. Resistance
○ E. Transference

28. A 26-year-old man fell from a ladder and landed on his neck and shoulder. His arm now hangs at the side of his body, and he is unable to move the arm sideways away from the body (abduct). He notices weakness when he flexes the elbow. His forearm is pronated, with the palm of his hand directed posteriorly. He can move his fingers and oppose his thumb normally. Which of the following could account for these symptoms?

○ A. Dislocation of the shoulder causing injury to the axillary nerve
○ B. Injury to the C5–C6 contributions to the brachial plexus
○ C. Injury to the lower brachial plexus
○ D. Injury to the ulnar nerve
○ E. Lesion of the posterior cord of the brachial plexus

29. A 65-year-old man has a history of an elevated red blood cell (RBC) count, frequent headaches, and pruritus after bathing. He now complains of a sudden onset of abdominal pain and bloody diarrhea. Physical examination shows a pulse of 150/min, blood pressure of 80/50 mm Hg, abdominal distention, and absent bowel sounds. Test for occult blood in the stool is positive. Which of the following sets of laboratory data would most likely represent this patient's hematologic disorder?

	RBC Mass	Plasma Volume	SaO$_2$	EPO Concentration
○ A.	Increased	Increased	Normal	Decreased
○ B.	Increased	Normal	Decreased	Increased
○ C.	Increased	Normal	Normal	Increased
○ D.	Normal	Decreased	Normal	Normal

EPO, Erythropoietin; *SaO$_2$*, oxygen saturation.

30. A 26-year-old woman who is a close household contact of a child with active tuberculosis (TB) is given the purified protein derivative (PPD) test and found to have a positive result. The woman is prescribed an appropriate drug for TB prophylaxis. Because she has risk factors for a potential adverse effect of the prophylactic drug, she is also instructed to take pyridoxine (vitamin B$_6$). The adverse effect that would be minimized by concurrent pyridoxine therapy is

○ A. discoloration of body fluids
○ B. hepatotoxicity
○ C. optic neuritis
○ D. peripheral neuropathy
○ E. systemic lupus erythematosus (SLE)

31. A 19-year-old man who recently returned from a camping trip to North Carolina suddenly develops chills, a headache, myalgia, and fever. Four days later, he develops a petechial rash on his wrists and ankles. The rash rapidly spreads to the palms and soles and then becomes generalized. He says he remembers being bitten several times by ticks just before he returned home. A blood sample produces no growth on standard microbiologic media, but small gram-negative coccobacilli are grown in mammalian cell cultures inoculated with the blood. Which of the following organisms is the most likely cause of the disease?

○ A. *Borrelia burgdorferi*
○ B. *Borrelia recurrentis*
○ C. *Ehrlichia chaffeensis*
○ D. *Rickettsia rickettsii*
○ E. *Rickettsia typhi*

32. A 42-year-old woman with a history of asthma and nasal polyps begins therapy with aspirin. This patient at increased risk for which adverse effect associated with aspirin?

○ A. Gastric ulceration
○ B. Hypersensitivity to aspirin
○ C. Increased bleeding
○ D. Renal dysfunction
○ E. Reye's syndrome

33. A 1-year-old boy is admitted to the hospital and diagnosed with enteroviral meningitis. His medical records indicate that he has failed to thrive and has had severe and recurrent respiratory tract infections caused by extracellular and intracellular pathogens. Immune competence tests show defective cells. Despite intensive treatment, the boy dies of an intractable infection. The figure below depicts purine catabolism; enzymes are labeled with the letters A through E. The most likely underlying cause of the boy's medical problems is a deficiency of which enzyme?

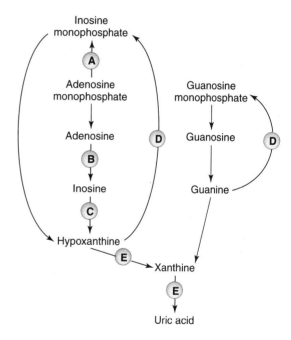

○ A. Enzyme A
○ B. Enzyme B
○ C. Enzyme C
○ D. Enzyme D
○ E. Enzyme E

34. A febrile 19-year-old African-American man with sickle cell disease develops pain in the right thigh. A radionuclide bone scan shows a lytic lesion with poorly defined borders in the metaphyseal area of the proximal right femur. The pathogenesis of the femoral bone lesion is most likely associated with which of the following conditions?

○ A. Aseptic necrosis related to ischemia
○ B. Metastatic cancer from an undetermined site
○ C. Osteomyelitis secondary to *Salmonella paratyphi* septicemia
○ D. Primary malignancy of bone

35. A 35-year-old woman with a history of progressive hearing loss and tinnitus in her left ear complains of frequent headaches that have increased in number and severity during the past 3 months. She has an ataxic gait and falls to the left. Which of the following is the most likely cause of her symptoms?

○ A. Acoustic neuroma
○ B. Acute lateral medullary syndrome
○ C. Demyelinating lesion in the basilar pons
○ D. Posterior communicating artery aneurysm
○ E. Weber syndrome

36. A 9-year-old girl whose dental x-rays show a significant loss of alveolar bone is presumed to have juvenile periodontitis. A complete blood cell count yields normal results. The child's disease may be associated with a defect in polymorphonuclear leukocyte (PMN) chemotaxis. In this patient, it would be helpful to check the level of which of the following components of the complement system?

○ A. C2b
○ B. C3a
○ C. C3b
○ D. C5a
○ E. C5b,6,7

37. A 53-year old black man with a history of type 2 diabetes mellitus has hypertension. Although his blood pressure is well controlled when he is treated with captopril, he is unable to tolerate a side effect of this drug. Captopril treatment is stopped, and losartan treatment is initiated.
When the patient's serum levels are subsequently checked, a decrease is most likely to be found in

○ A. aldosterone
○ B. angiotensin II
○ C. bradykinin
○ D. potassium
○ E. renin

38. While undergoing a routine examination, a lump is found in the testis of a 25-year-old man. Biopsy specimen confirms a diagnosis of carcinoma of the testis. Cells from this cancer would first spread via lymphatics to which of the following lymph nodes?

○ A. Deep inguinal
○ B. Horizontal group of superficial inguinal
○ C. Internal iliac
○ D. Lumbar (para-aortic)
○ E. Vertical group of superficial inguinal

39. Which of the following best describes the significance of the bicarbonate (HCO_3^-) buffer system?

○ A. HCO_3^- ions form irreversible complexes with free H^+ ions
○ B. It buffers more than 99% of the total H^+ concentration in the body
○ C. It is an open system that communicates with the environment through the lungs and kidneys
○ D. It is unlikely to be depleted of its acid (CO_2) or base (HCO_3^-) components
○ E. Its pK_a is very near arterial plasma pH

40. A 60-year-old man has pneumonia, characterized by a fever, chest pain, and a cough productive of blood-tinged sputum. A Gram stain of the sputum shows the presence of numerous neutrophils and gram-positive cocci occurring in pairs. Exudate obtained by transtracheal aspiration is cultured on blood agar and grows a predominance of mucoid colonies consisting of an organism morphologically similar to the organism observed in the Gram-stained sputum. The organism produces an oxygen-sensitive hemolysin, is encapsulated, and is sensitive to optochin. The cause of this patient's disease is also the most common cause of which of the following diseases in young children?

○ A. Croup
○ B. Meningitis
○ C. Otitis media
○ D. Pharyngitis
○ E. Pneumonia

41. A 42-year-old woman with AIDS complains of impaired vision in both eyes. Ophthalmoscopic examination shows perivascular hemorrhage and retinal scarring. Laboratory studies show a white blood cell count of $1300/mm^3$, with a differential of 26% neutrophils. Renal function is within normal limits. The patient's records indicate that she is seropositive for cytomegalovirus (CMV) and her last CD4+ count was 85 cells/mm^3. She has been unable to tolerate the hematologic manifestations of zidovudine or trimethoprim-sulfamethoxazole and is currently taking lamivudine, zalcitabine, indinavir, and atovaquone. Which drug would be preferred for the management of this patient's ophthalmologic problems?

○ A. Acyclovir
○ B. Amantadine
○ C. Foscarnet
○ D. Ganciclovir
○ E. Pentamidine

42. A 20-year-old man complains of progressive muscle weakness. Neurologic studies show a neuromuscular conduction defect, and diagnostic studies with an intravenous injection of edrophonium are found to rapidly increase his muscle strength. When the patient is treated with neostigmine, his status improves. The most probable target molecule in this treatment is

○ A. acetylcholinesterase
○ B. choline acetyltransferase
○ C. monoamine oxidase
○ D. muscarinic acetylcholine receptor
○ E. nicotinic acetylcholine receptor

43. A 45-year-old woman has a fever, joint and muscle pain, several suppurating cutaneous nodules on her hands, a productive cough, and pulmonary densities (noncalcified suppurating granulomas). A sputum sample cultured at room temperature grows a filamentous fungus that produces smooth-walled microconidia and macroconidia. The fungus is cultured at 37° C and grows a thick-walled yeast with broad-based buds. Which of the following fungi is the most likely cause of the disease?

○ A. *Blastomyces dermatitidis*
○ B. *Coccidioides immitis*
○ C. *Histoplasma capsulatum*
○ D. *Paracoccidioides brasiliensis*
○ E. *Sporothrix schenckii*

44. A 28-year-old woman with Hodgkin's disease was always driven to her chemotherapy treatments by a friend. Several months later when the friend picks her up for a social outing, the woman becomes nauseated when she gets into the car. Based on the principles of classical conditioning, the car now represents which of the following?

○ A. Conditioned response
○ B. Conditioned stimulus
○ C. Negative reinforcer
○ D. Unconditioned response
○ E. Unconditioned stimulus

45. A neonate is transferred to an intensive care unit because of neurologic abnormalities. Blood studies show a 3-fold increase in glutamine, no detectable citrulline, and a 2-fold decrease in arginine. Hyperammonemia is present, although the blood urea nitrogen (BUN) level is below the normal range. Urine tests show a 100-fold increase in orotic acid. The disease is most likely due to a deficiency of

○ A. arginase
○ B. argininosuccinate lyase
○ C. argininosuccinate synthase
○ D. carbamoyl phosphate synthetase I (CPSI)
○ E. ornithine carbamoyltransferase

46. A 54-year-old man has been taking hydrochlorothiazide for the management of hypertension and cisapride for gastroesophageal reflux disease (GERD). When diagnosed with pneumococcal pneumonia, he begins treatment with an antimicrobial drug. Five days later, he becomes so dizzy that his wife takes him directly to the emergency department, where an ECG is immediately performed. The figure below compares the normal ECG pattern with the P-QRS-T pattern seen on the patient's ECG:

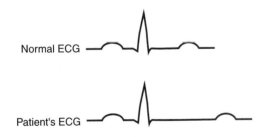

The patient loses consciousness while the ECG is being completed, and the ECG displays a polymorphic ventricular tachycardia. Antimicrobial therapy with which of the following drugs could cause the patient's dizziness and cardiac problem?

○ A. Erythromycin
○ B. Ketoconazole
○ C. Penicillin V
○ D. Rifampin
○ E. Streptomycin

47. A normotensive 49-year-old woman complains of fatigue, weight loss, and a dragging sensation in her right upper quadrant. She mentions that she works in a factory where she is exposed to benzene. Physical examination shows generalized, nontender lymphadenopathy and massive hepatosplenomegaly. Laboratory studies show her hemoglobin is 6.4 g/dL, leukocyte count is 130,000/mm^3, and platelet count is 90,000/mm^3. The peripheral smear shows neutrophils at various stages of development, including myeloblasts (1%), mature and immature eosinophils, basophils, and numerous myelocytes, bands, and segmented neutrophils. A bone marrow examination shows hypercellular marrow with a differential count similar to that observed in the peripheral blood. Which of the following additional laboratory findings is most likely in this patient?

○ A. Auer rods in myeloblasts
○ B. High leukocyte alkaline phosphatase score
○ C. Myeloblasts positive for CD_{10} antigen
○ D. Positive Philadelphia chromosome study
○ E. Positive tartrate-resistant acid phosphatase stain

48. A 20-year-old man displays no fear, rage, or aggression when provoked. He is hypersexual. He examines all objects with his hands and mouth and has visual agnosia. Which of the following conditions is the most likely cause of these findings?

○ A. Dandy-Walker syndrome
○ B. Jacksonian seizures
○ C. Kallmann syndrome
○ D. Klüver-Bucy syndrome
○ E. Tumor in the cingulate gyrus

49. Investigators studying the physiologic role of two low-abundance proteins in mammalian cells begin by overexpressing the two proteins in mammalian cells. The cDNAs of the two proteins are inserted into two mammalian expression vectors (plasmids), and these constructs are used to transfect human fibroblasts in tissue culture. After 48 hours, cells are collected and lysed. Which of the following techniques would be used to confirm that the transfections worked and that the proteins were produced?

○ A. DNA sequencing
○ B. Restriction mapping
○ C. Southern blot technique
○ D. Southwestern blot technique
○ E. Western blot technique

50. A febrile 22-year-old woman complains of crampy right upper quadrant pain. Physical examination shows scleral icterus, right upper quadrant tenderness to palpation, and mild splenomegaly. Laboratory studies show:

Leukocyte count	18,000/mm^3
Hemoglobin	9.5 g/dL
Reticulocyte count, corrected	6%
Mean corpuscular volume (MCV)	81 μm^3
Mean corpuscular hemoglobin concentration (MCHC)	38% Hgb/cell
Bilirubin, total//direct	3.6 mg/dL// 0.3 mg/dL
Serum alanine aminotransferase (ALT)	20 U/L

Many of the red blood cells (RBCs) in the peripheral blood lack central areas of pallor. An ultrasound shows numerous stones in the gallbladder. The patient states that there is a family history of gallbladder disease and anemia at an early age. Which of the following additional studies is most likely to be reported for this patient?

○ A. Abnormal hemoglobin electrophoresis
○ B. Increased RBC osmotic fragility
○ C. Low serum ferritin concentration
○ D. Positive direct Coombs' test
○ E. Positive Heinz body preparation

ANSWERS AND DISCUSSIONS

1. **E** (weight loss syndrome) is correct. When the body fat of a female is less than 15% of normal for her size and weight, hypothalamic secretion of gonadotropin-releasing hormone (GnRH) decreases. This results in decreased stimulation of anterior pituitary release of the gonadotropins FSH and LH. Loss of gonadotropins results in insufficient synthesis of estrogen by the ovaries, with subsequent development of amenorrhea. Amenorrhea may be secondary to disorders involving the hypothalamic/pituitary axis in producing gonadotropins, the ovaries in synthesizing estrogen, or anatomic defects (end-organ disease) that prevent the normal egress of blood out of the vagina (e.g., cervical stenosis, imperforate hymen). A progesterone challenge is an excellent test used to evaluate the cause of amenorrhea once pregnancy is ruled out. Withdrawal bleeding, when progesterone levels decrease, indicates adequate estrogen stimulation of the endometrial mucosa and absence of end-organ disease. Absence of withdrawal bleeding can indicate inadequate levels of estrogen or an end-organ problem. Measuring the levels of serum gonadotropins can help determine which of the three areas is responsible. In hypothalamic-pituitary axis disorders, gonadotropin levels are decreased; in ovarian disorders, gonadotropin levels are increased (loss of the estrogen and progesterone negative feedback on FSH and LH, respectively); and in end-organ disease, gonadotropin levels are normal. This patient's gonadotropin levels are decreased, indicating that the cause of this patient's amenorrhea lies in the hypothalamic-pituitary axis (i.e., excessive weight loss). An important clinical point to remember about weight loss syndromes, including anorexia nervosa, is that there is danger of osteoporosis related to the long-term loss of estrogen and its effect on maintaining normal bone density.

A (acromegaly) is incorrect. The increase in growth hormone is related to the stress of weight loss. This patient has none of the classic findings of acromegaly (e.g., prominent jaw, enlarged hands and feet).
B (Cushing's syndrome) is incorrect. The physical examination shows none of the classic findings of Cushing's syndrome (e.g., truncal obesity). Like growth hormone, cortisol is also a stress hormone that is increased in weight loss syndromes.
C (hypopituitarism) is incorrect. Levels of cortisol and growth hormone are increased and serum TSH is normal in hypopituitarism.
D (primary ovarian disease) is incorrect. Gonadotropin levels are low.

2. **B** (after integration into the host chromosome) is correct. The clinical and laboratory findings are consistent with the diagnosis of AIDS, a disease caused by the human immunodeficiency virus (HIV). Like other retroviruses, HIV replicates its genome after it has incorporated itself into the host genome. Once integrated, it is called a provirus. Viral RNA is transcribed in the cytoplasm, and the virus buds from the host cytoplasmic membrane.

A (after enclosure in a new viral capsid) is incorrect. Hepatitis B virus, but not HIV, continues genome synthesis after being enclosed in a new viral capsid.
C (freely within the host nucleus) is incorrect. Although HIV does not replicate its genome freely within the host nucleus, many other viruses do. These viruses include herpesviruses and most other DNA viruses.
D (in the cytoplasm of host cells) is incorrect. HIV does not replicate in the cytoplasm, but most RNA viruses do.
E (in the endoplasmic reticulum of host cells) is incorrect. Viruses are not known to replicate in the endoplasmic reticulum.

3. **D** (ophthalmic division of the left trigeminal nerve) is correct. The ophthalmic division is one of three divisions of the trigeminal nerve (CN V), the others being the maxillary and mandibular divisions. The ophthalmic division serves the skin around the eye, as well as the nasal area and cornea. The cornea has only pain afferents. Thus, damage to the ophthalmic division of CN V could be responsible for the patient's symptoms.

A (left frontal lobe) is incorrect. The perception of pain (or its loss) is a function of the somatosensory cortex, which is located in the parietal lobe, not the frontal lobe.
B (left motor nucleus of the trigeminal nerve) is incorrect. The motor nucleus of CN V innervates the muscles of mastication. Damage to this nerve would result in a "frozen jaw" (as seen in tetanus), not the symptoms reported for this patient.
C (left ventral posterolateral nucleus of the thalamus) is incorrect. The VPL nucleus of the thalamus receives pain sensations from the body, not from the face.
E (right nucleus of CN V) is incorrect. Although the right spinal nucleus of CN V carries pain sensations, damage affecting the entire nucleus would block the sensation of pain from the entire face, not just the portion served by the ophthalmic division of this nerve. Additionally, pain afferents from the left side of the face would synapse in the left spinal nucleus of CN V, not the right.

4. *A* (arteriosclerotic narrowing of a renal artery) is correct. Sudden onset of hypertension in an asymptomatic elderly person suggests renal vascular hypertension. The abdominal bruit is consistent with a renal arterial lesion, which can cause renovascular hypertension.

B (benign aldosterone-secreting tumor) is incorrect. Primary aldosteronism leads to hyperkalemia and metabolic alkalosis with changes in serum electrolytes.
C (coarctation of the aorta) is incorrect. Patients with coarctation of the aorta have reduced blood pressure below the coarctation (i.e., blood pressure is lower in the legs than in the arms).
D (essential hypertension) is incorrect. The onset of essential hypertension ordinarily occurs earlier in life and does not explain the abdominal bruit.
E (increased aortic compliance due to normal aging) is incorrect. Aortic compliance decreases with aging, leading to systolic hypertension with little or no elevation in diastolic pressure.

5. *E* (language is seriously impaired and warrants further evaluation) is correct. This child's language skills are consistent with a two-word message stage often seen in children between the ages of 12 and 24 months. She can respond to simple directions, follow action commands, understand pronouns, use two-word utterances, imitate sounds, refer to herself by name, and appears to know about 100 words. Further evaluation is clearly indicated since this child does not exhibit higher order language skills expected of a 4-year-old.

A (expressive skills are intact but receptive language is impaired) and B (receptive language is intact but expressive skills are impaired) are incorrect. Receptive language refers to an ability to comprehend language, whereas expressive language refers to an ability to speak language. Impairment is present in both domains.
C (language is progressing as expected) is incorrect. By age 4, children are typically in the grammar development stage and are able to understand and use many words. This girl should be able to understand prepositions, cause and effect, and analogies. She should also be able to rhyme and speak intelligibly more than 90% of the time.
D (language is within 1 year of her expected level) is incorrect. Even children between the ages of 2 and 3 years have more highly developed language skills than this child. For example, children 2 to 3 years of age understand body parts, family names, sizes, functions, and most adjectives. They also express themselves through the use of sentences with nouns and verbs, converse with other children in a simplified fashion, and typically know approximately 270 words at age 2, and up to 895 words at age 3.

6. *E* (positive heterophile antibody test) is correct. The patient most likely has infectious mononucleosis (IM), which is caused by the Epstein-Barr virus (EBV). The virus infects B cells ini-

tially by attaching to CD_{21} receptors on the cell surface. Circulating T lymphocytes interact with the infected B cells and become antigenically stimulated, resulting in atypical lymphocytosis. The key screening test for IM is the Monospot test, which detects heterophile antibodies in the patient's serum. Heterophile antibodies unique to IM are IgM antibodies directed against horse red blood cells (RBCs). An agglutination reaction against horse RBCs is the basis for a positive Monospot test.

A   (low total iron-binding capacity) is incorrect. In young women, iron deficiency anemia secondary to menorrhagia is the most common cause of microcytic anemia. Hence, the total iron-binding capacity should be increased due to increased synthesis of transferrin (binding protein for iron) by the liver whenever iron stores in the bone marrow are decreased.
B   (normal serum ferritin) is incorrect. The patient most likely has iron deficiency anemia and a low serum ferritin level. Serum ferritin reflects the amount of iron stored in macrophages in the bone marrow.
C   (normal serum transaminases) is incorrect. IM produces an anicteric viral hepatitis. The primary enzymes that are elevated in diffuse liver cell necrosis are serum transaminases, aspartate aminotransferase (AST), and alanine aminotransferase (ALT).
D   (positive hepatitis B surface antigen) is incorrect. The clinical history and physical findings are more compatible with IM-induced hepatitis than hepatitis due to the hepatitis B virus.

7. **B**   (antiparkinsonian effect of levodopa given concurrently with carbidopa *[curve X]* or levodopa given alone *[curve Y]*) is correct. Carbidopa is a drug that inhibits aromatic amino acid decarboxylase (dopa decarboxylase) and prevents the conversion of levodopa to dopamine in peripheral tissue but not in the brain. This action increases the apparent potency of levodopa, thereby causing a parallel shift to the left in the dose-response curve. By decreasing the peripheral formation of dopamine, carbidopa also minimizes nausea, vomiting, and arrhythmias, which are associated with the use of levodopa and are due to the stimulation of dopamine receptors by dopamine in the chemoreceptor trigger zone (CTZ) and by β_1-adrenergic receptors in the heart.

A   (analgesic effect of morphine given concurrently with naltrexone *[curve X]* or morphine given alone *[curve Y]*) is incorrect. Naltrexone is a competitive inhibitor of morphine at the opium mu (μ) receptor. All competitive inhibitors cause a parallel shift to the right in the dose-response curve.
C   (chronotropic effect of isoproterenol given concurrently with metoprolol *[curve X]* or isoproterenol given alone *[curve Y]*) is incorrect. Metoprolol is a competitive inhibitor of isoproterenol and other β_1-adrenergic receptor agonists. All competitive inhibitors cause a parallel shift to the right in the dose-response curve.

D (hypnotic effect of lorazepam given concurrently with fluma-zenil *[curve X]* or lorazepam given alone *[curve Y]*) is incorrect. Flumazenil is a competitive inhibitor of lorazepam at the benzodi-azepine BZ_1 and BZ_2 receptors. All competitive inhibitors cause a parallel shift to the right in the dose-response curve.

E (sedative effect of diazepam given to an individual who is physically dependent on ethanol but is sober and drug-free at the time of taking the diazepam *[curve X]* or diazepam given to an individual who is not physically dependent on ethanol and is so-ber and drug-free at the time of taking the diazepam *[curve Y]*) is incorrect. An individual who is physically dependent on etha-nol will exhibit tolerance to the effects of ethanol. There is cross-tolerance between benzodiazepines (such as diazepam) and ethanol. Thus, the alcoholic, when sober, would be less sensitive to a given dose of a benzodiazepine. Drug tolerance causes a paral-lel shift to the right in the dose-response curve, reflecting a de-crease in apparent potency.

8. **B** (third lumbar) is correct. The third lumbar spinal nerve (L3) exits the vertebral canal via the intervertebral foramen between the third and fourth lumbar vertebrae. (Spinal nerves exit the vertebral canal inferior to their named vertebrae, except for cervical spinal nerves, which exit through the intervertebral fo-ramina superior to their named vertebrae.) Therefore, a pos-terolateral herniation exerts pressure on L3 as the third spinal nerve exits through the intervertebral foramen.

Intervertebral disks consist of a rim of fibrocartilage, the anu-lus fibrosis, which surrounds a gelatinous center, the nucleus pulposis. The anulus fibrosis is reinforced by two sets of longitu-dinal ligaments. The anterior longitudinal ligament, which runs the length of the vertebral column anterior to the vertebral bodies and associated intervertebral disks, is a strong, broad liga-ment that seldom, if ever, permits anterior herniation of the nucleus pulposis. The posterior longitudinal ligament, which is situated against the posterior aspect of the vertebral bodies within the vertebral canal, also runs the length of the vertebral column. Although this ligament becomes wider at the interverte-bral disks, it is narrow and not very strong. Herniations of the intervertebral disks typically occur lateral to the posterior longi-tudinal ligament, but they also may occur through the ligament.

A (second lumbar) is incorrect. Lumbar spinal nerves exit infe-rior to their named vertebrae; accordingly, the second lumbar spi-nal nerve (L2) exits the vertebral canal through the intervertebral foramen between L2 and L3. Therefore, L2 would have exited the vertebral canal superior to the herniation.

C (fourth lumbar) is incorrect. The fourth lumbar spinal nerve (L4) exits the vertebral canal between the fourth and fifth lumbar vertebrae. If the hernial sac were situated more medially, it might put pressure on the cauda equina. In that case, the nerve roots most likely to be involved would be those that contribute to L4, since these are next in line to exit the vertebral canal and the most laterally situated. Posterolateral herniation is more common.

D   (fifth lumbar) is incorrect. The fifth lumbar spinal nerve (L5) should not be compromised by the herniation. If the hernial sac were situated more medially, it might put pressure on the cauda equina. In that case, the nerve roots most likely to be involved would be those that contribute to L5, since these are next in line to exit the vertebral canal and the most laterally situated. Posterolateral herniation is more common.

E   (first sacral) is incorrect. More medial herniations below the second lumbar vertebra can involve the cauda equina, which gives rise to the first sacral spinal nerve (S1). The posterolateral herniation is lateral to the cauda equina, but if the cauda equina should become affected, L4 would most likely be involved.

9. *A*   (cones) is correct. Macular degeneration refers to changes in the macula lutea. Many cone cells are found in the middle zone of the macula (the fovea centralis); color vision is adversely affected in patients with macular degeneration. It is without sex predilection and occurs more often in whites than in blacks. Age-related macular degeneration may be hereditary; an association appears to exist between smoking and age-related macular degeneration.

B   (endothelial cells) is incorrect. Endothelial cells are the major cell type affected in glaucoma, not in macular degeneration. The sinuses of the trabecular meshwork are lined with endothelial cells, which export aqueous humor to the canal of Schlemm. In patients with glaucoma, aqueous humor accumulates in the anterior and posterior chambers of the eye and causes an increase in the intraocular pressure.

C   (keratocytes) is incorrect. Keratocytes are the major cell type affected in corneal ulcers, not in macular degeneration. Keratocytes are special fibrocytes that maintain the structural integrity of the cornea. Corneal ulceration (usually due to infections) leads to the localized destruction of keratocytes.

D   (lens fibers) is incorrect. Lens fibers are the major cell type affected in cataracts, not in macular degeneration. Cataracts are cloudy spots in the lens. The spots result in part from excessive cross-linking of proteins in lens fibers.

E   (rods) is incorrect. Rods are the major cell type affected in retinitis pigmentosa, not in macular degeneration. Because rods are affected, defective night vision is one of the most common and earliest complaints of patients who suffer from retinitis pigmentosa.

10. *C*   (heat-stable enterotoxin) is correct. The manifestations described are consistent with the diagnosis of staphylococcal food poisoning. *Staphylococcus aureus* produces several enterotoxins that are heat-stable (resistant to heating at 100° C for 30 minutes). Consumption of enterotoxin-contaminated food results in the abrupt onset of symptoms, generally without a fever.

A (alpha toxin) and E (toxic shock syndrome toxin 1) are incorrect. *S. aureus* produces alpha toxin and TSST-1. Alpha toxin is cytotoxic for many cell types, but it is not responsible for the gastrointestinal and other manifestations described. TSST-1 is responsible for toxic shock syndrome but not for food poisoning.

B (heat-labile enterotoxin) is incorrect. *S. aureus* and other cocci do not produce heat-labile enterotoxins.

D (pyrogenic exotoxin) is incorrect. *S. aureus* does not produce pyrogenic exotoxins. *Streptococcus* species produce pyrogenic exotoxins, but streptococci do not cause food poisoning.

11. *E* (suppression of ADH secretion due to polydipsia) is correct. Extreme polydipsia causes complete suppression of ADH secretion and extreme polyuria, evidenced by a urine volume of 7.8 L in 24 hours.

A (acute attack of diabetes mellitus without glucosuria) is incorrect. The polyuria associated with diabetes mellitus is caused by glucosuria.

B (acute renal failure with a severe decrease in glomerular filtration rate) is incorrect. A severe decrease in GFR is likely to decrease urine flow.

C (cerebrovascular accident damaging the anterior pituitary gland) is incorrect. Damage to the anterior pituitary does not cause a major change in water metabolism; the posterior pituitary secretes ADH.

D (renal supersensitivity to the effects of antidiuretic hormone) is incorrect. Increased sensitivity to the effects of ADH decreases urine flow and elevates urine osmolality above normal levels.

12. *E* (severe atherosclerosis) is correct. The patient has the classic triad of a ruptured abdominal aortic aneurysm: sudden onset of left flank pain, hypotension, and a pulsatile abdominal mass. Atherosclerotic damage of the abdominal aorta weakens the vessel wall, leading to outpouching of the aorta and the potential for rupture as the expansion increases wall stress.

A (genetic defect in collagen) is incorrect. Ehlers-Danlos syndrome has multiple inheritance patterns and is characterized by defects in synthesis and structure of collagen. Clinical abnormalities include hyperextensibility, vascular instability, and a predisposition for dissecting aortic aneurysms, the most common cause of death in these patients. Dissecting aortic aneurysms usually are associated with a sudden onset of chest pain radiating into the back. Those extending distally are less likely to rupture than those extending proximally. This patient does not have Ehlers-Danlos syndrome.

B (genetic defect in fibrillin) is incorrect. Marfan's syndrome has an autosomal dominant inheritance and is associated with a defect on chromosome 15 involving the synthesis of a fibrillin component in elastic tissue. Eunuchoid proportions, lens dislocation, arachnodactyly, mitral valve prolapse, and a propensity for dissecting aortic aneurysms are common in these patients. Elastic tissue fragmentation and cystic medial necrosis occur in the wall of the aorta, leading to structural weakness of the vessel. An intimal tear allows blood to dissect through the weak areas. As discussed in A, the clinical findings in this patient do not support the diagnosis of a dissecting aortic aneurysm.

C (immunocomplex-mediated disease) is incorrect. Immunocomplex types of vasculitis are more often associated with small vessel vasculitis involving venules, arterioles, or with capillaries and vasculitis involving muscular arteries (e.g., coronary arteries) rather than elastic arteries such as the aorta.

D (normal changes associated with aging) is incorrect. The aorta is not structurally weakened in older age; it becomes less distensible, but is not prone to rupture.

13. *E* (reduced slow wave sleep of stages 3 and 4) is correct. Abnormalities in delta sleep, or deep sleep, are common in individuals with depression. Delta sleep begins in sleep stage 3, and by sleep stage 4 delta waves make up more than 50% of the EEG recording. This disturbance in delta sleep may not allow a depressed individual ample opportunity to physically restore the body.

A (decreased awakenings) is incorrect. In depression, multiple awakenings are common.

B (decreased length of first period of rapid eye movement sleep) is incorrect. The first REM period for patients with depression is often longer than for individuals who are not suffering from depression.

C (increased period of REM latency) is incorrect. Patients with depression have shown a shortened (not increased) period of REM latency. REM latency is the elapsed time between onset of sleep and the first REM sleep.

D (REM sleep onset) is incorrect. Initial and terminal insomnia are common symptoms of depression and are included as vegetative signs of the disorder. It is rare for a depressed person to fall asleep easily, although many patients with depression show both hyposomnia and hypersomnia.

14. *A* (epidermis and dermis) is correct. Blister formation occurs in second-degree burns. Blisters are the result of damage to small blood vessels (venules) in the papillary layer of the dermis. When the damaged vessels leak, fluid moves through their walls and flows into the surrounding connective tissue proper. Pressure caused by the increased fluid in the connective tissue proper ruptures hemidesmosomes that attach cells in the stratum basale to the subjacent papillary layer of the dermis. Once this occurs, excess fluid separates the epidermis from the dermis and causes a blister to form.

B (hypodermis and deep fascia) and C (hypodermis and dermis) are incorrect. The junction between the hypodermis and deep fascia and the junction between the hypodermis and dermis are deep. They would not be affected until many other more superficial tissues are severely damaged.

D (papillary layer and reticular layer of the dermis) is incorrect. Because of the absence of physical barriers at the junction between the papillary layer and the reticular layer of the dermis, fluid formation would not create pockets (blisters). Instead, the entire area would swell.

E (stratum corneum and stratum granulosum) is incorrect. Edema is dependent on vasculature. There is no vasculature in any portion of the epidermis, including the stratum corneum and stratum granulosum.

15. *D* (skin overlying the mandible just anterior to the insertion of the masseter muscle) is correct. The arterial pulse in the facial artery can be palpated just anterior to the insertion of the masseter muscle onto the angle and body of the mandible. Pressure at this point substantially reduces the flow of blood from the facial artery to the face. The facial artery, which arises at the tip of the greater horn of the hyoid bone as the third anterior branch of the external carotid artery, courses superiorly deep to the posterior digastric and stylohyoid muscles. It enters the face by ascending over the lateral surface of the body of the mandible.

A (internal carotid artery just inferior to the mandible) is incorrect. The common carotid artery bifurcates into external and internal carotid arteries at about the level of the upper border of the thyroid cartilage; the external branch is situated anteriorly, and the internal branch is situated posteriorly. The facial artery is a branch of the external carotid artery. There are no named branches of the internal carotid artery in the region of the injury near the upper lip.

B (medial angle of the eye) is incorrect. The facial artery angles across the face and courses toward the medial corner (angle) of the eye, giving rise to inferior and superior labial arteries along its course. Beside the nose, it becomes the angular artery after giving rise to the lateral nasal artery. Because the facial artery has been severed proximal to the angular artery, pressure at the corner of the eye would have little effect on the bleeding.

C (midpoint of the neck just posterior to the sternocleidomastoid muscle) is incorrect. The only way to stop the bleeding in the neck would involve putting pressure on the common carotid artery, which courses within the carotid sheath deep to the sternocleidomastoid muscle at this level. However, application of pressure posterior to the sternocleidomastoid would have no effect on the common carotid artery. The external jugular vein crosses the superficial surface of the sternocleidomastoid muscle to enter the posterior triangle of the neck at this point and would be susceptible to compression, but it would not slow the bleeding of the facial artery.

E (temporal region just anterior and superior to the ear) is incorrect. A pulse may be felt in the temporal region just anterior to the ear in the superficial temporal artery, one of the two terminal branches of the external carotid artery. Its purpose is to supply blood to the temporal region of the head and to the scalp. The superficial temporal artery gives rise to a transverse facial artery, which crosses the masseter muscle just superior to the parotid duct. It neither gives rise to the facial artery nor reaches the mouth.

16. *B* (poliovirus) is correct. The clinical, epidemiologic, and laboratory findings in this case are consistent with the diagnosis of paralytic poliomyelitis acquired via fecal-oral transmission of the poliovirus contained in the live oral vaccine. Although vaccine-acquired poliomyelitis is rare in the United States, it is now the most common form of poliomyelitis. Those at greatest risk are nonimmune individuals. The new polio vaccination schedule, which involves administering the inactivated polio vaccine for the first two doses, may help eliminate vaccine-acquired poliomyelitis.

A (mumps virus) and E (varicella-zoster virus) are incorrect. Mumps virus and varicella-zoster virus (VZV) can cause serious central nervous system manifestations. However, mumps virus is a member of the family *Paramyxoviridae,* while VZV is a member of the family *Herpesviridae.*

C (rubella virus) and D (rubeola virus) are incorrect. Rubella virus, the etiologic agent of rubella (German measles), is a member of the family *Togaviridae.* Rubeola virus, the etiologic agent of measles, is a member of the family *Paramyxoviridae.*

17. *C* (increased fraction of lidocaine in the ionized form) is correct. Local anesthetics are weak bases that act in their ionized form to block the Na^+ channel by binding to an intracellular site adjacent to the channel. In the presence of an acidic environment (e.g., in the presence of pus), a larger fraction of the drug would be in the ionized form and, as such, could not traverse the membrane. Consequently, there would be a longer time to onset and a reduced efficacy.

A (decrease in hepatic cytochrome P450 metabolism of lidocaine) is incorrect. In this patient, lidocaine was given by local injection (infiltration). Its metabolism by microsomal enzymes would have no impact on its time to onset. However, in patients with hepatic disease, the use of an amide-linked local anesthetic (such as lidocaine) is associated with an increased risk of systemic toxicity.

B (decrease in lipid solubility of lidocaine) is incorrect. It is not possible to change the lipid solubility of a drug.

D (rapid diffusion of lidocaine from the site of action) is incorrect. The rate of diffusion of a local anesthetic has an effect on the anesthetic's duration of action and its potential to cause systemic toxicity. To prolong its duration of action and reduce its toxicity, a local anesthetic is administered with a sympathomimetic drug that has α_1-agonist activity, such as epinephrine or phenylephrine.

E (rapid hydrolysis of lidocaine by pseudocholinesterases) is incorrect. There are two groups of local anesthetics. The amide-linked group includes bupivacaine, etidocaine, lidocaine, mepivacaine, and prilocaine (all drugs with the letter "i" in the syllables before "caine"). The ester-linked group includes benzocaine, chloroprocaine, cocaine, and procaine. Amide-linked local anesthetics are metabolized by the liver. Ester-linked local anesthetics are hydrolyzed by pseudocholinesterases. The hydrolysis yields *p*-aminobenzoic acid (PABA), the agent responsible for hypersensitivity reactions to ester-linked anesthetics.

18. *C* (impaired repetition) is correct. The highlighted area in the figure is the arcuate fasciculus. A lesion in this structure can lead to conduction aphasia, because it would disconnect Broca's area from Wernicke's area. The resulting aphasia would be characterized by an impaired ability to repeat what others have said.

A (akinetopsia) is incorrect. There is no mention here of the patient being unable to see moving objects.

B (bitemporal hemianopia) is incorrect. Bitemporal hemianopia is the inability to see in the temporal half of the visual field of one eye. It is caused by damage to the ipsilateral optic tract. The lesion in this figure does not appear in that structure.

D (ipsilateral deafness) is incorrect. Ipsilateral deafness can occur as a result of a lesion within the cochlear division of the vestibulocochlear nerve (CN VIII) somewhere between the cochlea and the cochlear nucleus in the brain stem. (After that point, axons carrying information about sound may or may not decussate so that information from both ears is found at, or above, the superior olive level.) These structures do not appear in this illustration.

E (nystagmus) is incorrect. The rapid back-and-forth movement of the eyes that characterizes nystagmus is caused by a lesion in the brain stem or cerebellum. The lesion highlighted in this figure is the arcuate fasciculus, which is in the cerebral cortex, not in the brain stem.

19. *D* (90%) is correct. Specificity is the accuracy of a test identifying healthy individuals. Specificity equals true negatives (360) divided by the sum of true negatives (360) and false positives (40), or in this case, 90% of the 500 patients who were tested.

A (20%) is incorrect. The prevalence of breast cancer in this population of 500 patients is 20% (i.e., 100 breast cancer patients divided by 500 total patients).

B   (66.67%) is incorrect. A positive predictive value in this example is the probability that a positive test actually means that an individual has breast cancer. The value is obtained by dividing true positives (80) by the sum of true positives (80) and false positives (40), which in this case equals 66.67%.
C   (80%) is incorrect. The test's sensitivity (ability to identify individuals with breast cancer) is 80%. Dividing true positives (80) by the sum of true positives (80) and false negatives (20) yields the test's sensitivity.
E   (94.7%) is incorrect. Negative predictive value in this example is the probability that a negative test actually means that an individual does not have breast cancer. The value is obtained by dividing true negatives (360) by the sum of true negatives (360) and false negatives (20), which in this case equals 94.7%.

20. *E*   (T lymphocytes) is correct. Transplants can be categorized as xenografts (from different species), allografts (from unrelated members of the same species), isografts (from an identical twin), and autografts (from a different part of the same person). Organ rejections can be categorized as hyperacute (occurring immediately after transplantation), acute (occurring 1–3 weeks after transplantation), and chronic (occurring months or years after transplantation). In this case, the patient's transplant is a xenograft, and he is suffering from acute rejection. Acute rejections are mediated by activation of T lymphocytes.

A   (action of complement and other serum mediators), B (action of neutrophils), and D (preformed antibodies) are incorrect. As discussed above, the patient is suffering from acute rejection. Only hyperacute rejections are mediated by the action of complement and other serum mediators, neutrophils, and preformed antibodies.
C   (combination of T lymphocytes and antibody-mediated mechanisms) is incorrect. The patient is suffering from acute rejection. Only chronic rejections are mediated by a combination of T lymphocytes and antibody-mediated mechanisms.

21. *C*   (filtration fraction falls to 0%) is correct. Complete renal failure can occur as a result of complete blockade of the ureters (e.g., by kidney stones) or renal tubules (by debris). Complete blocks are extremely rare, however. Renal failure is more likely to result from poor renal perfusion due to hypovolemic shock (low circulating fluid volume), congestive heart failure (low cardiac output), or renal artery stenosis (low renal perfusion pressure). Renal shutdown occurs before the renal perfusion pressure falls to 0 mm Hg; the vascular system of the kidney can still be perfused when the pressure within these blood vessels is too low to produce tubular flow. In this state, the kidney is in a self-protective mode: the renal parenchyma is kept alive, but urine does not flow. Therefore, the best definition of complete renal failure is when the filtration fraction (i.e., glomerular filtration rate [GFR] divided by renal plasma flow [RPF]) falls to 0%.

A (arterial pressure is too low to produce renal blood flow) is incorrect. Although poor renal perfusion is a very common cause of renal failure, the loss of renal function occurs before the renal perfusion pressure falls to 0 mm Hg. The blood pressure may be too low to support urine production, but it is still adequate to support perfusion of the functional tissue of the kidneys.

B (circulating levels of antidiuretic hormone are suppressed) is incorrect. ADH is secreted in response to a high osmolality of body fluids. It reduces urine flow by triggering the production of water channels in the distal tubules to promote the reabsorption of water. During renal failure, the osmolarity of body fluids rises, promoting an increase in ADH secretion.

D (tubuloglomerular feedback is maximally stimulated) is incorrect. Tubuloglomerular feedback, a mechanism designed to reduce the GFR during high tubular flow rates, is inhibited as the tubular flow rate approaches 0 mL/min.

E (water clearance is 0 mL/min) is incorrect. Water clearance is typically negative in that the body is producing a concentrated urine. When water clearance is 0 mL/min, however, the urine flow is copious and the urine osmolarity matches that of the blood (i.e., not concentrated).

22. D (21α-hydroxylase) is correct. The patient's clinical and laboratory findings are consistent with the diagnosis of congenital adrenal hyperplasia. In about 90% of cases, this disorder is attributable to 21α-hydroxylase deficiency, which causes a serious metabolic imbalance. Aldosterone and cortisol are not produced, and their precursors enter androgen synthesis pathways, thereby causing female genital abnormalities.

A (11β-hydroxylase) is incorrect. About 5% of cases of congenital adrenal hyperplasia are attributable to 11β-hydroxylase deficiency. Aldosterone is not produced, but its precursor, 11-deoxycorticosterone, acts as a mineralocorticoid and causes hypokalemia and hypertension. An overproduction of androgens causes masculinization similar to that found in 21α-hydroxylase deficiency.

B (16α-hydroxylase) is incorrect. 16α-Hydroxylase converts estradiol to estriol in the placenta. It is not produced in infants.

C (17α-hydroxylase) is incorrect. In 17α-hydroxylase deficiency, sex hormones and cortisol are not produced. Mineralocorticoid synthesis is increased.

E (3β-hydroxysteroid dehydrogenase) is incorrect. 3β-Hydroxysteroid dehydrogenase catalyzes the formation of pregnenolone, a common precursor for all steroid hormones. A deficiency of this enzyme results in early death due to the lack of steroid hormones.

23. C (inhibition of Na^+,K^+-ATPase) is correct. The drug described is digoxin. Digoxin is a cardiac glycoside that acts by inhibiting Na^+,K^+-ATPase (the "sodium pump") in the cell membrane of cardiac myocytes. Inhibition of the sodium pump causes an increase in the concentration of Na^+ in the myocyte, and this in turn increases the activity of the Ca^{2+},Na^+ antiporter (the calcium-sodium exchanger). As a result, more Ca^{2+} enters the myocyte. This Ca^{2+} (along with the Ca^{2+} that is trigger-released from the sarcoplasmic reticulum) binds to troponin and produces a conformational change in the tropomyosintroponin complex. This "frees" actin to interact with myosin and to thereby produce a positive inotropic response (i.e., an increase in the force of contraction). The binding of digoxin to Na^+, K^+-ATPase is increased by conditions leading to hypokalemia (e.g., diuretic therapy).

A   (inhibition of Ca^{2+} reuptake into the sarcoplasmic reticulum) is incorrect. No drug produces its positive inotropic action by inhibiting Ca^{2+} reuptake into the sarcoplasmic reticulum.
B   (inhibition of cyclic adenosine monophosphate phosphodiesterases) is incorrect. Amrinone and milrinone are drugs that produce their inotropic effect via inhibition of cyclic nucleotide phosphodiesterases (PDEs). The inhibition of PDEs causes an increase in cAMP, and thus can be said to mimic the stimulation of β_1-adrenergic receptors.
D   (stimulation of β_1-adrenergic receptors) is incorrect. The inotropic response to β_1-adrenergic receptor agonists occurs via an increase in cAMP. Phosphorylation of Ca^{2+} channels by cAMP-dependent protein kinase increases the influx of calcium. The increase in intracellular calcium leads to an increase in the force of contraction (see the discussion of C).
E   (stimulation of phospholipase C) is incorrect. Many drugs, including α_1-adrenergic receptor agonists, serotonin receptor agonists, muscarinic M_3 receptor agonists, and histamine, cause contraction of smooth muscle by activating phospholipase C. The subsequent increase in the inositol triphosphate (IP_3) level causes an increase in the release of Ca^{2+} from the sarcoplasmic reticulum. After calcium binds to calmodulin, the calcium-calmodulin complex activates myosin light chain kinase (MLC kinase), the enzyme that phosphorylates MLCs. Phosphorylated MLCs then interact with actin to cause smooth muscle contraction.

24. *E*   (positive Heinz body preparation) is correct. The patient has glucose-6-phosphate dehydrogenase (G6PD) deficiency, a sex-linked recessive disorder. G6PD deficiency leads to decreased synthesis of glutathione (GSH), which is necessary to neutralize peroxide in RBCs. The hemolysis is predominantly intravascular, leading to hemoglobinuria. Infection and therapy with oxidant drugs (e.g., primaquine and dapsone) precipitate hemolysis. In the Mediterranean variant, which is common in individuals of Mediterranean descent, fava beans can precipitate hemolysis. In G6PD deficiency, oxidant damage to RBCs leads to an accumulation of peroxide that cannot be neutralized by GSH. Peroxide damages the RBC membrane (intravascular hemolysis) and denatures hemoglobin, which forms discrete inclusions called Heinz bodies. Splenic macrophages often remove damaged RBC

membranes, leaving cells with membrane defects, called "bite cells," circulating in the peripheral blood. The screening test of choice in acute hemolysis is a Heinz body preparation, which requires a special supravital stain to identify the Heinz bodies. Enzyme analysis for G6PD is the confirmatory test and must be performed when active hemolysis has subsided. African-Americans have a milder variant of G6PD deficiency.

A (abnormal hemoglobin electrophoresis) is incorrect. The patient does not have an increase in normal hemoglobin (e.g., hemoglobin A_2 or F) or the presence of abnormal hemoglobin (e.g., hemoglobin S).
B (low mean corpuscular hemoglobin concentration) is incorrect. Patients with G6PD deficiency have normal hemoglobin synthesis, hence a normal MCHC.
C (low serum ferritin concentration) is incorrect. The patient does not have iron deficiency anemia, which is associated with an inadequate reticulocyte response to the anemia.
D (positive direct Coombs' test) is incorrect. Use of primaquine is not associated with an autoimmune hemolytic anemia.

25. **B** (tracing B) is correct. Because of dynamic changes in thoracic volume, which is controlled by the muscles of breathing, alveolar pressure (P_{alv}) changes with changes in intrapleural pressure (P_{pl}). That is, when intrapleural pressure is stable, alveolar pressure is stable and equal to atmospheric pressure (0 cm H_2O); when the intrapleural pressure falls, alveolar pressure falls to a subatmospheric level; and when the intrapleural pressure rises, alveolar pressure becomes supra-atmospheric. In the tracing shown, this recording of P_{alv} is the only one that correctly follows the fluctuation of P_{pl}.

A (tracing A) is incorrect. In the second breath for this tracing, P_{alv} and P_{pl} move in opposite directions.
C (tracing C) is incorrect. In the first breath for this tracing, P_{alv} and P_{pl} move in opposite directions.
D (tracing D) is incorrect. Throughout the entire recording, P_{alv} and P_{pl} move in opposite directions.
E (tracing E) is incorrect. In the second breath for this tracing, P_{alv} fails to return to 0 cm H_2O.

26. **D** (middle cerebral) is correct. The patient's stroke has caused Wernicke's aphasia, which is characterized by poor comprehension and grammatical expression. Wernicke's area lies in the postcentral gyrus, which is served by the middle cerebral artery. The somatosensory area is also in this region. A stroke that damages the postcentral gyrus may also result in diminished sensations.

A (anterior cerebral) is incorrect. The anterior cerebral artery supplies the medial aspect of the frontal and parietal lobes. If this ar-

tery had been involved in the stroke, the patient's leg and trunk would have been involved, but not speech.
B (callosomarginal) is incorrect. The callosomarginal artery serves the cingulate gyrus, which is in the limbic area. A stroke involving this artery may affect memory, emotions, and motivation-related behaviors, but not speech.
C (lenticulostriate) is incorrect. The lenticulostriate artery supplies the internal capsule. Damage to this artery would disrupt normal somatosensory transmission between the thalamus and the postcentral gyrus. It would not affect Wernicke's area. However, damage to Wernicke's area is suggested by problems with comprehension and grammatical expression.
E (posterior cerebral) is incorrect. The posterior cerebral artery supplies the occipital lobe, which is primarily involved with vision. A stroke involving this artery would affect vision, not speech.

27. **B** (countertransference) is correct. Countertransference is the thoughts and feelings a physician has toward a patient. This attitude is based on both conscious and unconscious factors and is heavily influenced by the physician's past relationships, especially those with significant authority figures. For example, the physician was experiencing countertransference because the patient reminded him of his deceased grandmother. Physicians should routinely monitor their feelings about patients to ensure objectivity.

A (codependency) is incorrect. Codependency describes an unhealthy relationship in which an individual circumvents personal needs to care for and support the needs of another. This pattern of behavior often develops in relationships in which one or both partners are abusing substances.
C (projection) is incorrect. Projection is a defense mechanism in which an individual unconsciously attributes unacceptable impulses and thoughts to another person.
D (resistance) is incorrect. Resistance characterizes barriers demonstrated by a patient, typically unconsciously, towards helpful interventions.
E (transference) is incorrect. Transference represents the unconscious projection of thoughts, feelings, and impulses a patient displays toward a physician based on the patient's past experiences. The feelings may be positive or negative. Transference is the reverse of countertransference.

28. **B** (injury to the C5–C6 contributions to the brachial plexus) is correct. C5 and C6 contribute to the upper portion of the brachial plexus by sending fibers to the lateral and posterior cords. Branches from the brachial plexus to muscles of the shoulder and arm receive the majority of fibers from spinal nerves C5–C6; muscles of the arm from C5, C6, and partially from C7; muscles of the forearm from C6–C8; and intrinsic muscles of the

hand from C8–T1. Therefore, injury to C5–C6 contributions to the brachial plexus could produce the patient's symptoms.

A good rule of thumb for determining motor innervation to the upper limb is that the more proximal the position of a muscle, the higher its source of innervation in the brachial plexus. Therefore, most of the symptoms exhibited by injury to the upper brachial plexus occur in muscles of the shoulder and arm. Loss of abduction of the upper limb movement away from the body results from loss of the deltoid muscle, whose fibers come from C5–C6 and are carried by the axillary nerve. Other muscles of the scapula, including the rotator cuff, would also be involved. Weakness in flexion and a pronated forearm would result from loss of the biceps brachii; loss of flexion would also include damage to the brachialis muscle. Both the biceps brachii and the brachialis receive innervation from C5–C6 via the musculocutaneous nerve.

A (dislocation of the shoulder causing damage to the axillary nerve) is incorrect. Damage to the axillary nerve would affect two muscles: the deltoid, which is the prime mover in the first 90 degrees of abduction; and the teres minor, one of the rotator cuff muscles. Damage to the axillary nerve would have no effect on flexion of the elbow or supination of the forearm.

C (injury to the lower brachial plexus) is incorrect. Injury to the lower brachial plexus would involve contributions from C8 and T1 spinal nerves. Therefore, the most noticeable loss of function would be in the hand, not the shoulder and arm. C8 and T1 contribute to three major nerves of the upper limb: the radial, which supplies primarily sensory nerves from C8–T1; the median, which supplies motor innervation to the thenar eminence of the hand and to the first two lumbricals; and the ulnar, which provides the remainder of the motor innervation to intrinsic muscles of the hand. Opposition of the thumb and fifth digits is possible, indicating that C8 and T1 have not been damaged.

D (injury to the ulnar nerve) is incorrect. The ulnar nerve, a nerve of the distal upper extremity, innervates the flexor carpi ulnaris and the ulnar half of the flexor digitorum profundus muscles in the forearm as well as the intrinsic muscles of the hand—the hypothenar muscles, third and fourth lumbricals, all interossei, and the adductor pollicis. A branch of the medial cord of the brachial plexus, the ulnar nerve originates from the spinal cord at C8 and T1. Motor innervation to intrinsic muscles of the hand occurs at spinal levels C8 and T1. Because the patient has normal movement in his hand, the ulnar nerve is undamaged.

E (lesion of the posterior cord of the brachial plexus) is incorrect. Such a lesion would involve the contributions from the upper trunk (C5–C6). Most of these fibers leave the posterior cord with nerves destined to innervate muscles of the shoulder (subscapular nerves, axillary nerve). Such a lesion could account for at least some of the symptoms of loss of movement to the shoulder. Such a lesion to the posterior cord would appreciably affect supination, but not flexion, of the elbow.

29. **A** (increased RBC mass; increased plasma volume; normal SaO_2; decreased EPO concentration) is correct. The patient has polycythemia rubra vera (PRV), which is a myeloproliferative disease involving a neoplastic proliferation of trilineage myeloid stem cells in the bone marrow. PRV is an absolute type of polycythemia, meaning there is an increase in the total number of RBCs in the body in mL/kg (RBC mass) as well as an increase in the RBC count (RBCs per µL of blood). Unlike other causes of polycythemia, the increase in RBC mass is accompanied by an increase in plasma volume. Because PRV is a stem cell disease, the bone marrow synthesis of RBCs is inappropriate, meaning that the increase in RBC production is not an EPO-mediated response to a hypoxic stimulus. The patient's SaO_2 is normal, and the EPO concentration is low. The increase in RBC mass increases the overall O_2 content of blood, suppressing EPO release from endothelial cells in peritubular capillaries in the kidneys. The patient's headaches and pruritus are due to histamine released into the blood by increased numbers of peripheral blood basophils and mast cells in skin. The abdominal pain and bloody diarrhea are secondary to thrombosis of the superior mesenteric vein, leading to a hemorrhagic infarction of the small bowel.

   B (increased RBC mass; normal plasma volume; decreased SaO_2; increased EPO concentration) is incorrect. This pattern of laboratory findings represents an appropriate type of absolute polycythemia related to a hypoxic stimulus for EPO release. Examples include obstructive and restrictive lung disease, cyanotic congenital heart disease, and living at high altitudes.
   C (increased RBC mass; normal plasma volume; normal SaO_2; increased EPO concentration) is incorrect. This pattern of findings represents an inappropriate type of absolute polycythemia (normal SaO_2) related to ectopic or inappropriate secretion of EPO. Examples include renal disease (e.g., cancer, cystic disease, hydronephrosis) and ectopic secretion of EPO from a hepatocellular carcinoma.
   D (normal RBC mass; decreased plasma volume; normal SaO_2; normal EPO concentration) is incorrect. This pattern represents a relative type of polycythemia where a loss of plasma hemoconcentrates RBCs in the peripheral blood, increasing the RBC count without affecting RBC mass. Any cause of volume depletion (e.g., excessive sweating, severe diarrhea) leads to this type of polycythemia.

30. **D** (peripheral neuropathy) is correct. Isoniazid (isonicotinic acid hydrazide, or INH) is the appropriate drug for TB prophylaxis in the patient described. Some individuals treated with INH develop peripheral neuropathy, characterized by tingling or numbness of the hands and feet. This adverse effect is attributed to INH-induced pyridoxine deficiency, and is more likely to occur in persons suffering from alcoholism, malnourishment, or diabetes. Concomitant administration of pyridoxine can reduce the incidence of this adverse effect from 20% to less than 1%.

A (discoloration of body fluids) is incorrect. Treatment with INH does not discolor body fluids. However, treatment with rifampin can cause orange-red discoloration of saliva, tears, sweat, and urine, and it can also cause permanent discoloration of contact lenses. The side effects of rifampin cannot be prevented by concurrent administration of pyridoxine.

B (hepatotoxicity) is incorrect. Hepatotoxicity sometimes occurs with the use of INH or other antitubercular drugs, such as pyrazinamide and rifampin. Drug-induced hepatotoxicity is unaffected by concomitant administration of pyridoxine.

C (optic neuritis) is incorrect. Ethambutol is sometimes associated with loss of visual acuity and loss of green-color vision. INH-induced optic neuritis has also been reported. These optic effects cannot be prevented by concomitant administration of pyridoxine.

E (systemic lupus erythematosus) is incorrect. INH undergoes acetylation more rapidly in some individuals than in others. INH-induced SLE, which occurs more frequently in slow acetylators (i.e., genetic polymorphism in *N*-acetyltransferase), is unaffected by concomitant administration of pyridoxine.

31. *D* *(Rickettsia rickettsii)* is correct. The clinical and laboratory findings are consistent with the diagnosis of Rocky Mountain spotted fever caused by *R. rickettsii*. Hard ticks are the major reservoirs and vectors of this organism, and most cases of the disease now occur in the southeast Atlantic and south central states. *R. rickettsii* produces no known toxins, and all of the clinical manifestations appear to be related to the organism's growth within endothelial cells.

A *(Borrelia burgdorferi)* is incorrect. *B. burgdorferi* is the cause of Lyme disease. Although the organism is transmitted to humans via tick bites, it is a spirochete, not a coccobacillus.

B *(Borrelia recurrentis)* is incorrect. *B. recurrentis* is a spirochete that is transmitted by lice and causes epidemic (louse-borne) fever.

C *(Ehrlichia chaffeensis)* is incorrect. *E. chaffeensis* is the cause of human monocytic ehrlichiosis. Although the organism is transmitted to humans via tick bites, it causes a rash in only about 20% of infected patients. Culture of the organism is extremely difficult. Diagnosis is confirmed serologically.

E *(Rickettsia typhi)* is incorrect. *R. typhi* causes murine (endemic) typhus. Infection is transmitted by fleas, and rodents are the reservoir.

32. *B* (hypersensitivity to aspirin) is correct. The incidence of hypersensitivity to aspirin (acetylsalicylic acid, or ASA) is increased in patients with a history of asthma or nasal polyps. Hypersensitivity is believed to be due to the "shunting" of arachidonic acid to the lipoxygenase pathway. This shunting causes an increase in the formation of leukotrienes. A patient who is hyper-

sensitive to ASA can be given nonacetylated salicylates but should not be treated with other nonsteroidal antiinflammatory drugs (NSAIDs).

A (gastric ulceration) is incorrect. ASA and other NSAIDs are believed to cause gastric ulceration by inhibiting cyclooxygenase (COX), thereby decreasing the production of "cytoprotective" gastric prostaglandins (PGE and PGI). Misoprostol, a PGE analogue, prevents NSAID-induced gastric ulcers.
C (increased bleeding) is incorrect. Increased bleeding is attributed to the inhibition of platelet COX and a subsequent decrease in the production of thromboxane A_2. Because ASA increases bleeding, it can be used to prevent myocardial infarction (MI) in patients with a history of MI or unstable angina. Selective COX-2 inhibitors (such as celecoxib) and nonacetylated salicylates have minimal effect on platelet hemostasis.
D (renal dysfunction) is incorrect. ASA and other NSAIDs are believed to cause renal dysfunction by inhibiting COX, thereby decreasing the production of prostaglandins that are necessary for the homeostatic regulation of renal perfusion. Individuals who are at increased risk for NSAID-induced renal dysfunction include patients with congestive heart failure, ascites, or hypovolemia. In these patients, treatment with sulindac (a drug whose active metabolite does not reach the kidney) or with a selective COX-2 inhibitor (such as celecoxib) would be preferred to treatment with an NSAID.
E (Reye's syndrome) is incorrect. Reye's syndrome has been associated with the use of ASA in children with antecedent viral illnesses. To avoid the risk of Reye's syndrome, children should be given acetaminophen instead of ASA.

33. *B* (enzyme B) is correct. The boy's medical history and findings are consistent with the diagnosis of severe combined immunodeficiency disease (SCID), an X-linked or autosomal recessive disorder characterized by abnormalities in both T cells and B cells. Affected children are prone to severe infections with extracellular and intracellular pathogens and usually die before their second birthday. SCID is caused by a deficiency of adenosine deaminase (enzyme B in the figure). In healthy individuals, adenosine deaminase catalyzes the conversion of adenosine to inosine (as shown in the figure) and also catalyzes the conversion of deoxyadenosine to deoxyinosine (not shown in the figure). Recently, bone marrow transplantation has been curative in these patients.

A (enzyme A) is incorrect. In the figure, enzyme A is adenylate deaminase, also called adenosine monophosphate (AMP) deaminase. This enzyme is responsible for converting AMP to inosine monophosphate (IMP). A deficiency of the enzyme results in a relatively benign muscle disorder that is characterized by easy fatigability and exercise-induced muscle aches.

C (enzyme C) is incorrect. Enzyme C is purine-nucleoside phosphorylase (PNP), the enzyme that converts inosine to hypoxanthine and also converts guanosine to guanine. A deficiency of this enzyme causes abnormalities only in T cells. In affected patients, recurrent infections are usually caused by extracellular organisms, because these patients are deficient in serum opsonins necessary for phagocytosis.

D (enzyme D) is incorrect. Enzyme D is hypoxanthine-guanine phosphoribosyltransferase (HGPRT). A deficiency of this enzyme causes Lesch-Nyhan syndrome.

E (enzyme E) is incorrect. Enzyme E is xanthine oxidase. A deficiency of this enzyme results in hypouricemia, increased urinary excretion of hypoxanthine and xanthine, and formation of xanthine stones.

34. *C* (osteomyelitis secondary to *Salmonella paratyphi* septicemia) is correct. The most common pathogen causing osteomyelitis in patients with sickle cell disease is *Salmonella paratyphi* (75% of cases). *Staphylococcus aureus* septicemia is the most common cause of osteomyelitis in children; however, in patients with sickle cell disease, the loss of splenic function due to repeated infarctions predisposes them to sepsis caused by *Salmonella* species and not by other pathogens. The metaphysis is the most common location for osteomyelitis associated with sepsis, because it is the most vascular part of bone. A radionuclide bone scan has much greater sensitivity than a routine radiograph in detecting osteomyelitis in its earliest stages. A bone biopsy is the confirming test for osteomyelitis.

A (aseptic necrosis related to ischemia) is incorrect. Aseptic necrosis most commonly occurs in the femoral head rather than the metaphysis of bone. Furthermore, the bone in aseptic necrosis shows increased density due to reactive bone formation after the ischemic event. Aseptic necrosis of the femoral head is a common complication of sickle cell disease.

B (metastatic cancer from an undetermined site) is incorrect. The femoral head is a more common location for metastasis than the metaphyseal area. Furthermore, the clinical presentation of a febrile patient with sickle cell disease and a lytic lesion in bone is more likely to be diagnostic of osteomyelitis than of primary or metastatic cancer.

D (primary malignancy of bone) is incorrect. The most common bone cancer found in the metaphysis of the femur is an osteogenic sarcoma. As the name implies, it is a bone-producing sarcoma; hence increased density of bone, rather than bone lysis, is expected.

35. *A* (acoustic neuroma) is correct. An acoustic neuroma is a tumor that develops from Schwann cells. It can affect both divisions of the vestibulocochlear nerve (CN VIII) and can grow large enough to press against the cerebellum and brain stem. Cerebellar damage is indicated in this patient by ataxia (loss of

muscle coordination); falling to the left indicates the side on which the lesion is growing. Patients with this type of tumor may also have tinnitus, papilledema, and nystagmus.

B   (acute lateral medullary syndrome) is incorrect. The lateral medullary syndrome (Wallenberg's syndrome) is caused by occlusion of the posterior inferior cerebellar artery. The main features of this syndrome are dysphagia, dysphonia, dizziness, ipsilateral Horner's syndrome, and ipsilateral loss of pain and temperature sensations in the face accompanied by contralateral loss of pain and temperature sensations in the body. The glossopharyngeal (CN IX) or vagal (CN X) nerve may be involved. CN VIII is not affected, however, because it enters the brain stem at a higher level. Therefore, unlike the patient described, a patient with Wallenberg's syndrome would retain the senses of hearing and balance.
C   (demyelinating lesion in the basilar pons) is incorrect. Fibers carrying auditory information cross in the lower pontine tegmentum, not in the basilar pons.
D   (posterior communicating artery aneurysm) is incorrect. The posterior communicating artery connects the internal carotid artery with the posterior cerebral artery (which serves much of the occipital lobe), as well as the parahippocampal gyrus and the medial and inferior surfaces of the temporal lobe. Since it does not serve structures that are directly involved in hearing or balance, an aneurysm in the posterior communicating artery would not be responsible for this patient's symptoms.
E   (Weber syndrome) is incorrect. Weber syndrome is caused by a lesion in the cerebral peduncle that causes ipsilateral CN III paralysis and contralateral hemiparesis. It does not affect structures involved in hearing or balance.

36. *D*   (C5a) is correct. C5a is a complement component involved in the chemotaxis and margination of PMNs. It also functions as an anaphylatoxin.

A   (C2b), B (C3a), and C (C3b) are incorrect. C2b, C3a, and C3b are not involved in the chemotaxis of PMNs. C2b is part of the classic complement pathway C3 convertase. C3a is an anaphylatoxin that binds to basophils and mast cells. C3b binds to factor B as part of the alternative pathway or binds to C4b2b as part of the classic pathway to form C5 convertase.
E   (C5b,6,7) is incorrect. C5b,6,7 is not involved in the chemotaxis of PMNs. It is part of the membrane attack complex, which is usually deficient in individuals who have difficulty dealing with infection with *Neisseria gonorrhoeae* or *Neisseria meningitidis*.

37. *C*   (bradykinin) is correct. Captopril and other "pril" drugs are inhibitors of angiotensin-converting enzyme (ACE). Bradykinin is inactivated by ACE. Consequently, when the patient was

taking captopril, bradykinin levels would increase. The increased bradykinin levels are thought to contribute to a dry cough, a common side effect that may have been the cause of the patient's intolerance of captopril. When treatment with losartan (an angiotensin II receptor antagonist that blocks AT_1 receptors) was initiated, the serum levels of bradykinin would decrease and the dry cough would be likely to stop.

A (aldosterone) is incorrect. Angiotensin II stimulates the release of aldosterone. ACE inhibitors and AT_1 receptor antagonists both block this effect, so there would be no change in serum aldosterone levels when the patient was switched from captopril to losartan. The inhibition of aldosterone release accounts for the hyperkalemia commonly associated with the use of these two types of drugs.

B (angiotensin II) is incorrect. ACE inhibitors block the conversion of angiotensin I to angiotensin II. This would increase the serum level of angiotensin I and decrease the serum level of angiotensin II. Switching to therapy with an AT_1 antagonist would cause the opposite effect, decreasing the serum level of angiotensin I and increasing that of angiotensin II.

D (potassium) is incorrect. As discussed in A, hyperkalemia is commonly associated with the use of ACE inhibitors and AT_1 receptor antagonists. Thus, there would probably be no change in the serum potassium level when the patient was switched from captopril to losartan.

E (renin) is incorrect. Renin levels are controlled by the negative feedback of angiotensin II. ACE inhibitors and AT_1 receptor antagonists would both block the feedback. Thus, there would probably be no change in serum aldosterone levels when the patient was switched from captopril to losartan.

38. D (lumbar [para-aortic]) is correct. The lumbar (para-aortic) lymph nodes are found on either side of the abdominal aorta, between it and the lumbar vertebrae. The testis (and ovary) drains to the para-aortic nodes because of its embryologic origin: it develops in the upper abdominal region at about the L1–L2 vertebral level and subsequently descends with blood supply and lymph vessels to its place in the scrotum. Therefore, infections or cancer metastases from the testis first spread to these upper para-aortic lymph nodes. Similarly, although the ovary is not situated in the perineum, it has the same embryologic origin as the testis and therefore the same lymphatic drainage.

A (deep inguinal) is incorrect. The deep inguinal lymph nodes receive lymph from the deeper structures of the lower extremity, as well as from the superficial inguinal nodes. Although the penis and clitoris do send a few lymph vessels directly to the deep inguinal nodes, most lymph from these structures drains first to the superficial inguinal nodes. Efferents from the deep inguinal nodes first drain into the external iliac nodes, then to the common iliac nodes, and eventually to the para-aortic nodes.

B (horizontal group of superficial inguinal) is incorrect. The horizontal group of superficial inguinal lymph nodes, which is situated just inferior to the inguinal ligament, runs parallel to the ligament in the proximal thigh. This group of nodes receives lymph from much of the perineum, including the external genitalia (i.e., the scrotum, labia majora, penis, clitoris, and vestibule) as well as the anus and anal canal below the pectinate line, but not the testis. In addition, structures in the anterior abdominal wall below the umbilicus and from the gluteal region also drain into the superficial inguinal nodes.

C (internal iliac) is incorrect. The internal iliac lymph nodes lie along the internal iliac artery, and the internal iliac lymph vessels and associated nodes receive lymph from much of the pelvic viscera. Most of the pelvic structures drain either to internal or external iliac nodes. Typically, the more superior aspects of the pelvic viscera (e.g., fallopian tube) drain, in part, to the external iliac nodes.

E (vertical group of superficial inguinal) is incorrect. The vertical group of superficial inguinal lymph nodes runs roughly perpendicular to the horizontal group, generally following the great saphenous vein. The vertical group receives lymph primarily from the superficial lower extremity. Both the vertical and horizontal groups of superficial inguinal nodes drain to the deep inguinal nodes.

39. C (it is an open system that communicates with the environment through the lungs and kidneys) is correct. The bicarbonate buffer system is completely bidirectional:

$$CO_2 + H_2O \longleftrightarrow H_2CO_3 \longleftrightarrow HCO_3^- + H^+$$

When H^+ ions begin to accumulate, the reaction can move in reverse, with the resulting excess CO_2 being blown off by the lungs. Conversely, when CO_2 levels rise in blood, the system will move forward, producing more H^+ ions that are secreted by the kidney along with enhanced HCO_3^- reabsorption.

A (HCO_3^- ions form irreversible complexes with free H^+ ions) is incorrect. In the bicarbonate system, HCO_3^- ions interact reversibly with free H^+ ions, according to the acid-base challenge at hand.

B (it buffers more than 99% of the total H^+ concentration in the body) is incorrect. Much of the H^+ ions in blood are also buffered by hemoglobin, which is a closed system.

D (it is unlikely to be depleted of its acid (CO_2) or base (HCO_3^-) components) is incorrect. There are limits to effectiveness of the bicarbonate buffer system. For example, in patients with severe metabolic acidosis (e.g., ketoacidosis of diabetes), the HCO_3^- ion concentration can almost be depleted to the point that it becomes virtually impossible for the pulmonary system to compensate by means of secondary respiratory alkalosis.

E (its pK_a is very near as arterial plasma pH) is incorrect. Buffer systems are most effective when their characteristic pK_a values are within a single pH unit of the environmental pH. The pK$_a$ for the bicarbonate system is 6.1—far below the arterial plasma pH of 7.40. However, the importance of the open-ended nature of the bicarbonate system far outweighs its non-optimal pK$_a$.

40. *C* (otitis media) is correct. This patient's clinical and laboratory findings are consistent with the diagnosis of pneumonia caused by *Streptococcus pneumoniae*. This organism is the leading bacterial cause of otitis media in children. Other bacterial causes of otitis media include *Haemophilus influenzae* and *Streptococcus pyogenes*. Acute otitis media is one of the most prevalent childhood diseases, affecting more than two thirds of all children by the age of 3 years.

A (croup) is incorrect. Croup is usually caused by viruses. It is not caused by *S. pneumoniae*.
B (meningitis) is incorrect. Meningitis due to *S. pneumoniae* is more common in adults than in children.
D (pharyngitis) is incorrect. *S. pneumoniae* is not a major cause of pharyngitis.
E (pneumonia) is incorrect. In older individuals, most cases of pneumonia are caused by bacteria. In young children, most cases of pneumonia are caused by viruses.

41. *C* (foscarnet) is correct. The patient has symptoms consistent with CMV retinitis, the most common presentation of CMV infection in patients with CD4+ counts <100 cells/mm^3. Foscarnet directly inhibits viral DNA polymerases and sometimes causes nephrotoxicity. Ganciclovir is a prodrug that undergoes nonspecific triphosphorylation and is associated with bone marrow suppression (neutropenia). Since this patient has a low absolute neutrophil count and has exhibited intolerance to myelosuppressive drugs in the past, foscarnet would be preferable to ganciclovir for the treatment of her CMV retinitis.

A (acyclovir) is incorrect. Acyclovir is ineffective against CMV, since this virus lacks thymidine kinase. The drug is efficacious in the treatment of herpesvirus and varicellazoster virus infections.
B (amantadine) is incorrect. Amantadine is ineffective against DNA viruses. It is indicated for the management of Parkinson's disease and for the prevention and early treatment of viral A influenza.
D (ganciclovir) is incorrect. Ganciclovir is used to treat CMV retinitis, but it would not be the drug of choice for a patient with a low absolute neutrophil count (see the discussion of C).
E (pentamidine) is incorrect. Pentamidine is used in the management of *Pneumocystis carinii* pneumonia. It is not active against viruses.

42. *A* (acetylcholinesterase) is correct. The patient's clinical manifestations and test results are consistent with the diagnosis of myasthenia gravis, a disease in which autoantibodies are directed against the acetylcholine receptor. Patients with myasthenia gravis are treated with acetylcholinesterase inhibitors to increase the concentration of acetylcholine in the synapse. A higher concentration increases the probability that acetylcholine will bind to its receptors.

B (choline acetyltransferase) is incorrect. Choline acetyltransferase is an enzyme that catalyzes the formation of acetylcholine from acetyl CoA and choline in the cytoplasm of the presynaptic nerve terminal.
C (monoamine oxidase) is incorrect. Monoamine oxidase is an enzyme that degrades monoamines (such as catecholamines). It is not present in the neuromuscular junction.
D (muscarinic acetylcholine receptor) is incorrect. In myasthenia gravis, the antibodies are not formed against the muscarinic receptors. These receptors, found only on autonomic effectors, are not affected.
E (nicotinic acetylcholine receptor) is incorrect. In myasthenia gravis, the nicotinic acetylcholine receptors of the neuromuscular junctions are affected, but they are not a target for therapy with neostigmine.

43. *A* (*Blastomyces dermatitidis*) is correct. The clinical and laboratory findings are consistent with the diagnosis of chronic cutaneous and pulmonary blastomycosis caused by the dimorphic fungus *B. dermatitidis*. This disease is endemic in the Ohio and Mississippi river valley regions and is initiated by the inhalation of conidia. Most cases are asymptomatic or characterized by mild pulmonary symptoms.

B (*Coccidioides immitis*) is incorrect. *C. immitis* causes respiratory tract infections. However, at 37° C, it forms spherules containing endospores.
C (*Histoplasma capsulatum*) is incorrect. While the clinical manifestations of histoplasmosis are similar to those described, *H. capsulatum* usually produces tuberculate macroconidia at room temperature and small budding yeasts at 37° C.
D (*Paracoccidioides brasiliensis*) is incorrect. *P. brasiliensis* can cause both pulmonary and cutaneous manifestations of disease. However, when grown at room temperature, *P. brasiliensis* forms hyphae without macroconidia. At 37° C, it grows as large yeasts with multiple buds.
E (*Sporothrix schenckii*) is incorrect. The laboratory findings are not consistent with *S. schenckii* infection, because this fungus produces only microconidia at room temperature.

44. *B* (conditioned stimulus) is correct. Classical conditioning occurs when a neutral stimulus is repeatedly paired with one that naturally evokes a response until the neutral stimulus gener-

ates the same response. In this case, the car is a neutral stimulus and would not lead to nausea except that riding in it has now been paired with going to a clinic for chemotherapy.

A (conditioned response) is incorrect. The conditioned response is also nausea when it occurs in response to the car (i.e., the conditioned stimulus). In classical conditioning paradigms, the conditioned and unconditioned response are always the same response. The defining difference is which stimulus (conditioned or unconditioned) evokes the response.
C (negative reinforcer) is incorrect. A negative reinforcer is a term used in operant conditioning. Negative reinforcers increase the likelihood that a behavior will occur by the removal of an aversive or unwanted event.
D (unconditioned response) and E (unconditioned stimulus) are incorrect. The unconditioned response is nausea, since nausea occurs naturally in response to chemotherapy. Chemotherapy is both the unconditioned response and the unconditioned stimulus.

45. *E* (ornithine carbamoyltransferase) is correct. Hyperammonemia in a neonate is characteristic of a defect in the urea cycle. The most common defect in this cycle is a deficiency of ornithine carbamoyltransferase (also called ornithine transcarbamoylase), which causes type II hyperammonemia. In an enzymatic defect of the urea cycle, levels of the immediate substrate of the deficient enzyme are elevated in blood and urine. Ornithine carbamoyltransferase catalyzes the formation of citrulline from carbamoyl phosphate and ornithine. Thus, a deficiency of this enzyme results in elevated levels of ornithine and the absence of citrulline. Glutamine levels are often elevated because excess ammonia is metabolized to glutamine. Accumulated carbamoyl phosphate is converted into orotic acid in the cytoplasm and excreted in the urine.

A (arginase), B (argininosuccinate lyase), and C (argininosuccinate synthase) are incorrect. In arginase deficiency, plasma arginine levels are high. In argininosuccinate lyase deficiency, argininosuccinate levels are extremely high. In argininosuccinate synthase deficiency, citrulline levels are extremely high.
D (carbamoyl phosphate synthetase I) is incorrect. CPSI catalyzes the first step of the urea cycle, which is the synthesis of carbamoyl phosphate. Laboratory findings in CPSI deficiency are similar to those in ornithine carbamoyltransferase deficiency, but there is no increase in orotic acid excretion and the CPSI deficiency results in type I hyperammonemia.

46. *A* (erythromycin) is correct. The patient is experiencing torsade de pointes, a polymorphic ventricular tachycardia associated with prolonged repolarization and a prolonged QT interval. By blocking cardiac potassium channels, cisapride can produce this arrhythmia. The CYP3A4 isozyme of cytochrome P450 normally

inactivates cisapride. By inhibiting CYP3A4, erythromycin would increase the serum levels of cisapride and thereby increase the risk of torsade de pointes, contraindicating concomitant use of cisapride and erythromycin. Hydrochlorothiazide-induced hypokalemia is another predisposing factor for torsade de pointes. It should be noted that although cisapride is still manufactured, it has limited clinical availability today.

B (ketoconazole) is incorrect. Ketoconazole is ineffective for the treatment of pneumococcal pneumonia, and would not have been used to treat this patient. Ketoconazole and other "-azole" antifungal agents are inhibitors of CYP3A4. Consequently, their concomitant use with cisapride is contraindicated.
C (penicillin V) is incorrect. In the absence of hypersensitivity to penicillin, penicillin V is the preferred drug for the treatment of pneumococcal pneumonia. Penicillin V would not have contributed to the development of torsade de pointes in the patient described.
D (rifampin) is incorrect. Rifampin, a potent inducer of cytochrome P450 enzymes, is ineffective in the treatment of pneumococcal pneumonia. When used to treat tuberculosis, it has not been associated with the development of torsade de pointes.
E (streptomycin) is incorrect. Streptomycin is ineffective in the treatment of pneumococcal pneumonia. When used to treat other infections, it has not been associated with the development of torsade de pointes.

47. **D** (positive Philadelphia chromosome study) is correct. The patient has chronic myelogenous leukemia (CML). Like all leukemias, CML is a malignancy arising from stem cells in the bone marrow. Predisposing factors include exposure to radiation or benzene. The classic chromosome abnormality is a t(9;22) translocation of the *abl* oncogene (which is responsible for non-receptor tyrosine kinase activity) from chromosome 9 to chromosome 22 (the Philadelphia chromosome) with fusion at the break cluster region (bcr). The presence of the bcr-c-*abl* fusion gene is 100% specific for CML, whereas the Philadelphia chromosome has high sensitivity for CML, but it is not 100% specific. CML and acute myelogenous leukemia are the most common leukemias in persons 39–60 years of age. CML progresses in ~3 years into a blast crisis, which usually ends in the patient's death. The Philadelphia chromosome is not lost in therapy for CML; t(9;22) is still present.

A (Auer rods in myeloblasts) is incorrect. Auer rods are seen only in acute myelogenous leukemias. Auer rods are red, splinter- or rod-shaped inclusions (fused lysosomes) in the cytosol of neoplastic myeloblasts or progranulocytes.
B (high leukocyte alkaline phosphatase score) is incorrect. In CML, the leukocyte alkaline phosphatase (LAP) score is usually low. LAP is normally present in nonneoplastic neutrophils from the myelocyte stage to segmented neutrophils. Because the

neutrophils of CML are neoplastic, a stain for LAP is usually negative; hence the stain intensity in neutrophils is usually very low or zero. The LAP score is increased in patients whose neutrophil elevations are associated with inflammation.

C   (myeloblasts positive for CD_{10} antigen) is incorrect. The CD_{10} antigen refers to the common acute lymphoblastic leukemia antigen (CALLA), which is positive in most cases of acute lymphoblastic leukemia.

E   (positive tartrate-resistant acid phosphatase stain) is incorrect. This stain identifies the neoplastic B cells of hairy cell leukemia.

48. *D*   (Klüver-Bucy syndrome) is correct. Klüver-Bucy syndrome is characterized by emotional blunting, hypersexual activity, visual agnosia (inability to recognize objects by sight), and hyperorality. It is caused by damage to the amygdala and temporal lobe. Damage to the amygdala can result in hyperorality, hypersexuality, and blunted emotions. Since the temporal lobe contains visual association areas, damage to this region can result in visual agnosia.

A   (Dandy-Walker syndrome) is incorrect. Dandy-Walker syndrome is caused by obstruction of the foramina of Luschka and Magendie, which causes all four ventricles to expand. This condition is associated with hydrocephalus, which is not reported for this patient.

B   (jacksonian seizures) is incorrect. Jacksonian seizures are simple partial motor seizures that affect the motor cortex of the brain. They begin in one hand and progress up the arm or begin in the face and spread downward, eventually involving an arm and a leg.

C   (Kallmann syndrome) is incorrect. Kallmann syndrome is associated with male hypogonadism, which results from a deficiency in gonadotropin-releasing hormone (GnRH). Patients with this condition often have color blindness and skeletal structural defects (e.g., midline facial defects or a cleft palate or cleft lip). They do not develop the personality changes observed in this patient.

E   (tumor in the cingulate gyrus) is incorrect. The cingulate gyrus, which surrounds the corpus callosum, is a major component of the limbic system. A tumor in this structure could cause symptoms of limbic damage but not the visual agnosia reported for this patient.

49. *E*   (Western blot technique) is correct. Western blotting is an immunoblotting technique used to identify specific proteins (specific antigens) recognized by polyclonal or monoclonal antibodies. The technique has several steps. First, proteins are separated on a gel called SDS-PAGE (sodium dodecyl sulfate for polyacrylamide gel electrophoresis) and transferred to a membrane. Second, the membrane is probed with the primary antibody. Third, the membrane is washed and treated with the secondary antibody coupled to horseradish peroxidase or alka-

line phosphatase. Finally, chromogenic or luminescent sub-strates are used to visualize the activity of the identified antibody-antigen complexes.

A   (DNA sequencing) is incorrect. DNA sequencing shows only the sequence of a particular fragment of DNA. In the experiment described, the investigators had cDNAs of the two proteins, so the gene must have been sequenced before.
B   (restriction mapping) is incorrect. In restriction mapping, DNA is cut with one or more restriction endonucleases. Digested DNA fragments of different sizes can be visualized on an agarose gel by electrophoresis, and restriction maps of DNA can be created. Restriction maps allow for the detection of deletions or other rear-rangements in the gene. In the experiment described, this tech-nique is unnecessary.
C   (Southern blot technique) is incorrect. A Southern blot is used to analyze DNA. DNA is run on an agarose gel and transferred to a membrane. After the DNA is immobilized in the membrane, the DNA can be subjected to hybridization analysis, enabling the identification of bands that have sequences similar to those of a labeled probe. A Southern blot would show whether cDNAs had been successfully inserted into cells, but it would not indicate whether proteins had been produced.
D   (Southwestern blot technique) is incorrect. A Southwestern blot is used to study interactions between proteins and DNA.

50. *B*   (increased RBC osmotic fragility) is correct. The patient has congenital spherocytosis complicated by acute cholecystitis sec-ondary to calcium bilirubinate stones. Congenital spherocyto-sis is an autosomal dominant disease associated with a spectrin defect in the RBC membrane. Spherocytes are easily rec-ognized because they lack central areas of pallor. Normal RBCs are biconcave disks with a central area of pallor where hemoglo-bin is less concentrated. Splenic macrophages extravascularly remove spherocytes, which results in anemia and an increase in serum levels of unconjugated bilirubin (end product of hemoglo-bin metabolism in macrophages). Liver conjugation of exces-sive unconjugated bilirubin supersaturates the bile, predisposing to the formation of jet-black calcium bilirubinate stones in the gallbladder. The RBC osmotic fragility test will confirm spherocy-tosis; spherocytes hemolyze earlier than normal RBCs when placed in saline solutions ranging from 0.85% to 0.20% in con-centration. Splenectomy is the treatment of choice.

A   (abnormal hemoglobin electrophoresis) is incorrect. The pa-tient does not have a hemoglobinopathy, such as β-thalassemia, where there is an increase in hemoglobins A_2 and F, or sickle cell disease, where there is abnormal hemoglobin and sickled RBCs in the peripheral blood.
C   (low serum ferritin concentrations) is incorrect. The patient does not have iron deficiency anemia. Unlike the hemolytic anemias, iron deficiency anemia does not have an elevated,

corrected (for the degree of anemia) reticulocyte count. An increased reticulocyte count indicates an appropriate bone marrow response (e.g., increased RBC synthesis) to the anemia, which eliminates bone marrow disease (e.g., aplastic anemia) as the cause of the patient's disorder. Iron deficiency anemia is associated with a low corrected reticulocyte count, because iron is necessary for the synthesis of hemoglobin and proper development of RBCs in the bone marrow. Furthermore, in iron deficiency anemia, the RBCs are microcytic and contain less hemoglobin. This results in a low MCV and a decreased MCHC. In spherocytosis, the MCV is normal and the MCHC is increased, the latter due to increased concentration of hemoglobin in the spherocytes.

D (positive direct Coombs' test) is incorrect. The patient does not have an autoimmune hemolytic anemia. A direct Coombs' test identifies IgG or complement on the surface of RBCs. The patient has a family history of gallbladder disease and anemia, indicating a genetic rather than acquired basis for RBC hemolysis.

E (positive Heinz body preparation) is incorrect. The patient does not have glucose-6-phosphate dehydrogenase deficiency, which is a sex-linked recessive disease predominantly seen in males.

Test 5

TEST 5

DIRECTIONS: Each numbered item or incomplete statement is followed by options arranged in alphabetical or logical order. Select the best answer to each question. Some options may be partially correct, but there is only **ONE BEST** answer.

1. A 68-year-old woman has a 10-year history of type 2 diabetes mellitus. She is approximately 15–20% above her desired weight, and despite dieting is unable to lose weight. Her blood glucose had been fairly well controlled by a sulfonylurea medication, although the dose has been increased over the years to maintain control. About 3 years ago, the patient began taking a thiazide diuretic for hypertension. Since that time, her blood glucose control has deteriorated, and she has developed blurred vision, polyuria, nocturia, and fatigue. Her blood pressure is 126/82 mm Hg. Funduscopic examination shows non-proliferative retinopathy. Decreased pulses in the lower extremities and a right femoral bruit are heard on auscultation. Neurologic examination shows absent ankle reflexes and diminished vibratory sensation. Touch sensation is normal. The next step in managing this patient is

○ A. consider adding a second oral agent
○ B. continue the diet and exercise program for 3 more months
○ C. monitor blood pressure for 24 hours
○ D. obtain a 24-hour urine output to determine the calcium level
○ E. order a series of pancreatic function tests

2. A 49-year-old man is brought to the emergency department about 6 hours after the onset of crushing chest pain. An ECG is suggestive of acute myocardial infarction (MI), and a troponin-I test is positive. He suddenly develops ventricular arrhythmia and despite appropriate treatment dies 1 hour after admission. At autopsy, the heart shows an area of scarring in the posterior wall of the left ventricle, but no new focus of infarction. For the usual signs of coagulation necrosis to become evident, the patient would have had to survive the recent MI for

○ A. 20–40 minutes
○ B. 2 hours
○ C. 8–12 hours
○ D. 24–48 hours
○ E. 72 hours

3. A 21-year-old female college student has been uncharacteristically tired for the past 3 days and has fallen asleep in class several times. Enlarged cervical lymph nodes are found on physical examination. Testing of blood samples is most likely to show

○ A. decrease in lymphocyte count
○ B. high titer of IgG antibody to Epstein-Barr virus (EBV)
○ C. high titer of IgM antibody to EBV
○ D. increase in cholesterol levels
○ E. increase in platelet count

185

4. A 4-year-old boy who had developmental delays during infancy now demonstrates social impairment and stereotypies. His language is intact, and he can use age-appropriate self-care skills. Which of the following is the most likely diagnosis?

- ○ A. Asperger's syndrome
- ○ B. Autistic disorder
- ○ C. Childhood disintegrative disorder
- ○ D. Fragile X syndrome
- ○ E. Rett's syndrome

5. A 72-year-old man can speak only with great effort. Although right-handed, he is now unable to use his right arm and hand. This patient most likely has a lesion in which of the labeled areas in the figure below?

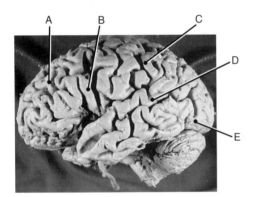

- ○ A. Area A
- ○ B. Area B
- ○ C. Area C
- ○ D. Area D
- ○ E. Area E

6. A 43-year-old woman with a history of intravenous drug abuse is being treated with lamivudine, nevirapine, and indinavir. At a follow-up visit, she says that she feels tired, has frequent night sweats, and has been coughing and having chest pains for 3 months. The cough has recently become productive. A sputum sample shows the presence of acid-fast bacilli. The most appropriate presumptive treatment for this patient would be

- ○ A. azithromycin
- ○ B. isoniazid
- ○ C. rifampin and isoniazid
- ○ D. rifampin, isoniazid, pyrazinamide, and ethambutol
- ○ E. trimethoprim-sulfamethoxazole (TMP-SMX)

7. A 68-year-old man complains of feeling lethargic and mentally confused. Laboratory studies show high plasma creatinine levels, low urinary output, and metabolic acidosis. Radiographic studies show no evidence of renal artery stenosis or inadequate renal perfusion. Which of the following physiologic variables would be closest to the normal range in this patient?

- ○ A. Blood urea nitrogen (BUN)
- ○ B. Glomerular filtration rate (GFR)
- ○ C. Plasma levels of renin
- ○ D. Proton secretion rate
- ○ E. Renal plasma flow (RPF)

8. A 58-year-old woman complains of epigastric pain, weight loss, vomiting of coffee ground–like material, and dark black, sticky stools. Physical examination shows epigastric pain on deep palpation and enlarged, nontender left supraclavicular lymph nodes. Both ovaries are enlarged and firm on bimanual pelvic examination. Test for occult blood in the stool is positive. Which of the following clinical scenarios best explains the signs and symptoms in this patient?

- ○ A. Primary malignant lymphoma of the stomach with ovarian metastasis
- ○ B. Primary ovarian cancer with metastasis to the left supraclavicular lymph nodes
- ○ C. Primary ovarian cancer with metastasis to the stomach
- ○ D. Primary pancreatic cancer with ovarian metastasis
- ○ E. Primary stomach cancer with ovarian metastasis

9. A 42-year-old man weighs over 180 kg (400 lb), primarily because he has an insatiable appetite, loves to cook, and continues to consume a high-fat diet. Which of the following processes would be most likely to occur in the medium-sized arteries and place him at increased risk for a heart attack?

○ A. Excessive secretion of elastin by fibroblasts throughout the intima
○ B. Fibrosis throughout the adventitia
○ C. Local proliferation of endothelial cells
○ D. Local proliferation of smooth muscle cells in the intima and media
○ E. Reduplication of the internal elastic lamina

10. A 29-year-old woman with a cough, dyspnea, and wheezing is found to have eosinophilia. Which of the following organisms is the most likely cause of the disease?

○ A. *Ascaris lumbricoides*
○ B. *Diphyllobothrium latum*
○ C. *Enterobius vermicularis*
○ D. *Taenia saginata*
○ E. *Trichuris trichiura*

11. A 72-year-old man is embarrassed by unexpected dribbling of urine. During voluntary urination, he produces only a weak urine stream. A cystometrogram shows suppressed bladder tonus at 300 mL volume, a lack of spontaneous micturition contractions when the bladder volume is 500 mL, and fluid eventually leaking around the catheter when the volume exceeds 700 mL. He experiences no discomfort during the entire test. Which of the following mechanisms best explains this patient's condition?

○ A. Pelvic afferents from the bladder are nonfunctional
○ B. Pontine descending inhibitory inputs are blocked
○ C. Psychological factors dominate the loss of bladder control
○ D. Pudendal nerve efferents to the external sphincter are severed
○ E. Sympathetic innervation of the bladder via the hypogastric nerve is disrupted

12. A 33-year-old woman with HIV infection says she has had severe headaches for the past several days. There is no evidence of focal neurologic deficits. Blood tests and chest x-rays are unremarkable. A cerebrospinal fluid sample shows a cryptococcal antigen titer of 1:28. Which drug would provide appropriate therapy directed against the synthesis of ergosterol?

○ A. Amphotericin B
○ B. Fluconazole
○ C. Flucytosine
○ D. Griseofulvin
○ E. Ketoconazole

13. A 54-year-old man with a history of gastroesophageal reflex disease (GERD) is prescribed a proton pump inhibitor. He says he cannot afford the medication and is unable to adhere to the recommended treatment regimen but instead relies on over-the-counter medications such as antacids and herbal remedies. Brush cytology of the esophagus shows marked reactive changes of the squamous cells as well as the presence of reactive glandular cells consistent with origin in the body of the stomach. This patient is most seriously at risk of developing

○ A. adenocarcinoma
○ B. esophageal candidiasis
○ C. esophageal stenosis
○ D. esophageal varices
○ E. ulceration of the esophageal mucosa

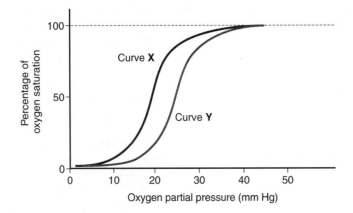

14. The figure above shows two curves for oxygen binding to hemoglobin. *Curve Y* represents the findings in a healthy individual under normal conditions, and *curve X* represents the findings in which of the following?

○ A. Healthy individual living in the high Rocky Mountains
○ B. Patient with chronic anemia
○ C. Patient with increased levels of 2,3-bisphosphoglycerate
○ D. Patient with obstructive pulmonary emphysema
○ E. Patient who is depleted of 2,3-bisphosphoglycerate

15. A 31-year-old man complains of left unilateral ptosis and pupillary constriction in the left eye. Which of the following should be considered when developing a differential diagnosis?

○ A. Destruction of celiac ganglion
○ B. Destruction of postganglionic neurons in the ciliary ganglion
○ C. Loss of innervation of the superior tarsal muscle (Muller's muscle)
○ D. Mesothelioma of the diaphragmatic surface of the left lung
○ E. Papilledema of the left optic disc

16. A 3-year-old girl has pharyngitis, a fever, and vesicular lesions distributed throughout her mouth. A Tzanck smear of material from the base of a lesion yields positive results. Which of the following agents is the most likely cause of the disease?

○ A. Coxsackievirus A2
○ B. Coxsackievirus A16
○ C. Enterovirus 71
○ D. Herpes simplex virus 1
○ E. Mumps virus

17. A 60-year-old man with a history of liver disease complains of chronic skin lesions. Physical examination shows blisters and pigmented scarring on his arms and other body parts that are exposed to sunlight. The patient's urine sample has a light brown color. Urinalysis would be most likely to indicate an elevated level of

○ A. γ-aminolevulinic acid
○ B. bilirubin
○ C. porphobilinogen
○ D. urobilinogen
○ E. uroporphyrinogen

18. A 16-year-old boy is found to have hypogonadotropic hypogonadism, extreme obesity, and cor pulmonale. His history indicates that at 14 months of age, he had short stature for his age, upslanting, almond-shaped eyes, and full cheeks; and at 7 years of age, his IQ was 50 and he was a voracious eater. This patient most likely has which of the following disorders?

○ A. Growth hormone–secreting tumor
○ B. Pheochromocytoma
○ C. Prader-Willi syndrome
○ D. Sturge-Weber syndrome
○ E. Williams syndrome

19. A highly agitated 23-year-old woman is admitted to a psychiatric unit complaining that "dead people" are telling her that she is going to be buried alive. She also claims that Tom Brokaw has been reading her mind and telling everyone her intimate secrets on the "NBC Nightly News." Organic causes for the patient's behavior are ruled out, and a thorough psychiatric evaluation indicates that her current behavior did not arise secondary to a mood disorder. The patient is treated with a drug considered to be appropriate for her condition. Two days later, she complains of severe pain in the eyes and neck and is found to have a fixed upward gaze and a twisting upward torsion of the head. Treatment with which drug would most likely cause the patient's eye and neck problems?

○ A. Amitriptyline
○ B. Chlorpromazine
○ C. Fluphenazine
○ D. Lithium
○ E. Risperidone

20. A 62-year-old man who has smoked three packs of cigarettes daily for 40 years has shortness of breath on exertion. He is thin with a slightly expanded barrel-shaped chest and ribs that tend to be somewhat horizontal. He breathes through pursed lips. He is not cyanotic. Forced expiratory volume in 1 second (FEV_1) is 16% of predicted value. His oxygen saturation is 80%. Which of the following is the most likely cause of this patient's reduced FEV_1?

○ A. Airway obstruction due to a reduction in elastic recoil of the lung
○ B. Airway obstruction due to severe bronchospasm
○ C. Bronchiolar obstruction due to mucous gland hyperplasia and mucous secretion
○ D. Inability to adequately use accessory muscles of respiration in expiration
○ E. Ventilation/perfusion ratio <1.0

21. Laboratory studies indicate that two patients are carriers of *Helicobacter pylori*. Patient X has signs and symptoms consistent with peptic ulcer disease, while patient Y has no physical complaints. In managing these two patients, the physician should

○ A. treat each patient with a single antibiotic
○ B. treat each patient with combination antibiotic therapy
○ C. treat patient X with a single antibiotic and monitor patient Y
○ D. treat patient X with an acid blocker and monitor patient Y
○ E. treat patient X with combination antibiotic therapy and monitor patient Y

22. A routine eye examination of a 31-year-old woman shows an elevated intraocular pressure in both eyes and cupping of both optic discs. The patient is diagnosed with primary open-angle glaucoma. A direct-acting cholinomimetic drug useful for this condition is

○ A. atropine
○ B. dipivefrin
○ C. echothiophate
○ D. pilocarpine
○ E. timolol

23. Respiratory distress syndrome (RDS) commonly causes death in premature infants because at least one cell type in the lung is incompletely differentiated when infants are born prematurely. Which of the following cell types is incompletely differentiated?

- ○ A. Alveolar macrophage
- ○ B. Goblet cell
- ○ C. Granule cell
- ○ D. Type I pneumocyte
- ○ E. Type II pneumocyte

24. A 68-year-old man complains of steadily decreasing mobility. When asked to walk, he takes very short steps and often freezes when he attempts to turn. The physician notes that the patient's blink rate is decreased. The most likely cause of these findings is

- ○ A. decreased output from the putamen to the globus pallidus externa
- ○ B. decreased output from the substantia nigra pars reticulata to the ventrolateral nucleus
- ○ C. decreased output from the subthalamic nucleus to the internal segment of the globus pallidus
- ○ D. decreased output from the ventrolateral nucleus to the cerebral cortex
- ○ E. increased output from the putamen to the substantia nigra pars reticulata

25. A 28-year-old woman consults her physician because she has been experiencing involuntary muscle contractions in the vagina that prohibit sexual intercourse with her husband. This disorder would be classified in which of the following categories of sexual dysfunction?

- ○ A. Orgasm disorders
- ○ B. Paraphilias
- ○ C. Sexual arousal disorders
- ○ D. Sexual desire disorders
- ○ E. Sexual pain disorders

26. A 51-year-old man with a history of alcoholism and Wernicke-Korsakoff syndrome is taken to the hospital suffering from confusion and oculomotor disturbances. He is found to have severe dehydration and is treated intravenously with dextrose solution. After treatment is initiated, his symptoms become worse. The most likely explanation for this response is

- ○ A. alcohol oxidation is under tight control, and control is lost when dextrose or other sugars are introduced
- ○ B. dextrose infusion can cause lactic acidosis and thereby worsen the patient's condition
- ○ C. the patient has an inherited form of dextrose intolerance
- ○ D. the patient has been taking disulfiram to help him abstain from alcohol, and he should not have been given any intravenous fluids
- ○ E. the patient is suffering from ethanol poisoning, and dextrose competes with ethanol for the same enzymes to reverse the poisoning

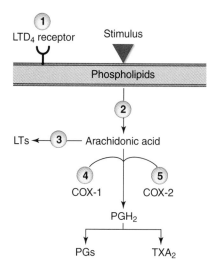

Abbreviations: LT = leukotriene; COX = cyclooxygenase; PG = prostaglandin; and TX = thromboxane.

27. In the figure above, the numbers 1 through 5 represent potential sites of action for drugs that affect eicosanoid metabolism. When aspirin is used in the management of rheumatoid arthritis, its efficacy is attributed to an action at

○ A. site 1
○ B. site 2
○ C. site 3
○ D. site 4
○ E. site 5

28. A 7-year-old boy has a high fever and dysentery. Microscopic examination of a stool sample shows the presence of leukocytes and a preponderance of curved rods. Which of the following organisms is the most likely cause of the disease?

○ A. *Campylobacter jejuni*
○ B. *Clostridium difficile*
○ C. Enteroinvasive *Escherichia coli*
○ D. *Shigella flexneri*
○ E. *Vibrio cholerae*

29. A 28-year-old man has a family history of sudden cardiac death at a young age (<45 years of age). Physical examination shows a systolic murmur that decreases in intensity when the patient is lying down and increases in intensity when he is sitting up. An echocardiogram shows abnormal movement of the anterior mitral valve leaflet against an asymmetrically thickened interventricular septum. The mechanism for sudden cardiac death in this patient's family is most closely attributed to which of the following conditions?

○ A. Acute myocardial infarction (MI)
○ B. Congenital bicuspid aortic valve
○ C. Conduction system defects
○ D. Dissecting aortic aneurysm
○ E. Mitral valve prolapse

30. When evaluating a 67-year-old woman for dementia, the physician conducts a thorough examination of all elements of memory. Which of the following statements is most appropriate to ask this patient to measure remote memory?

○ A. Name the last four presidents of the United States
○ B. Repeat after me, "No ifs, ands, or buts"
○ C. Starting with the number 100, count backwards by 7s
○ D. State the day, month, year, and time of day
○ E. Tell me how a cat and a dog are alike

31. A 24-year-old bicyclist severely injures his right leg after colliding with an automobile. He is hemorrhaging from the wound but is stabilized, with a blood pressure of 90/40 mm Hg and a heart rate of 100/min. He was not wearing protective head gear at the time of the accident but shows no evidence of head trauma. His breathing is rapid and shallow. Blood pressure and urine flow could best be improved in this patient by

○ A. administration of an oral diuretic
○ B. administration of physiologic saline solution
○ C. blood transfusion
○ D. indirect cardiac massage
○ E. intravenous injection of norepinephrine

32. A pregnant woman contracted rubella (German measles) at approximately 8 weeks' gestation. Which malformation resulting from this infection may be found in her infant?

○ A. Detachment of the retina
○ B. Discoloration of permanent teeth
○ C. Failure of the cochlea and spiral ganglia to develop
○ D. Failure of the semicircular canals to develop
○ E. Pulmonary stenosis

33. A 23-year-old man had his third injection of hepatitis B vaccine, and the next day he says that his arm is sore. He says that he experienced some pain after the first injection, more pain after the second, and the most pain after the third. This progression is most likely the result of

○ A. allergic reaction to a component of the vaccine
○ B. tissue destruction associated with any injection
○ C. type I hypersensitivity reaction
○ D. type II hypersensitivity reaction
○ E. type III hypersensitivity reaction

34. A 35-year-old woman complains of progressive muscle weakness that has lasted for the past 2 months. Her symptoms usually begin in the face and throat and have not been accompanied by muscle atrophy. Based on these symptoms, which type of receptor would most likely be affected?

○ A. Cholinergic
○ B. Dopaminergic
○ C. GABAergic
○ D. Glutaminergic
○ E. Serotonergic

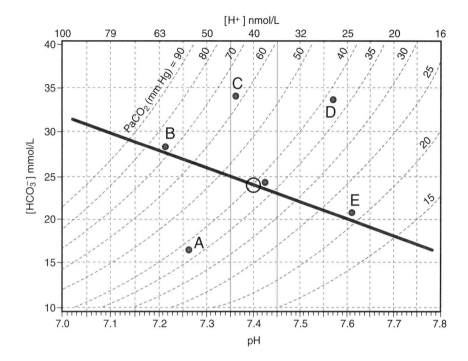

35. An arterial blood sample (filled circle near the center of the Davenport diagram above) is obtained from a hospitalized patient who has been on a ventilator for 2 weeks because of severe chronic obstructive pulmonary disease (COPD). A few minutes after the sample was taken, the respirator failed. Within 30 seconds, the tubing was disconnected, but the patient's breathing was notably labored. A second arterial blood sample was taken within 5 minutes after the tubing was removed. Which point on the diagram above (letters A-E) is consistent with the acid-base relationship in the second blood sample?

○ A. Point A
○ B. Point B
○ C. Point C
○ D. Point D
○ E. Point E

36. A 45-year-old woman complains of weight gain, thirst, polyuria, and leg weakness. Physical examination shows hypertension; obesity in the face, neck, trunk, and abdomen; red-purple striae over the abdomen and breasts; and hirsutism over the face, abdomen, and breasts. A glucose tolerance test is abnormal. Measurement of free cortisol in a 24-hour urine specimen shows excess cortisol excretion. She undergoes a dexamethasone suppression test, and serum cortisol levels are measured the following morning. Which of the following results would be expected in this patient?

○ A. Decreased serum cortisol and below normal serum adrenocorticotrophic hormone (ACTH)
○ B. Elevated corticotrophin-releasing hormone (CRH), low ACTH, and unaffected serum cortisol
○ C. Elevated serum cortisol and serum ACTH
○ D. Increased serum ACTH
○ E. Low serum CRH and ACTH and increased serum cortisol

37. When a 5-year-old girl returns from a day-care center, her cheeks look intensely red as if they had been slapped. The mother suspects child abuse and takes her to a pediatric clinic. Examination of the girl shows a slight fever, intense erythema on the cheeks, and a blanching, lacy, reticulate maculopapular rash on the upper extremities. The most likely diagnosis is

○ A. child abuse with hand-foot-and-mouth disease
○ B. child abuse with heat rash
○ C. erythema infectiosum
○ D. exanthema subitum
○ E. measles

38. A 69-year-old man complains of episodes of "squeezing" substernal chest pain, which began 3 weeks ago and occur when he physically exerts himself. He says that he sometimes feels the pain in his jaw, and it often radiates down his left arm. After thorough evaluation, he is diagnosed with chronic stable angina (exertional angina) and instructed to take nitroglycerin. The mechanism by which nitroglycerin exerts its beneficial effects in angina is by

○ A. blocking α_1-adrenergic receptors and reducing myocardial oxygen consumption by decreasing cardiac preload and afterload
○ B. blocking β_1-adrenergic receptors and reducing myocardial oxygen consumption by preventing an increase in heart rate and contractility
○ C. blocking slow Ca^{2+} channels and reducing myocardial oxygen consumption by decreasing cardiac contractility, heart rate, and arterial pressure
○ D. causing smooth muscle relaxation by stimulating the formation of nitric oxide, thereby causing an increase in the level of cyclic guanosine monophosphate (cGMP)
○ E. preventing platelet aggregation by inhibiting platelet cyclooxygenase activity

39. A 40-year-old man has a 4-month history of unilateral headaches accompanied by miosis, ptosis, lacrimation, rhinorrhea, and eyelid edema. His headaches occur 1 to 8 times a day and last 15 minutes to 2 hours. They also occur within 45 minutes after he consumes alcohol. Which of the following conditions is the most likely diagnosis?

○ A. Atypical facial pain
○ B. Cervicogenic headache
○ C. Cluster headache
○ D. Temporal arteritis
○ E. Trigeminal neuralgia

40. Physical examination of a 22-year-old woman with leg pain shows a mass in the proximal aspect of the anterior thigh in the lateral aspect of the femoral triangle. The mass appears to lie within the anterior fascia of the iliacus muscle as the muscle passes posterior to the inguinal ligament. It is putting pressure on specific structures of the femoral triangle. Which of the following would most likely be associated with these findings?

○ A. Loss of extension of the leg
○ B. Necrosis of the femoral head
○ C. Occlusion of the femoral vein
○ D. Paralysis of the adductor muscles of the thigh
○ E. Weakness of extension of the hip

41. An 8-year-old boy has a defect in the extracellular steps of collagen synthesis. Which of the following processes is most likely to be impaired in this patient?

○ A. Cleavage of terminal propeptides from procollagen
○ B. Degradation of improperly coiled collagen molecules
○ C. Formation of interchain and intrachain disulfide bonds
○ D. Glycosylation of selected hydroxylysines
○ E. Hydroxylation of prolines and lysines

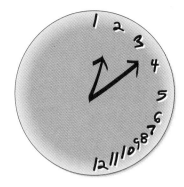

42. A patient undergoing a neurologic examination is asked to illustrate 2:20 PM on a clock face. Which of the following deficits is reflected in this patient's drawing (see figure above)?

○ A. Central dysarthria
○ B. Constructional apraxia
○ C. Parietal agraphia
○ D. Spatial neglect
○ E. Visual agnosia

43. A 25-year-old man who sustains facial injuries in a bar brawl waits 1 week before seeking medical care. He is found to have inflamed gums and sinus tracts that drain to the exterior of his cheek. A Gram stain of exudate from the draining tract is most likely to show

○ A. gram-negative diplococci
○ B. gram-negative rods
○ C. gram-positive cocci in chains
○ D. gram-positive cocci in clusters
○ E. gram-positive filamentous rods

44. A 75-year-old woman slipped and fell on her hand while getting off the train. X-ray examination shows a fracture of the surgical neck of the humerus, which may have resulted in laceration of the nerve from the posterior cord of the brachial plexus. Which of the following deficits may occur as a result of this injury?

○ A. Impaired abduction of the shoulder
○ B. Inability to flex the elbow
○ C. Loss of sensation over the lateral side of the forearm
○ D. Loss of sensation over the medial side of the forearm
○ E. Weakness of pronation

45. A febrile 12-year-old boy complains of joint pains and abdominal pain with associated bloody stools, which began 1 week after an upper respiratory tract infection. Physical examination shows a palpable purpuric rash limited to the buttocks and lower extremities. Laboratory studies show occult blood in the stool, red blood cells (RBCs) and RBC casts in the urine, mild proteinuria, and a normal complete blood cell count. Which of the following mechanisms is most closely associated with this patient's condition?

○ A. Genetic vascular disorder
○ B. Immunocomplex vasculitis
○ C. Infectious type of vasculitis
○ D. Previous group A streptococcal infection
○ E. Type II hypersensitivity vasculitis

46. A 60-year-old man develops sepsis after undergoing choledocholithotomy and choledochoduodenostomy. Therapy appropriate for a mixed aerobic and gram-negative infection is instituted. The patient then experiences several side effects, including muscular weakness, dysphagia, dysarthria, ataxia, and vertigo. Which drug was most likely used to treat the patient's mixed infection?

○ A. Aztreonam
○ B. Ceftriaxone
○ C. Gentamicin
○ D. Metronidazole
○ E. Piperacillin

47. A 2-year-old girl with a history of severe hypoglycemia, vomiting, and jaundice undergoes oral tolerance tests for several disaccharides. The tests show that her metabolism of lactose and maltose is normal, but her metabolism of saccharose is abnormal. The girl most likely has a deficiency of

○ A. aldolase
○ B. fructokinase
○ C. fructose-1,6-bisphosphatase
○ D. hexokinase
○ E. phosphofructokinase

48. A 33-year-old man with no previous psychiatric history has just discovered that his sexual partner has AIDS. He immediately asks to be tested for HIV and tells his physician that he intends to commit suicide if the test is positive. Which of the following is the most ethical action for the physician to take?

○ A. Conduct the requested test and report the results regardless of findings
○ B. Initiate proceedings for involuntary psychiatric hospitalization
○ C. Provide HIV/AIDS counseling and education and initiate testing
○ D. Provide HIV/AIDS counseling and education and postpone testing
○ E. Refuse to conduct the HIV test and discontinue the interview

49. An afebrile 72-year-old man has fatigue and substernal chest pain with exertion that is relieved by resting. Physical examination shows a blood pressure of 110/88 mm Hg, pulse of 102/min, pale conjunctiva and palmar creases, and a grade IV systolic ejection murmur heard best in the right second intercostal space. The murmur radiates into the carotid arteries and increases in intensity with expiration. Laboratory studies show:

Hemoglobin	7.0 g/dL
Leukocyte count	6500/mm^3
Mean corpuscular volume (MCV)	77 μm^3
Platelet count	580,000/mm^3
Partial thromboplastin time (activated, aPTT)	Normal
Prothrombin time (PT)	Normal
Reticulocyte count, corrected	4%
Direct Coombs' test	Negative
Urine dipstick	Positive for blood

The peripheral smear shows numerous schistocytes (fragmented red blood cells, RBCs). RBCs are not present in the sediment. Which of the following mechanisms best explains these clinical and laboratory findings?

○ A. Autoimmune destruction of RBCs
○ B. Disseminated intravascular coagulation (DIC)
○ C. Genetic defect in the RBC membrane
○ D. Iron deficiency unrelated to the valvular defect
○ E. Valvular defect leading to intravascular hemolysis

50. A 51-year-old woman requires drug therapy for major depression. Her records indicate that she is currently being treated with guanethidine for hypertension. Which agent would be appropriate for the patient's mood disorder but would most likely interfere with or antagonize her antihypertensive therapy?

○ A. Carbamazepine
○ B. Haloperidol
○ C. Midazolam
○ D. Nortriptyline
○ E. Sertraline

ANSWERS AND DISCUSSIONS

1. **A** (consider adding a second oral agent) is correct. Type 2 diabetes mellitus is a progressive disease, and individuals with a 10-year history of the disease commonly require treatment with more than one agent.

   B (continue the diet and exercise program for 3 more months) is incorrect. It has already been demonstrated that diet, exercise, and a sulfonylurea agent are inadequate for the control of diabetes mellitus in this patient. Further observation with the same treatment would be inappropriate.

   C (monitor blood pressure for 24 hours) is incorrect. The blood pressure reading obtained during the initial clinic visit indicates that her blood pressure is adequately controlled. Thus, it would be inappropriate to order 24-hour blood pressure monitoring. An angiotensin-converting enzyme (ACE) inhibitor would be the drug of choice to control the patient's blood pressure, since these drugs have both cardiovascular and renal benefits.

   D (obtain a 24-hour urine output to determine the calcium level) is incorrect. Nothing (other than the patient's sex and age) indicates the possibility of calcium or bone dysfunction. Therefore, there is no reason to obtain a 24-hour urine output for calcium.

   E (order a series of pancreatic function tests) is incorrect. This would be justified if there were evidence of diminished insulin production or signs that the patient had type 1 diabetes mellitus. However, the patient has a long history of controlling blood glucose with a single oral agent, which is consistent with type 2 diabetics. At this point, she is more likely to need a change in her blood pressure medication as well as the addition of a second oral agent to control the diabetes and its complications (cardiovascular abnormalities, peripheral neuropathy, and vision problems) that were detected during her most recent examination.

2. **C** (8–12 hours) is correct. The typical signs of coagulative necrosis, including nuclear pyknosis, karyolysis, karyorrhexis, and increased cytoplasmic eosinophilia, appear 8–12 hours after infarction occurs.

   A (20–40 minutes) is incorrect. The changes that occur in such a short period of time are only ultrastructural (e.g., mitochondrial swelling).

   B (2 hours) is incorrect. In 2 hours, a few "wavy" fibers are visible at the margin of the infarct.

   D (24–48 hours) is incorrect. At 24 hours, both the microscopic and gross changes of necrosis would be discernible. At 48 hours, an influx of neutrophils would also be present.

E   (72 hours) is incorrect. At 72 hours, the influx of neutrophils would be at its height, and signs of dissolution of the necrotic heart muscle would be evident.

3. *C*   (high titer of IgM antibody to Epstein-Barr virus) is correct. Acute infectious mononucleosis occurs most frequently in adolescents and young adults. The patient most often has malaise and lymphadenopathy; acute infection is characterized by a high titer of IgM antibody to Epstein-Barr virus (human herpesvirus 4).

A   (decrease in lymphocyte count) is incorrect. In patients with acute infectious mononucleosis, the lymphocyte count is usually increased, rather than decreased.
B   (high titer of IgG antibody to Epstein-Barr virus) is incorrect. Titers of IgG antibody to Epstein-Barr virus are not increased during the acute phase of infectious mononucleosis. As discussed, titers of IgM antibody are increased.
D   (increase in cholesterol levels) and E (increase in platelet count) are incorrect. In infectious mononucleosis, there is no increase in cholesterol levels or in the platelet count.

4. *A*   (Asperger's syndrome) is correct. A 4-year-old boy who demonstrates social impairment and stereotypies with language intact most likely has Asperger's syndrome. Asperger's syndrome is similar to autistic disorder since developmental delays are associated with both conditions. Social impairment, stereotypies, and a restricted repertoire of activities characterize both conditions. However, in patients with Asperger's syndrome, language skills are preserved.

B   (autistic disorder) is incorrect. Children with autistic disorder display impairments in social interactions and communication and show either a restricted range of activities or stereotypies. Onset of the disorder occurs before 3 years of age, with abnormalities in development usually noted before 6 months of age.
C   (childhood disintegrative disorder) is incorrect. In childhood disintegrative disorder, normal development occurs for at least 2 years, followed by a functional decline prior to age 10. Abnormalities are seen in social interactions, communication, and behavior.
D   (fragile X syndrome) is incorrect. The first evidence of fragile X syndrome usually appears after 2 years of age. Affected children usually show physical abnormalities, including elongated faces, large ears, prominent foreheads, midfacial hypoplasia, protruding jaws, and hands that hyperextend. Varying degrees of mental impairment accompany the disorder.
E   (Rett's syndrome) is incorrect. Rett's syndrome is a rare X-linked syndrome seen only in females. Deficits usually develop after 5 months of normal development. Progressive deterioration ensues, and death typically occurs prior to adolescence.

5. *B* (area B, precentral gyrus and Broca's area) is correct. The patient has a lesion involving Broca's area, which provides motor information required for speech. The lesion lies approximately midway between the circumferential midline and the most superior aspect of the postcentral gyrus, placing it in the portion of the motor homunculus that regulates movement in the hands. When Broca's area is affected, the lesion will be on the left side of the brain in about 95% of patients. Since most corticospinal fibers project to the contralateral spinal cord, this lesion could also account for the paralysis in the patient's right arm and hand.

A (area A, prefrontal association area) is incorrect. Association areas are concerned with functions of a higher order than the primary motor activity described for this patient.
C (area C, posterior parietal lobe) is incorrect. The posterior parietal cortex coordinates somatic sensation and vision and integrates these perceptions with movement. It is not a primary motor area; therefore, it does not control speech or arm movement.
D (area D, Wernicke's area) is incorrect. Damage to this area results in Wernicke's aphasia, which is characterized by impaired comprehension (rather than execution) of speech. This is not a primary motor area; therefore, it does not regulate motor activity required for speech or arm movement.
E (area E, occipital lobe) is incorrect. The occipital cortex receives information about vision. It is a sensory area, not a primary motor area. Therefore, lesions in this area will not affect motor activity required to move the arm or to speak.

6. *D* (rifampin, isoniazid, pyrazinamide, and ethambutol) is correct. Treatment with lamivudine, nevirapine, and indinavir indicates that the patient is infected with HIV. Chest pains and other recent symptoms and laboratory results are consistent with a diagnosis of active tuberculosis (TB) caused by *Mycobacterium tuberculosis.* A patient who is HIV-positive and has a history of intravenous drug abuse is at increased risk of infection with drug-resistant strains of *M. tuberculosis,* so initial therapy for this patient should include **r**ifampin, **i**soniazid, **p**yrazinamide, and **e**thambutol (**RIPE** therapy).

A (azithromycin) is incorrect. Azithromycin is ineffective against *M. tuberculosis* but is used frequently to treat pneumonia caused by *Chlamydia* species, *Legionella pneumophila,* or *Mycoplasma pneumoniae.* Azithromycin and other macrolides are also active against the *Mycobacterium avium-intracellulare* complex (MAC) and are used in combination with either rifampin or ethambutol to treat MAC diseases.
B (isoniazid) is incorrect. Single-drug therapy is inappropriate for the treatment of TB. However, single-drug therapy with isoniazid can be used for the prevention of TB in individuals who are

considered at risk for the disease but have no known or suspected resistance to isoniazid.

C (rifampin and isoniazid) is incorrect. Treatment with rifampin plus isoniazid is not appropriate for the patient described, but it is appropriate for patients in whom the infecting strain of *M. tuberculosis* is unlikely to be a drug-resistant strain.

E (trimethroprim-sulfamethoxazole) is incorrect. TMP-SMX is ineffective against *M. tuberculosis*. It is frequently used to treat *Pneumocystis carinii* pneumonia in patients with AIDS. The presenting symptoms of *P. carinii* pneumonia include fever, chest pain, and a nonproductive cough.

7. *E* (renal plasma flow) is correct. The patient's symptoms are consistent with poor tubular flow and decreased urinary output (e.g., due to glomerular nephritis), which results in the accumulation in plasma of substances normally cleared by the glomerular apparatus—including creatinine, H^+ ions (leading to metabolic acidosis), and urea (leading to mental confusion). The lack of renal artery stenosis or reduced renal perfusion suggests that RPF is adequate in this patient. Therefore, a decrease in the filtration fraction (GFR/RPF) is much more likely to be responsible for the accumulation of substances in the blood than inadequate blood flow to the kidneys.

A (blood urea nitrogen) is incorrect. When the GFR is compromised, all major substances that are normally filtered by the glomerular apparatus, including urea, accumulate in plasma. Therefore, the BUN would be expected to rise.

B (glomerular filtration rate) is incorrect. The elevated creatinine level suggests that the creatinine clearance rate is inadequate. This, in addition to the low tubular flow rate, is consistent with a suppressed GFR.

C (plasma levels of renin) is incorrect. A low tubular flow rate, which is suggested by the increased concentration of creatinine in plasma, would induce the release of renin from the juxtaglomerular apparatus. Renin, in turn, would initiate the pathway leading to the release of aldosterone to adjust the blood pressure to increase tubular flow. Therefore, plasma levels of renin would be elevated.

D (proton secretion rate) is incorrect. H^+ ions normally are secreted, not reabsorbed. With a fall in GFR, the decreased tubular flow cannot carry sufficient H^+, causing it to back up in the blood and cause metabolic acidosis.

8. *E* (primary stomach cancer with ovarian metastasis) is correct. The patient has a primary stomach cancer that has metastasized hematogenously to both ovaries (called Krukenberg tumors). Stomach cancer is the most common primary site for metastasis to the left supraclavicular nodes. The signet-ring cell type of stomach cancer usually is associated with Krukenberg tumors of the ovaries. This high-grade cancer diffusely infiltrates the wall of the stomach, giving it a firm, nonpliable consistency, hence

the term "linitis plastica" or "leather bottle" stomach. Signet-ring cells are malignant cells filled with mucin; the mucin pushes the nucleus to the periphery of the cell, giving the cell a signet-ring appearance.

A (primary malignant lymphoma of the stomach with ovarian metastasis) is incorrect. Gastric lymphomas are uncommon and rarely metastasize to the ovaries.
B (primary ovarian cancer with metastasis to the left supraclavicular lymph nodes) is incorrect. This does not explain the patient's epigastric distress and black, tarry stools.
C (primary ovarian cancer with metastasis to the stomach) is incorrect. Ovarian cancers rarely metastasize to the stomach or to the left supraclavicular lymph nodes.
D (primary pancreatic cancer with ovarian metastasis) is incorrect. Most pancreatic cancers involve the head of the pancreas and are associated with obstructive jaundice and light-colored stools. Pain usually radiates to the back, because the pancreas is retroperitoneal. Pancreatic cancers do metastasize to the left supraclavicular lymph nodes.

9. **D** (local proliferation of smooth muscle cells in the intima and media) is correct. Medium-sized arteries, such as the anterior descending interventricular artery, are rich in intimal foam cells and smooth muscle cells. These smooth muscle cells are induced to divide in atherosclerosis. This is one of the major reasons why the intima thickens in patients who eat a diet high in fats.

A (excessive secretion of elastin by fibroblasts throughout the intima) is incorrect. There is very little elastin in the intima of blood vessels, especially medium-sized arteries.
B (fibrosis throughout the adventitia) is incorrect. Chronic vascular disease seldom affects the adventitia of blood vessels.
C (local proliferation of endothelial cells) is incorrect. Endothelial cells are damaged, but they do not proliferate in response to this type of injury.
E (reduplication of the internal elastic lamina) is incorrect. Reduplication of the elastic lamina is a normal consequence of aging.

10. **A** *(Ascaris lumbricoides)* is correct. *A. lumbricoides* is a free-swimming nematode. Migration of its larvae to the lungs of infected persons can produce the respiratory tract symptoms described, and the heavy antigenic burden results in eosinophilia. Ascaris is prevalent in areas where sanitation is poor and where human feces is used as a fertilizer. The disease is transmitted by food contaminated with soil containing the eggs. Although the disease occurs worldwide, it is endemic in the tropics. Humans are the only hosts.

B *(Diphyllobothrium latum)* and D *(Taenia saginata)* are incorrect. *D. latum* and *T. saginata* are tapeworms that can cause eosinophilia but do not generally produce respiratory tract symptoms.

C *(Enterobius vermicularis)* is incorrect. *E. vermicularis* is called the pinworm. It is not associated with respiratory tract symptoms.
E *(Trichuris trichiura)* is incorrect. *T. trichiura* is called the whipworm. Although eosinophilia may be present in patients with whipworm infection, there are few if any associated respiratory tract problems.

11. *A* (pelvic afferents from the bladder are nonfunctional) is correct. Poor innervation is suggested by the flaccid or atonic bladder and the fact that the patient can hold large volumes of urine without pain. The latter symptom points specifically to denervation of sensory afferent nerves. "Dribbling" also suggests abnormal neural activity, specifically the lack of an operative micturition reflex, which makes it impossible to excrete urine, except by overflow dribbling at higher bladder volumes and pressures. Bladder stimulation techniques will provide the best solution to this patient's problem. An alternative is urine drainage by urethral/bladder catheterization; however, abdominal pressure would have to be raised to help collapse the bladder.

B (pontine descending inhibitory inputs are blocked) is incorrect. Blocked descending inputs from the brainstem may play a role in this patient's inability to produce a stream of urine, but would not suppress bladder tone or spontaneous micturition contractions.
C (psychological factors dominate in the loss of bladder control) is incorrect. Psychological factors are rejected because the micturition reflex can be neither voluntarily nor involuntarily suppressed.
D (pudendal nerve efferents to the external sphincter are severed) and E (sympathetic innervation of the bladder via the hypogastric nerve is disrupted) are incorrect. Impaired functioning of pudendal nerves or disrupted sympathetic efferents are each precluded as a cause of the patient's symptoms because they have little effect on the micturition reflex, the lack of which may explain the loss of bladder tonus and suppressed bladder sensation.

12. *B* (fluconazole) is correct. The patient's symptoms and laboratory findings are consistent with cryptococcal meningitis, a disease that occurs primarily in HIV-positive and other immunocompromised individuals. The patient's low cryptococcal antigen titer and lack of neurologic deficits portend a good outcome if appropriate treatment is instituted. Azole antifungals act by inhibiting 14α-demethylase (a fungal P450 enzyme), thereby blocking the conversion of lanosterol to ergosterol. Unlike other azole drugs, fluconazole is able to penetrate the cerebrospinal fluid (CSF) well, causing the drug level in the CSF to become as high as 50%–90% of the drug level in the plasma.

A (amphotericin B) is incorrect. Amphotericin B is a polyene antifungal agent that acts by binding to ergosterol and forming pores or channels. This results in leakage of the intracellular contents of the fungus. Although amphotericin B does not penetrate the CSF, it is formulated for intrathecal use and can be employed to treat serious fungal meningeal infections.

C (flucytosine) is incorrect. Flucytosine is not directed against the synthesis of ergosterol. Flucytosine is a prodrug that is converted by fungal cytosine deaminase to 5-fluorouracil (5-FU). The 5-FU is in turn converted to 5-fluorodeoxyuridine monophosphate (5-FdUMP) and 5-fluorodeoxyuridine triphosphate (5-FdUTP). The 5-FdUMP inhibits thymidylate synthase and thereby blocks DNA synthesis, whereas the FdUTP inhibits RNA synthesis.

D (griseofulvin) is incorrect. Griseofulvin is inactive against *Cryptococcus neoformans* and is used to treat dermatophytoses (such as tinea corporis and tinea capitis).

E (ketoconazole) is incorrect. Ketoconazole acts in the same manner as fluconazole, but it has no CSF bioavailability and is not available in an intrathecal formulation. Consequently, it would not be appropriate for the management of cryptococcal meningitis.

13. *A* (adenocarcinoma) is correct. The presence of glandular cells in the esophageal brushing indicates that the patient has glandular metaplasia of the esophageal mucosa, or Barrett's esophagus (metaplastic columnar epithelium), a complication of chronic GERD. Adenocarcinoma of the esophagus is 30–40 times more likely to occur in patients with Barrett's esophagus.

B (esophageal candidiasis) is incorrect. Esophageal candidiasis is not a complication of GERD or Barrett's esophagus. It would tend to be found in immunocompromised or debilitated patients.

C (esophageal stenosis) is incorrect. Although esophageal stenosis is a frequent complication of GERD and Barrett's esophagus, it is not a life-threatening condition.

D (esophageal varices) is incorrect. Development of varices is not a complication of GERD.

E (ulceration of the esophageal mucosa) is incorrect. Although ulceration of the esophageal mucosa is not an uncommon complication of GERD or Barrett's esophagus, it is not life threatening unless serious bleeding, an unusual event, occurs.

14. *E* (patient who is depleted of 2,3-bisphosphoglycerate) is correct. In normal blood cells, 2,3-bisphosphoglycerate (2,3-BPG) binds to the T conformation of hemoglobin and stabilizes it. The T conformation has a low oxygen-binding affinity, and the 2,3-BPG is a negative allosteric effector. The 2,3-BPG does not affect oxygenation in the lung, but it enhances unloading of oxygen in tissues. Therefore, a decreased level of 2,3-BPG shifts the curve to the left. Transfusions with blood stored in acid-citrate dextrose can result in 2,3-BPG depletion.

A (healthy individual living in the high Rocky Mountains), B (patient with chronic anemia), C (patient with increased levels of 2,3-bisphosphoglycerate), and D (patient with obstructive pulmonary emphysema) are incorrect. Any circumstance or condition that increases the 2,3-BPG level would shift the curve to the right. The 2,3-BPG level is increased in healthy individuals who have adapted to a high altitude, and it is also increased in patients with chronic anemia or obstructive pulmonary emphysema.

15. *C* (loss of innervation of the superior tarsal muscle) is correct. Carcinoma in the apex of the left lung can destroy the superior cervical sympathetic ganglion, whose postganglionic sympathetic fibers innervate both the dilator muscle of the iris and Muller's muscle (the smooth muscle component of the levator palpebrae superioris muscle). Contraction of Muller's muscle raises the upper eyelid. Its function is overruled by contraction of the orbicularis oculi muscle. The activity of both muscles is seen during a blink.

A (destruction of the celiac ganglion) is incorrect. The celiac ganglion is a sympathetic ganglion located in the abdomen. Its postganglionic fibers do not innervate the eye.
B (destruction of postganglionic neurons in the ciliary ganglion) is incorrect. The ciliary ganglion is a parasympathetic ganglion. The clinical signs described for this patient strongly suggest a defect in sympathetic innervation of the eye, not parasympathetic innervation.
D (mesothelioma of the diaphragmatic surface of the left lung) is incorrect. Mesothelioma is a neoplasm that arises from the pleural mesothelium. A mesothelioma on the diaphragmatic surface of the lung would not be positioned correctly to destroy the superior sympathetic ganglion.
E (papilledema of the left optic disc) is incorrect. Papilledema of the optic disc indicates increased intracranial pressure, not a loss of sympathetic innervation to the dilator muscle and Muller's muscle of the eye.

16. *D* (herpes simplex virus 1) is correct. In patients infected with herpes simplex virus 1 (HSV-1) or other herpesviruses, a Tzanck smear shows characteristic multinucleated giant cells (syncytia).

A (coxsackievirus A2), B (coxsackievirus A16), and C (enterovirus 71) are incorrect. Coxsackievirus A2 is an agent of herpangina, and coxsackievirus A16 and enterovirus 71 are agents of hand-foot-and-mouth disease. Both diseases affect children and are characterized by the presence of pharyngitis and vesicular lesions in the mouth. However, the lesions do not contain multinucleated giant cells.
E (mumps virus) is incorrect. Mumps virus causes parotid swelling. It does not cause pharyngitis or vesicular lesions in the mouth.

17. *E* (uroporphyrinogen) is correct. The patient's clinical manifestations are characteristic of porphyria cutanea tarda. This is the most common type of porphyria and is seen most frequently

in patients with alcoholism or chronic liver damage. In healthy individuals, the I and III isomers of uroporphyrinogen are converted to coproporphyrinogen isomers by uroporphyrinogen decarboxylase. In patients with alcoholism or chronic liver damage, a deficiency of this enzyme causes uroporphyrinogen to accumulate and be excreted in urine. The excretion of γ-aminolevulinic acid is usually normal. The urine may be pink, light brown, or yellow-brown.

A (γ-aminolevulinic acid) is incorrect. An increased level of γ-aminolevulinic acid is found in the urine of patients who have lead poisoning or a deficiency of uroporphyrinogen I synthase (also called porphobilinogen deaminase). Manifestations include nervous system disorders and blood disorders.
B (bilirubin) is incorrect. Bilirubin is a yellow pigment produced in heme catabolism. All types of bilirubinemia cause icterus. Only conjugated bilirubin can be excreted by the kidneys. Excess amounts of conjugated bilirubin cause the urine to be yellow-brown.
C (porphobilinogen) is incorrect. Both porphobilinogen and γ-aminolevulinic acid accumulate in patients with a deficiency of uroporphyrinogen I synthase. The resulting acute intermittent porphyria is characterized by neurologic and psychiatric symptoms. After a short period of time, the urine sample turns dark red-brown as a result of the formation of uroporphyrin and porphobilin. Patients with increased levels of porphobilinogen are not photosensitive.
D (urobilinogen) is incorrect. Urobilinogens are colorless and are formed during heme degradation. A small amount of urobilinogen is absorbed in the ileum, returned to the liver, and secreted in the bile. Only a small trace is excreted in the urine. Patients with increased levels of urobilinogens are not photosensitive.

18. C (Prader-Willi syndrome) is correct. Prader-Willi syndrome is caused by a mutation in one or more genes along the proximal long arm of chromosome 15. This syndrome is characterized by reduced fetal activity, obesity, mental retardation, and hypogonadotropism. Infants with this condition may develop failure to thrive, which usually improves by 12 months of age. During the next 6 months, they often develop hyperphagia and a consequent increase in the rate of weight gain. Rapid weight gain continues into adulthood and is accompanied by short stature.

A (growth hormone–secreting tumor) is incorrect. Growth hormone enhances skeletal growth. A growth hormone–secreting tumor would result in excessive growth, possibly acromegaly, rather than the short stature reported for this patient.
B (pheochromocytoma) is incorrect. Pheochromocytoma is a tumor of chromaffin cells, which are found primarily in the adrenal medulla and secrete catecholamines. These sympathetic agents increase the force and rate of contraction of the heart.

Pheochromocytomas are associated with hypertension, tachycardia, postural hypertension, and related symptoms; they do not affect bone structure or growth or influence intelligence. A pheochromocytoma would not be responsible for the symptoms reported for this patient.

D (Sturge-Weber syndrome) is incorrect. Sturge-Weber syndrome is a congenital disorder that begins during infancy and is characterized by developmental delay and mental impairment. Patients with this disorder have characteristic facial nevi and port-wine stains.

E (Williams syndrome) is incorrect. Williams syndrome is a rare disorder that consists of numerous congenital defects, including supravalvular aortic stenosis, mental retardation, and "elfin" facies. Children born with this disorder are often abnormally sensitive to vitamin D and, as a result, have hypercalcemia. Short stature is not a characteristic of this syndrome.

19. C (fluphenazine) is correct. The patient's clinical manifestations are consistent with the diagnosis of schizophrenia, so she would have been treated with an antipsychotic agent. Her eye and neck problems are examples of dystonic reactions. These reactions and other acute extrapyramidal side effects (e.g., akathisia and parkinsonism) often occur in the early months of therapy with antipsychotic drugs. The side effect profiles of "typical" and "atypical" antipsychotic drugs vary. The typical antipsychotic agents include phenothiazines (such as fluphenazine, thioridazine, and chlorpromazine) and haloperidol. The newer, atypical antipsychotic agents include azepines (such as clozapine and olanzapine) and risperidone. The typical drugs are more likely to produce acute extrapyramidal side effects than are the atypical drugs. Within the group of phenothiazines, fluphenazine is the drug most likely to produce acute extrapyramidal side effects; the drug least likely to produce side effects is chlorpromazine.

A (amitriptyline) and D (lithium) are incorrect. Amitriptyline is a tricyclic antidepressant, and lithium is a mood-stabilizing drug that is used to treat bipolar disorder. Neither of these agents would have caused acute extrapyramidal side effects, and neither of these agents would have been used to treat the patient described.

B (chlorpromazine) is incorrect. As discussed in C, chlorpromazine is a typical antipsychotic drug and a member of the phenothiazine class. Each phenothiazine has a piperazine, piperidine, or aliphatic group attached to the thiazine ring. Drugs with a piperazine group (such as fluphenazine) are the most potent and the most likely to cause acute extrapyramidal side effects. Drugs with either a piperidine group (such as thioridazine) or an aliphatic group (such as chlorpromazine) are less potent and less likely to cause acute these side effects.

E (risperidone) is incorrect. Risperidone is an atypical antipsychotic drug. Atypical drugs are less likely than typical drugs to cause extrapyramidal side effects.

20. *A*   (airway obstruction due to a reduction in elastic recoil of the lung) is correct. The patient has emphysema as a result of his history of cigarette smoking for 40 years. Smoking has resulted in the release of an excess of elastase by inflammatory cells (neutrophils and macrophages) in the lungs, causing destruction of the normal architecture of the pulmonary parenchyma. The result is a loss of normal lung elastance and an increase in compliance. Elastic recoil is one of the major sources of energy for movement of air out of the lung during expiration. When it is reduced, the pressure surrounding the small airways becomes greater than the pressure within them, resulting in dynamic collapse of the airway and hence obstruction to airflow in expiration. This normally occurs toward the end of expiration, but in patients with emphysema, it occurs too early, trapping air and increasing residual volume and reducing the FEV_1.

B   (airway obstruction due to severe bronchospasm) is incorrect. Bronchospasm is one of the major causes of airway obstruction in bronchial asthma and sometimes in chronic bronchitis. It does not play a role in patients with "pure" emphysema.
C   (bronchiolar obstruction due to mucous gland hyperplasia and mucous secretion) is incorrect. Excessive secretion of bronchial mucus would cause obstruction in a patient with chronic bronchitis.
D   (inability to adequately use the accessory muscles of respiration in expiration) is incorrect. Such inability might be a cause of respiratory difficulty in a patient with a neuromuscular problem, but would not be a factor in a typical patient with emphysema.
E   (ventilation/perfusion ratio <1.0) is incorrect. A change in $\dot{V}/\dot{Q}$ (ventilation/perfusion) would not explain the diminished FEV_1, which is a problem with lung mechanics.

21. *B*   (treat each patient with combination antibiotic therapy) is correct. *H. pylori* is a class I carcinogen; therefore anyone who tests positive for this organism should be treated. To avoid the rapid development of antibiotic resistance, combination therapy should be given and should consist of a minimum of three drugs (including, for example, bismuth subsalicylate, metronidazole, and either amikacin or tetracycline).

A, C, D, and E are incorrect. As discussed in B, both symptomatic and asymptomatic carriers of *H. pylori* should be treated with combination antibiotic therapy. An acid blocker will only alleviate the symptoms; it will not eradicate the organism.

22. *D*   (pilocarpine) is correct. Pilocarpine is a direct-acting muscarinic receptor agonist that can be used to treat primary open-angle glaucoma (POAG). The drug lowers intraocular pressure by increasing the outflow of aqueous humor. This action is attrib-

uted to the contraction of the ciliary muscle, which opens space in the trabecular meshwork. Carbachol, another direct-acting muscarinic receptor agonist, can also be used to treat primary open-angle glaucoma.

A   (atropine) is incorrect. Atropine is a muscarinic receptor antagonist. Its use would raise the intraocular pressure and likely precipitate an acute attack of glaucoma. Drugs that have antimuscarinic activity are contraindicated in patients with angle-closure glaucoma (also called narrow-angle glaucoma or closed-angle glaucoma) and should be used cautiously in patients with primary open-angle glaucoma.
B   (dipivefrin) is incorrect. Dipivefrin is a prodrug that undergoes hydrolysis in the eye and is converted to epinephrine. Dipivefrin lowers the intraocular pressure by decreasing the production and increasing the outflow of aqueous humor. The exact mechanisms by which these actions occur are poorly understood.
C   (echothiophate) is incorrect. Echothiophate and physostigmine are indirect-acting cholinomimetic drugs that reversibly inhibit acetylcholinesterase. These drugs act by increasing synaptic levels of acetylcholine. This in turn lowers the intraocular pressure by the same mechanism described in D for the direct-acting muscarinic agents.
E   (timolol) is incorrect. Timolol is a nonselective β-adrenergic receptor antagonist. It lowers the intraocular pressure by decreasing the production of aqueous humor. The exact mechanisms by which this occurs are poorly understood.

23. *E*   (type II pneumocyte) is correct. Type II pneumocytes (also called great alveolar cells) secrete surfactant, a phospholipid that decreases alveolar surface tension and thus allows alveoli to expand for normal gas exchange. The surfactant-containing lamellar bodies of type II pneumocytes are incompletely differentiated in premature infants. This impairs gas exchange in the lungs.

A   (alveolar macrophage), B (goblet cell), and C (granule cell) are incorrect. The function of alveolar macrophages, goblet cells, and granule cells is unrelated to respiratory distress syndrome. Alveolar macrophages eliminate particulate matter from the airways of the lungs. Goblet cells secrete mucus. Granule cells in the respiratory tract are presumed to have a neuroendocrine function similar to endocrine cells in the gut. (Endocrine cells in the gut are also called enteroendocrine cells, basal granular cells, APUD cells, and DNES cells. APUD is an acronym for amine precursor uptake and decarboxylation, and DNES is an acronym for diffuse neuroendocrine system.)
D   (type I pneumocyte) is incorrect. Type I pneumocytes are responsible for limiting the rate at which oxygen and carbon dioxide are exchanged between air and blood. The function of this type of pneumocyte is unrelated to RDS.

24. *D* (decreased output from the ventrolateral nucleus to the cerebral cortex) is correct. The decreased blink rate and rigid and shuffling gait are typical of Parkinson's disease. These problems result from a decreased input from the ventrolateral (VL) nucleus of the thalamus to the motor cortex of the brain. This input, which is modulated by the basal ganglia, normally modifies descending cortical motor output to allow the individual to initiate voluntary movements at an appropriate pace. Thalamic input is modulated by the basal ganglia via two basal ganglia pathways: direct and indirect. The extent to which the VL nucleus is inhibited depends on the balance of activity in each pathway.

A (decreased output from the putamen to the globus pallidus externa) is incorrect. The globus pallidus externa inhibits the subthalamic nucleus, which is a key structure in the indirect pathway. The globus pallidus externa is normally inhibited by GABAergic fibers projecting from the putamen (a component of the striatum). When striatal output decreases, output from the subthalamic nucleus increases. The subthalamic nucleus normally excites the globus pallidus interna, which projects GABAergic fibers (inhibitory) to the thalamic VL nucleus. As a result, the inhibitory pallidal fibers inhibit the thalamic VL.
B (decreased output from the substantia nigra pars reticulata to the ventrolateral nucleus) is incorrect. The substantia nigra pars reticulata projects inhibitory input to specific thalamic nuclei, including VL and ventroanterior. Nigrothalamic fibers are inhibitory; therefore, VL is normally tonically inhibited. If nigral input decreased, then a greater number of VL fibers would be able to fire, cortical motor output would be enhanced, and movement would be facilitated.
C (decreased output from the subthalamic nucleus to the internal segment of the globus pallidus) is incorrect. The subthalamic nucleus normally transmits excitatory signals to the globus pallidus interna.
E (increased output from the putamen to the substantia nigra pars reticulata) is incorrect. Output from the putamen to the substantia nigra pars reticulata (via the direct pathway) is normally inhibitory.

25. *E* (sexual pain disorders) is correct. Vaginismus is defined as involuntary vaginal muscle contractions during intercourse and is categorized as a sexual pain disorder. If the contractions are not caused by organic factors, the disorder is often linked to ambivalence about engaging in sex. In other words, the female may consciously desire coitus while being unconsciously inhibited.

A (orgasm disorders) is incorrect. Orgasmic disorders include disorders in which orgasm does not occur while adequate sexual stimulation is present or the orgasm occurs prematurely.
B (paraphilias) is incorrect. Paraphilias are defined as recurrent sexual fantasies, urges, and behaviors involving nonhuman

objects, the suffering of others, or nonconsenting individuals such as children.

C (sexual arousal disorders) is incorrect. Sexual arousal disorders result from an inability to maintain sufficient physical manifestations of sexual desire, such as erectile dysfunction in men and inadequate amounts of lubrication in women.

D (sexual desire disorders) is incorrect. Sexual desire disorders include two types of disorders. The first type reflects a deficiency or complete absence of sexual fantasies and interest in sexual activity. The second type refers to sexual aversion.

26. *B* (dextrose infusion can cause lactic acidosis and thereby worsen the patient's condition) is correct. Alcoholics with Wernicke-Korsakoff syndrome have thiamine deficiency. When dextrose is metabolized, a large amount of pyruvate is formed and cannot be cleared without an adequate supply of thiamine pyrophosphate. Pyruvate is converted to lactic acid. Lactic acidosis is a life-threatening condition.

A (alcohol oxidation is under tight control, and control is lost when dextrose or other sugars are introduced) is incorrect. Ethanol metabolism is not affected by feedback control or endocrine system control. Ethanol is oxidized by alcohol dehydrogenase to form acetaldehyde, and then acetaldehyde is oxidized by aldehyde dehydrogenase to form acetate. High levels of the reduced form of nicotinamide adenine dinucleotide ($NADH^+$) are produced, and the availability of NAD^+ drops.

C (the patient has an inherited form of dextrose intolerance) is incorrect. Inherited dextrose intolerance is an unlikely cause of the patient's deterioration.

D (the patient has been taking disulfiram to help him abstain from alcohol, and he should not have been given any intravenous fluids) is incorrect. Dextrose infusions would not have an effect on disulfiram.

E (the patient is suffering from ethanol poisoning, and dextrose competes with ethanol for the same enzymes to reverse the poisoning) is incorrect. Dextrose does not compete with ethanol, and it does not reverse ethanol poisoning.

27. *E* (site 5) is correct. Two isoforms of COX exist. COX-2 is inducible, with constitutive expression limited to the central nervous system. Lipopolysaccharides, cytokines (such as interleukin-1), and other factors (such as transforming growth factor and tumor necrosis factor) induce COX-2 synthesis, thereby giving rise to inflammation, pain, and fever. Thus, the anti-inflammatory, analgesic, and antipyretic effects of aspirin and other nonsteroidal anti-inflammatory drugs (NSAIDs) are thought to be due, in part, to inhibition of COX-2.

A (site 1) is incorrect. Zafirlukast acts at site 1. The drug's utility in the long-term management of asthma is thought to be due to its blockade of cysteinyl-leukotriene (LTD_4) receptors.

B (site 2) is incorrect. Glucocorticoids act at site 2. Release of arachidonic acid from membrane phospholipids is catalyzed by phospholipase A_2 (PLA_2). Glucocorticoids act to stimulate production of lipocortins, which inhibit PLA_2. This contributes, in part, to the anti-inflammatory activity of glucocorticoids.

C (site 3) is incorrect. Zileuton acts at site 3. The drug's utility in the long-term management of asthma is thought to be due to its inhibition of lipoxygenase, the enzyme that normally converts arachidonic acid to leukotrienes.

D (site 4) is incorrect. COX-1 is constitutively expressed and is ubiquitous. It functions to maintain adequate TXA_2 levels in the platelets and prostaglandin levels in the gastrointestinal tract and kidneys. When NSAIDs inhibit COX-1, they inhibit platelet hemostasis and cause gastrointestinal and renal side effects.

28. A *(Campylobacter jejuni)* is correct. The clinical and laboratory findings are consistent with the diagnosis of dysentery caused by *C. jejuni,* a curved (vibrio-shaped) bacterium. *C. jejuni* is a major cause of diarrhea in the United States. The major source of infection is food and water contaminated with animal feces.

B *(Clostridium difficile)* is incorrect. *C. difficile* is a rod rather than a curved bacterium. Because of the mechanism by which *C. difficile* produces diarrhea, stool samples do not contain many leukocytes.

C (enteroinvasive *Escherichia coli*) and D *(Shigella flexneri)* are incorrect. *S. flexneri* and enteroinvasive strains of *E. coli* can cause high fever and dysentery. However, these organisms are bacilli rather than curved bacteria.

E *(Vibrio cholerae)* is incorrect. *V. cholerae* is a curved bacterium, but it does not cause fever and dysentery. It produces profuse watery diarrhea with no blood or pus in the feces.

29. C (conduction system defects) is correct. The patient has hypertrophic cardiomyopathy (idiopathic hypertrophic subaortic stenosis), which is the most common cause of sudden cardiac death in young people. In some cases, there is an autosomal dominant inheritance pattern. Because of asymmetric hypertrophy of the interventricular septum, the anterior leaflet of the mitral valve is closer to the septum than normal. This narrows the outlet channel for blood flow through the aorta. When systole occurs, the anterior leaflet of the mitral valve is drawn against the interventricular septum, thus obstructing blood flow below the level of the aortic valve. This produces a systolic ejection murmur that is easily confused with aortic stenosis. Aberrant myofibers in the hypertrophied septum and conduction system abnormalities also occur; the latter are responsible for fatal ventricular arrhythmia and sudden death. The murmur intensity decreases (less obstruction) whenever left ventricular volume (preload) is increased. Hence, increased venous return to the right-sided heart (lying down) or drugs that decrease cardiac contractility and heart rate (e.g., β-blockers, calcium channel block-

ers) decrease murmur intensity. Sitting up reduces venous return to the heart (decreases preload) and intensifies the murmur (greater obstruction). Drugs that have an inotropic effect on the heart (e.g., digitalis) or the patient holding his breath against a closed glottis (Valsalva maneuver) have a similar effect.

A (acute myocardial infarction) is incorrect. Hypertrophic cardiomyopathy is not associated with coronary artery disease. Furthermore, conduction defects do not predispose patients to acute MIs.

B (congenital bicuspid aortic valve) is incorrect. This congenital anomaly is the most common cause of aortic stenosis in young to middle-aged patients. It predisposes patients to dystrophic calcification of the valve cusps and subsequent reduction in valve orifice area for blood flow out of the aorta. In aortic stenosis, increasing preload increases the intensity of the murmur (increases obstruction), and reducing preload decreases the intensity (lessens obstruction).

D (dissecting aortic aneurysm) is incorrect. Dissections do not cause sudden death and are not associated with systolic murmurs. Proximal dissections stretch the aortic valve ring, causing aortic regurgitation, which is a diastolic murmur heard after the second heart sound. Furthermore, the orifice to the left subclavian artery is often occluded, leading to a diminished pulse.

E (mitral valve prolapse) is incorrect. Mitral valve prolapse (MVP) is associated with a midsystolic ejection click followed by a murmur. Except for MVP associated with Marfan syndrome, MVP is not associated with sudden cardiac death.

30. *A* (name the last four presidents of the United States) is correct. Each statement listed is part of a mental status examination. However, the request to name the last four presidents is the only item that requires remote memory skills. If the patient cannot name the presidents, other questions about past significant events (e.g., wars), important people, or verifiable personal information (e.g., anniversaries, children's birthdays) can be asked.

B (repeat after me, "No ifs, ands, or buts") is incorrect. Repeating a statement such as "no ifs, ands, or buts" is used as a measure of language.

C (starting with the number 100, count backwards by 7s) is incorrect. Serial sevens is a measure of attention.

D (state the day, month, year, and time of day) is incorrect. A patient who is able to state the day, month, year, and time of day reflects intact orientation to time. Further questions about person, place, and purpose would be needed to ensure complete orientation.

E (tell me how a cat and a dog are alike) is incorrect. Asking a patient to state the similarities and differences between items is a measure of abstract reasoning. Interpretation of proverbs is another measure of abstract reasoning.

31. *C* (blood transfusion) is correct. This patient's blood pressure is low and his heart rate is high, signs that he is suffering from hypovolemic shock. The abnormally low pressure is exerted against the aortic and carotid sinus baroreceptors causing a reflex-mediated increase in sympathetic activity, which is responsible for the increased rate of breathing. It also causes arteriolar constriction, which helps prevent the arterial blood pressure from falling any lower. In the kidney, arteriolar constriction results in reduced renal perfusion and a lower glomerular filtration rate, both of which help the body conserve fluids and reduce urinary output. Increasing the blood volume will obviate the baroreceptor-mediated reflex and help maintain an adequate blood pressure and urinary output. Ideally, infusion of matched whole blood should be given; if there are time constraints, however, the next best choice is a plasma expander (e.g., dextran), which contains colloidal particles too large to cross the capillary endothelium. The osmotic force causes fluid to remain within the vascular space.

A (administration of an oral diuretic) is incorrect. A diuretic increases the amount of urine produced; thus, it would exacerbate the hypovolemia in this patient.
B (administration of physiologic saline solution) is incorrect. Physiologic saline solution is not as effective for fluid replacement as blood or a plasma expander, because it is not contained within the plasma space but leaks to the interstitium. Thus, large volumes of saline will be required to improve the patient's blood pressure.
D (indirect cardiac massage) is incorrect. Cardiac massage may help increase the cardiac output, but this effort is futile with insufficient fluid to pump.
E (intravenous injection of norepinephrine) is incorrect. The administration of norepinephrine (a sympathetic neurotransmitter) is contraindicated because it induces vascular constriction, which is already increased due to reflex-mediated sympathetic activity.

32. *C* (failure of the cochlea and spiral ganglia to develop) is correct. The rubella virus crosses the placenta and causes various types of malformation, depending on the stage of embryonic development at which infection occurs. Interruption of the *Pax-2* gene at 8 weeks' gestation by the virus results in malformation of the cochlea and spiral ganglia, resulting in congenital deafness.

A (detachment of the retina) is incorrect. Detachment of the retina refers to a separation of the retinal nervous layer from the pigmented layer. Congenital cataracts, not retinal detachment, is one of the triad of malformations resulting from exposure of the embryo to the rubella virus.
B (discoloration of permanent teeth) is incorrect. The effects of German measles, such as pits and fissures in enamel hypopla-

sia, may not be evident for several years after birth. Tetracycline taken during pregnancy crosses the placenta and attaches to active sites of calcification, discoloring tooth enamel. The defect becomes evident when the permanent teeth erupt.

D (failure of the semicircular canals to develop) is incorrect. Development of the inner ear is under separate genetic control. Semicircular canals, which are under the control of the homeobox containing the *Nkx5* genes, begin development at about 5 weeks' gestation.

E (pulmonary stenosis) is incorrect. Pulmonary stenosis is one component of the tetrad of cardiac anomalies referred to as the tetralogy of Fallot; the other three defects are ventricular septal defect, overriding aorta, and right ventricular hypertrophy. The most common cardiac malformation resulting from rubella infection is patent ductus arteriosus.

33. *E* (type III hypersensitivity reaction) is correct. Type III reactions are hypersensitivity reactions mediated by immune complexes. Examples of these reactions include serum sickness, immune complex disorders, and Arthus reactions. The worsening pain after each booster is most likely an Arthus reaction.

A (allergic reaction to a component of the vaccine) is incorrect. An allergic reaction to a component of the vaccine would be classified as a type I hypersensitivity reaction. Refer to the discussion of E.

B (tissue destruction associated with any injection) is incorrect. The type of tissue destruction associated with any injection would not account for the increasing level of pain associated with the boosters.

C (type I hypersensitivity reaction) is incorrect. Type I reactions are immediate hypersensitivity reactions that are mediated by IgE antibody. A topical manifestation, such as eczema, would be expected in addition to pain if the patient's response had been mediated by IgE antibody.

D (type II hypersensitivity reaction) is incorrect. Type II reactions are cytotoxic reactions that are mediated by antitissue antibodies, such as IgM and IgG. Vaccinations do not usually result in the production of autoantibodies.

34. *A* (cholinergic) is correct. These symptoms suggest myasthenia gravis, an autoimmune disease that develops when postsynaptic neuromuscular receptors are destroyed. The lack of muscle atrophy in this patient suggests that the muscle fibers in this patient have a reasonable supply of trophic factors and are not being overworked. The cause of muscle weakness is most likely a lack of innervation. Motor neurons activate their target muscles by releasing the neurotransmitter acetylcholine, which binds to postsynaptic cholinergic receptors (especially nicotinic receptors). If these receptors are destroyed, the muscle will not contract.

B   (dopaminergic) is incorrect. Dopamine is found primarily in central neurons (e.g., the substantia nigra, ventral tegmentum, hypothalamus, and retina) that extend to other central structures. These neurons do not extend directly to muscles. Instead, they modulate cortical motor signals before they reach the muscles.

C   (GABAergic) is incorrect. GABA is an inhibitory neurotransmitter.

D   (glutaminergic) is incorrect. In the peripheral nervous system, glutamine is produced primarily by afferent nerves. The symptoms described for this patient indicate damage to efferent nerves.

E   (serotonergic) is incorrect. Serotonin is involved primarily in the regulation of mood, sleep, and pain. Its receptors do not induce motor activity.

35. *B*   (point B) is correct. Point B is located near the respiratory line attributed to mass action shifts along the normal buffer line for hemoglobin. The pH is decidedly acidotic due to decreased ventilation and CO_2 accumulation. Since the renal system is so slow to respond to the elevated CO_2, there is no time for renal compensation.

A   (point A) is incorrect. Point A represents "pure" metabolic acidosis.

C   (point C) is incorrect. Point C lies in a region that suggests that metabolic alkalotic compensatory processes have come into play. This would probably have occurred if the patient had remained off the ventilator over the subsequent days (which he did not).

D   (point D) is incorrect. Point D represents "pure" metabolic alkalosis.

E   (point E) is incorrect. Point E represents "pure" respiratory alkalosis.

36. *C*   (elevated serum cortisol and serum ACTH) is correct. This patient's symptoms are typical of Cushing's syndrome, most often caused by an ACTH-secreting pituitary adenoma. Elevated ACTH levels stimulate cortisol production and prevent cortisol suppression by exogenous corticosteroids.

A   (decreased serum cortisol and below normal serum ACTH) is incorrect. A low serum cortisol level is unlikely to occur with increased urinary free cortisol excretion.

B   (elevated corticotrophin-releasing hormone, low ACTH, and unaffected serum cortisol) is incorrect. If CRH is elevated, ACTH should also be elevated.

D   (increased serum ACTH) is incorrect. Administration of an exogenous steroid inhibits ACTH secretion.

E   (low serum CRH and ACTH and increased serum cortisol) is incorrect. Serum CRH and ACTH could be low if there was ectopic production of cortisol, but administration of exogenous cortisol should not increase serum cortisol.

37. *C* (erythema infectiosum) is correct. A "slapped cheek" appearance in conjunction with a lacy rash on the trunk is consistent with the diagnosis of erythema infectiosum. This disease is also called fifth disease and is caused by parvovirus B19.

A (child abuse with hand-foot-and-mouth disease) and B (child abuse with heat rash) are incorrect. Lesions on the upper extremities are not characteristic of hand-foot-and-mouth disease, which can be caused by coxsackieviruses A9 and A16 or by enterovirus 71. The rash associated with heat rash would be more intense on covered areas of the body and would be more papillary in nature. D (exanthema subitum) is incorrect. Exanthema subitum, which is caused by human herpesvirus 6, is also called sixth disease and roseola infantum. The disease has a prodrome of high fever, and the distribution of the rash is less intense on the cheeks. E (measles) is incorrect. The rash of measles is florid and intensely erythematous. Patients with measles have a 3-day prodrome of cough, coryza, conjunctivitis, and Koplik's spots.

38. *D* (causing smooth muscle relaxation by stimulating the formation of nitric oxide, thereby causing an increase in the level of cyclic guanosine monophosphate) is correct. Acting via the formation of a nitrosothio intermediate, nitroglycerin and other nitrates increase the formation of nitric oxide. The nitric oxide activates guanylyl cyclase and thereby causes an increase in the level of cGMP. The cGMP activates its own kinase, which phosphorylates phosphatases. These phosphatases then dephosphorylate (inactivate) myosin light chains and cause smooth muscle relaxation. The relaxation of large veins and arteries reduces preload and afterload, respectively, and decreases the myocardial oxygen demand. Nitrates also redistribute blood flow along collateral vessels, and this could contribute to their beneficial effects. Nitroglycerin and other nitrates are useful in the management of Prinzmetal's angina (also called variant angina or vasospastic vasospasm) and chronic stable angina. Tolerance rapidly develops to the effects of nitrates because the drugs cause cellular depletion of sulfhydryl compounds.

A (blocking α_1-adrenergic receptors and reducing myocardial oxygen consumption by decreasing cardiac preload and afterload) is incorrect. This is a description of the mechanism for the beneficial effects of selective α_1-adrenergic receptor antagonists (such as doxazosin, prazosin, and terazosin) in patients with hypertension. While hypertension may contribute to angina, these drugs are not indicated for the treatment of angina per se. B (blocking β_1-adrenergic receptors and reducing myocardial oxygen consumption by preventing an increase in heart rate and contractility) is incorrect. This is a description of the mechanism for the beneficial effects of β-adrenergic receptor antagonists (such as propranolol and metoprolol) in patients with chronic stable angina. The β-blockers are not useful for the treatment of Prinzmetal's angina, because this form of angina has no catecholamine component.

C (blocking slow Ca^{2+} channels and reducing myocardial oxygen consumption by decreasing cardiac contractility, heart rate, and arterial pressure) is incorrect. This is a description of the mechanism for the beneficial effects of calcium channel blockers (such as diltiazem, nifedipine, and verapamil) in patients with chronic stable angina. These drugs are also used in the treatment of Prinzmetal's angina.

E (preventing platelet aggregation by inhibiting platelet cyclooxygenase activity) is incorrect. This is a description of the mechanism for the beneficial effects of aspirin in patients with chronic unstable angina. The irreversible inhibition of platelet cyclooxygenase blocks the formation of thromboxane A_2. This prevents the aggregation of platelets and the formation of platelet plugs that are responsible for coronary occlusion.

39. *C* (cluster headache) is correct. Cluster headache is a severe, unilateral headache that occurs around the eye or in the temporal region of the head. It lasts 15 minutes to 2 hours and occurs up to 8 times a day. It may be accompanied by tearing, redness, a stuffy nose, facial sweating, and ptosis or miosis. It is more common in men than women and may be triggered by alcohol, sleep, or a change in barometric pressure. The cause is unknown, although calcium channel blockers and serotonin antagonists have been used prophylactically. Associated autonomic findings include signs of an incomplete Horner's syndrome (e.g., miosis, ptosis, and sweating), which are evident in this patient.

A (atypical facial pain) is incorrect. Atypical facial pain is often a chronic, fluctuating pain with no associated signs.

B (cervicogenic headache) is incorrect. Cervicogenic headache originates in the upper cervical spine and may be caused by rheumatoid arthritis, osteoarthritis, and other diseases of the cervical spine.

D (temporal arteritis) is incorrect. Temporal arteritis is a chronic inflammation of large blood vessels (especially cranial branches of the carotid artery) that results in arterial stenosis or occlusion. This condition often causes a severe headache, particularly in the temporal and occipital regions, but not around the eye. The accompanying symptoms (which include visual disturbances, pain on chewing, and sometimes blindness) are much more severe than those of a cluster headache.

E (trigeminal neuralgia) is incorrect. Trigeminal neuralgia is a severe pain that occurs when arteriolar or venous loops press against the trigeminal nerve root. The pain normally lasts no longer than 2 minutes, rather than 15 minutes to 2 hours, as in this case. Also, the pain often has trigger points.

40. *A*   (loss of extension of the leg) is correct. A tumor on the anterior iliacus would very likely involve the femoral nerve, which enters the anterior thigh on the anterior surface of the iliacus portion of the iliopsoas muscle. The femoral nerve, which supplies much of the cutaneous innervation to the anterior and medial thigh, also innervates the quadriceps femoris muscle, which includes four components whose major function is extension of the leg at the knee. Loss of the quadriceps femoris results in total loss of leg extension. In addition, the femoral nerve innervates other muscles, including the iliacus, sartorius, pectineus, and articularis genu (the iliacus muscle is innervated within the abdomen, before the muscle enters the thigh).

B   (necrosis of the femoral head) is incorrect. Necrosis of the femoral head might result from loss of the circumflex femoral arteries, particularly the medial circumflex femoral artery, which is the major source of blood to the head and neck of the femur. The medial circumflex femoral artery arises from the deep femoral artery in the femoral triangle and courses posteriorly between the iliopsoas and pectineus muscles. A tumor of the iliacus might eventually involve this artery, but a condition that involves the femoral nerve is more likely.
C   (occlusion of the femoral vein) is incorrect. A tumor on the iliacus would be situated lateral to the femoral sheath and would of necessity involve the femoral artery before affecting the femoral vein. The femoral sheath, which surrounds the femoral vessels when they enter the thigh, lies medial to the iliopsoas muscle and has three compartments. The femoral artery lies closest to the iliacus muscle in the lateral compartment of the femoral sheath. The femoral vein is next to the femoral artery and in the middle compartment of the femoral sheath. The medial compartment contains lymphatics from the deep inguinal lymph nodes crossing into the abdomen.
D   (paralysis of the adductor muscles of the thigh) is incorrect. The adductor muscles, which are located in the medial compartment of the thigh, receive innervation from the obturator nerve entering the thigh through the obturator foramen. The iliacus muscle, which originates from the anterior surface of the iliac fossa, enters the anterior compartment of the thigh, combining with the psoas major to form the iliopsoas muscle, the chief flexor of the thigh at the hip. Thus, a tumor in the muscle would not affect the adductor muscles, either directly or by involvement of the obturator nerve of the medial compartment of the thigh.
E   (weakness of extension of the hip) is incorrect. It could be argued that there would be weakness in flexion of the hip, either by involvement of the iliacus or by loss of innervation to the rectus femoris (the only muscle of the quadriceps femoris that crosses and acts on the hip joint). However, this would have no effect on extension of the thigh. The hamstring muscles of the posterior compartment of the thigh (tibial division of sciatic nerve innervation) or the gluteus maximus muscle (inferior gluteal nerve innervation) would produce such action.

41. *A* (cleavage of terminal propeptides from procollagen) is correct. The polypeptides of collagen, called preprocollagen molecules, are synthesized by ribosomes in the rough endoplasmic reticulum (ER). The preprocollagen contains propeptides, which are additional sequences at the amino and carboxyl ends. Some of the prepropeptide chains from the amino end are removed cotranslationally by signal peptidase, and this converts preprocollagen to procollagen. Procollagen molecules secreted into the extracellular space have *N*- and *C*-terminal propeptides. These terminal propeptides are cleaved extracellularly from procollagen by *N*- and *C*-procollagen peptidases. After cleavage, triple helix collagen molecules are formed.

B (degradation of improperly coiled collagen molecules) is incorrect. Only properly coiled procollagen molecules are secreted into the extracellular matrix. The improperly coiled molecules are degraded intracellularly.
C (formation of interchain and intrachain disulfide bonds) is incorrect. Interchain and intrachain disulfide bonds are formed in the ER.
D (glycosylation of selected hydroxylysines) is incorrect. After hydroxylation, some of the hydroxylysines (but not hydroxyprolines) are modified by glycosylation in the ER.
E (hydroxylation of prolines and lysines) is incorrect. Proline and lysine molecules found in the Y position of -Gly-X-Y- can be hydroxylated in the lumen of the ER. This step requires vitamin C.

42. *D* (spatial neglect) is correct. The drawing reflects spatial neglect (visual inattention), which is a visual-spatial impairment in performing tasks contralateral to a lesion. The patient who produced this drawing was asked to illustrate 2:20 PM on a clock and is most likely to have a lesion in the right posterior parietal lobe, since the left side of the clock has been neglected.

A (central dysarthria) is incorrect. Central dysarthria refers to difficulty in articulation. Language skills remain intact, but speech is slurred or incoherent because of a dysfunction in muscle movements associated with speech. If the patient cannot articulate words, including "clock," dysarthria would be present.
B (constructional apraxia) is incorrect. Constructional apraxia is associated with parietal lobe lesions and reflects difficulty in putting together one-dimensional units to form two-dimensional figures. The disorder is detected by asking patients to copy a design (e.g., interlocking figures) or to construct something (e.g., blocks). When copying a design, patients might crowd the drawing into one corner of a page, superimpose their drawing on the original, reverse the drawing in mirror image fashion, or distort the drawing in an obvious manner.
C (parietal agraphia) is incorrect. Parietal agraphia, also known as alexia with agraphia, is the inability to read or write. To test for

parietal agraphia, the patient would be asked to write or read the word "clock."
E (visual agnosia) is incorrect. Individuals who fail to recognize familiar objects (including people) by sight are displaying visual agnosia. If this patient had been shown a clock and asked to name it, but could not, visual agnosia would be present.

43. *E* (gram-positive filamentous rods) is correct. The patient's history and clinical findings are consistent with the diagnosis of actinomycosis, a disease caused by *Actinomyces israelii* and other *Actinomyces* species. These species are part of the normal flora of the mouth and appear as gram-positive filamentous rods.

A (gram-negative diplococci) is incorrect. Gram-negative diplococci, such as *Moraxella catarrhalis,* are part of the normal flora of the nasopharynx. However, disease caused by these organisms is principally limited to otitis media.
B (gram-negative rods) is incorrect. Gram-negative rods, such as *Prevotella gingivalis,* can be found in the mouth, especially if gingivitis or periodontal disease is present. However, these organisms tend to cause abscesses rather than lesions of the type found in the patient described.
C (gram-positive cocci in chains) is incorrect. Gram-positive cocci that grow in chains, such as *Streptococcus mutans,* are part of the normal flora of the mouth. However, the lesions caused by virulent *S. mutans* are principally limited to dental caries.
D (gram-positive cocci in clusters) is incorrect. Gram-positive cocci that grow in clusters, such as *Staphylococcus aureus,* tend to cause pyogenic abscesses.

44. *A* (impaired abduction of the shoulder) is correct. Fracture of the surgical neck of the humerus may result in laceration of the nerve from the posterior cord of the brachial plexus. The axillary nerve, which innervates two muscles, the deltoid and the teres minor, arises from the posterior cord of the brachial plexus and lies on the medial side of the surgical neck of the humerus. Fracture of the humerus in this area may damage the axillary nerve, thus affecting abduction of the shoulder. This commonly occurs in elderly individuals.

B (inability to flex the elbow) is incorrect. Flexion of the elbow is unaffected by a fracture of the surgical neck of the humerus, because the musculocutaneous and radial nerves do not relate to the surgical neck of the humerus. The brachialis and biceps brachii, which are both innervated by the musculocutaneous nerve from the lateral cord, and the brachioradialis, which is innervated by radial nerve, are flexors of the elbow.
C (loss of sensation over the lateral side of the forearm) is incorrect. The lateral antebrachial cutaneous nerve, a continuation of the musculocutaneous nerve from the lateral cord of the brachial plexus, is responsible for the sensation over the lateral side of the forearm.

D   (loss of sensation over the medial side of the forearm) is incorrect. The medial antebrachial cutaneous nerve from the medial cord is responsible for sensation over the medial side of the forearm.

E   (weakness of pronation) is incorrect. Pronation is unaffected by fracture of the surgical neck of the humerus because the median nerve (which arises from the lateral and medial cords) travels through the middle of the arm to innervate the pronator teres and pronator quadratus.

45. *B*   (immunocomplex vasculitis) is correct. The patient has Henoch-Schönlein purpura (HSP), an immunocomplex disease (type III hypersensitivity) involving small vessels primarily in the skin (palpable purpura), gastrointestinal (GI) tract, and glomeruli of the kidneys. HSP is the most common type of vasculitis in children. Increased circulating levels of polymeric IgA and immunocomplexes with IgA and C3 are present in the patient. The immunocomplexes deposit in small vessels and activate the alternative complement system, which produces complement components that are chemotactic for neutrophils. Hence, neutrophils are primarily responsible for tissue damage in this and all other immunocomplex diseases. The glomerulonephritis associated with HSP is similar to IgA glomerulonephritis (Berger's disease) in that IgA immunocomplexes deposit in the mesangium, resulting in hematuria, RBC casts, and proteinuria.

A   (genetic vascular disorder) is incorrect. The most common genetic vascular disorder is Osler-Weber-Rendu disease (hereditary hemorrhagic telangiectasia). It is an autosomal dominant disease associated with dilated vessels (telangiectasia) on the skin, in the mouth, and throughout the mucosa of the GI tract. When found in the GI tract, chronic iron deficiency anemia occurs.

C   (infectious type of vasculitis) is incorrect. The multisystem involvement and peculiar distribution of the vasculitis on the buttocks and lower extremities favor a diagnosis of HSP.

D   (previous group A streptococcal infection) is incorrect. The patient does not have acute rheumatic fever or poststreptococcal glomerulonephritis. In both conditions, neither bloody diarrhea nor vasculitis is part of the clinical presentation.

E   (type II hypersensitivity vasculitis) is incorrect. Most small vessel types of vasculitis are immunocomplex, type III hypersensitivity reactions. Refer to the discussion for C.

46. *C*   (gentamicin) is correct. Gentamicin, streptomycin, amikacin, and other aminoglycosides can inhibit the release of acetylcholine at the neuromuscular junction. The resulting adverse effects (muscle weakness, dysphagia, dysarthria, and respiratory depression) mimic competitive neuromuscular blockade and can be reversed by the administration of calcium gluconate or neostigmine. Other adverse effects of aminoglycosides include nephrotoxicity and ototoxicity. In the case of gentamicin, the ototoxicity tends to be irreversible and mainly causes symptoms

of vestibular dysfunction (vertigo, dizziness, and ataxia), although hearing loss may also occur. Ototoxicity is believed to be due to the destruction of sensory hair cells in the ear.

A (aztreonam), B (ceftriaxone), and E (piperacillin) are incorrect. Aztreonam is a monobactam antibiotic; ceftriaxone is a third-generation cephalosporin; and piperacillin is an antipseudomonal penicillin. Any of these drugs may have been an appropriate choice for treating a mixed aerobic and gram-negative infection. However, their use has not been associated with the adverse effects that occurred in the patient described.
D (metronidazole) is incorrect. Treatment with metronidazole would not be indicated for the patient described. Metronidazole is useful in the treatment of giardiasis, trichomoniasis, amebiasis, *Clostridium difficile* infection, and many other anaerobic bacterial infections. Adverse effects of metronidazole include paresthesias and peripheral neuropathy. A disulfiramlike reaction occurs with the concurrent ingestion of metronidazole and alcoholic beverages.

47. *A* (aldolase) is correct. Although lactose and maltose do not contain fructose, saccharose does. In the liver, fructokinase converts fructose to fructose 1-phosphate. After aldolase cleaves fructose 1-phosphate to dihydroxyacetone phosphate, the dihydroxyacetone phosphate enters the glycolytic pathway. In patients with aldolase deficiency, excessive fructose 1-phosphate tends to accumulate in the liver, where it can tie up the inorganic phosphate and deplete the cells of adenosine triphosphate. Hepatic cells then swell and undergo osmotic lysis.

B (fructokinase) is incorrect. A deficiency of fructokinase leads to fructosuria, which is a benign, asymptomatic metabolic anomaly.
C (fructose-1,6-bisphosphatase) is incorrect. Fructose-1,6-bisphosphatase converts fructose 1,6-bisphosphate to fructose 6-phosphate in the gluconeogenesis pathway.
D (hexokinase) is incorrect. Hexokinase catalyzes the conversion of glucose to glucose 6-phosphate.
E (phosphofructokinase) is incorrect. Phosphofructokinase (PFK) phosphorylates fructose 6-phosphate to fructose 1,6-bisphosphate in the glycolysis pathway. This reaction is specific for glycolysis.

48. *D* (provide HIV/AIDS counseling and education and postpone testing) is correct. The patient is making decisions while in a heightened emotional state since he has discovered his sexual partner has AIDS. Providing counseling and education decreases the patient's anxiety and increases rational decision-making. Having the patient postpone testing for HIV until he regains his emotional stability provides him time to reconsider and strengthens the physician's ability to prevent suicidal behavior in the patient.

A (conduct the requested test and report the results regardless of findings) is incorrect. The patient's frame of mind demonstrates that he is unable to appropriately deal with the test results without preventive intervention. Therefore, giving him the results simply because he requests them would be unethical and dangerous and would interfere with treatment planning.

B (initiate proceedings for involuntary psychiatric hospitalization) is incorrect. Since there is no immediate danger of suicide unless testing is conducted, involuntary commitment of this patient is unlikely to be achievable. Even if commitment is feasible, the approach unnecessarily impinges on patient autonomy and is an overreaction.

C (provide HIV/AIDS counseling and education and initiate testing) is incorrect. When a patient is highly emotional, counseling and education may need to be repeatedly provided. Rescheduling the testing within a reasonable time frame does not harm the patient and allows the physician an opportunity to reevaluate the patient's emotional stability.

E (refuse to conduct the HIV test and discontinue the interview) is incorrect. Fundamental duties of a physician include providing needed health care, guiding rational decision-making, and avoiding patient harm. Refusing testing without providing other services violates each of these duties.

49. *E* (valvular defect leading to intravascular hemolysis) is correct. The patient has classic aortic stenosis (systolic ejection murmur with radiation into the carotids) complicated by an intravascular hemolytic anemia due to RBC damage (schistocytes) by the stenotic valve. Chronic loss of hemoglobin in the urine produced iron deficiency (low MCV). Aortic stenosis is the most common cause of intravascular hemolysis associated with schistocytes. Thrombocytosis is secondary to chronic iron deficiency anemia. The classic angina seen in this patient is related to decreased filling of the coronary arteries in diastole due to decreased stroke volume in aortic stenosis plus the moderately severe anemia with concomitant reduced oxygen content of blood.

A (autoimmune destruction of RBCs) is incorrect. The direct Coombs' test is negative.

B (disseminated intravascular coagulation) is incorrect. The aPTT and PT are normal, and the platelet count is elevated. Consumption of coagulation factors and platelets in fibrin clots in the microvasculature prolongs the PTT and PT and lowers the platelet count.

C (genetic defect in the RBC membrane) is incorrect. Schistocytes are produced by extrinsic damage to the RBC membrane (e.g., stenotic valve, intravascular clots).

D (iron deficiency unrelated to the valvular defect) is incorrect. The stenotic aortic valve damaged RBCs, leading to hemoglobinuria and loss of iron in the urine.

50. *D* (nortriptyline) is correct. Nortriptyline is indicated for major depression but would antagonize the effects of guanethidine. Nortriptyline is a tricyclic antidepressant (TCA). Like other TCAs, it blocks the reuptake process in presynaptic adrenergic nerve terminals. If this process does not occur, guanethidine cannot exert its antihypertensive effects, which are attributed to the gradual depletion of intraneuronal stores of norepinephrine. In addition to antagonizing the antihypertensive effects of guanethidine, TCAs antagonize the centrally mediated antihypertensive effects of α_2-adrenergic receptor agonists such as methyldopa and clonidine.

A (carbamazepine) is incorrect. Carbamazepine has no efficacy for the treatment of major depression, and it would not antagonize the antihypertensive effects of guanethidine. Indications for the use of carbamazepine include bipolar disorder, tonic-clonic seizures, partial seizures, and trigeminal neuralgia.

B (haloperidol) is incorrect. Haloperidol is an antipsychotic agent that might have been used to treat this patient's depression if it were accompanied by hallucinations, delusions, or other symptoms of psychotic disorders. Haloperidol would not antagonize the antihypertensive effects of guanethidine, but it could potentiate the α_1-adrenergic receptor-blocking activity of the drug.

C (midazolam) is incorrect. Midazolam would not have been used to treat this patient. Midazolam is a benzodiazepine that is commonly employed for preoperative amnesia and sedation. The drug would not antagonize the antihypertensive effects of guanethidine.

E (sertraline) is incorrect. Sertraline is an agent used to treat major depression. However, because it is a selective serotonin reuptake inhibitor (SSRI), it would not be expected to antagonize the antihypertensive effects of guanethidine.

Test 6

TEST 6

DIRECTIONS: Each numbered item or incomplete statement is followed by options arranged in alphabetical or logical order. Select the best answer to each question. Some options may be partially correct, but there is only **ONE BEST** answer.

1. A 46-year-old man has paresis of upward gaze, defective convergence, and large pupils that respond more briskly to accommodation than to light. This man most likely has

○ A. Bell's palsy
○ B. cerebellar gaze palsy
○ C. internuclear ophthalmoplegia
○ D. one-and-a-half syndrome
○ E. Parinaud's syndrome

2. A routine physical examination of an asymptomatic, normotensive 21-year-old African-American woman is normal; however, a urinalysis shows red blood cells (RBCs) with no casts. The patient says that she occasionally has had blood in her urine in the past. A urine culture is negative. Laboratory studies show:

Serum blood urea nitrogen (BUN)	10 mg/dL
Serum creatinine	1.0 mg/dL
Hemoglobin	11.0 g/dL
Mean corpuscular volume	78 μm^3
Reticulocyte count, corrected	2%

The peripheral smear shows occasional hypochromic RBCs. Renal ultrasonography is normal. Which of the following is the next best step in the management of this patient?

○ A. Bone marrow examination
○ B. Cystoscopy
○ C. Renal biopsy
○ D. Sickle cell preparation
○ E. No further investigation is necessary

3. A 61-year-old woman with a 5-year history of type 2 diabetes mellitus is brought to the emergency department suffering from dizziness, confusion, and lethargy. She has noticeable tremors, is sweating, and has a blood pressure of 160/100 mm Hg and a pulse of 132/min. A member of her family reports that the patient recently began taking a "pill" to control her "sugar." The patient was most likely being treated for type 2 diabetes with

○ A. acarbose
○ B. glyburide
○ C. human insulin
○ D. metformin
○ E. rosiglitazone

4. A healthy 51-year-old man is given a skin test with purified protein derivative (PPD) and is found to have some erythema but no edema or induration at the site of testing. He is tested with *Candida* antigen, and his response is the same. Based on these results, this patient should be tested for

- ○ A. asymptomatic measles virus infection
- ○ B. HIV infection
- ○ C. reaction to cold agglutinins
- ○ D. reactivity to Hib
- ○ E. response to B cell mitogen

5. Which of the following sets of values represents an acid-base disturbance that is almost fully compensated?

	pH	Base/Acid Ratio	Acid Component [HA]
○ A.	7.31	Low	Above normal range
○ B.	7.37	Near normal	Above normal range
○ C.	7.40	Exactly normal	Exactly normal
○ D.	7.43	Near normal	Within normal range
○ E.	7.50	High	Below normal range

6. A 22-year-old man fell off his bicycle and fractured the medial epicondyle of the humerus. The physician must determine the integrity of the ulnar nerve. Which of the following pairs of muscles would allow the patient to hold a dollar bill between the fingers against resistance?

- ○ A. Abductor digiti minimi—dorsal interossei
- ○ B. Adductor pollicis—lumbricals
- ○ C. Dorsal interossei—palmar interossei
- ○ D. Lumbricals—palmar interossei

7. A 3-year-old girl is brought to the pediatrician's office by her mother, who gave birth to the child before moving to the United States. The mother says that the child has never been seen by a physician, and she is concerned because the child seems to be "slower" than other children in her age group. The girl has a peculiar odor about her. In comparison with the mother, the daughter looks very fair. Examination shows that the daughter is mentally retarded. The most likely diagnosis is

- ○ A. alkaptonuria
- ○ B. cystinuria
- ○ C. Down syndrome
- ○ D. homocystinuria
- ○ E. phenylketonuria (PKU)

8. A 19-year-old man with a genital herpes simplex virus (HSV-2) infection is treated with acyclovir but fails to respond to the drug. This therapy is stopped, and foscarnet treatment is begun. Within 1 week, the patient's condition improves. The most likely explanation for the patient's failure to respond to acyclovir was that the infecting HSV was a mutant strain that lacked

- ○ A. cytosine deaminase
- ○ B. DNA polymerase
- ○ C. reverse transcriptase
- ○ D. thymidine kinase
- ○ E. thymidylate synthase

9. A 55-year-old man has a history of rapidly progressive weakness in all extremities, plus muscle atrophy, fasciculations, and increased deep tendon reflexes. There is a familial history of such motor weakness. Chromosomal analysis shows a point mutation in exon 1 of the gene for superoxide dismutase (SOD) on chromosome 21. Which of the following is the most likely diagnosis?

- ○ A. Amyotrophic lateral sclerosis (ALS)
- ○ B. Brown-Séquard's syndrome
- ○ C. Charcot-Marie-Tooth disease
- ○ D. Duchenne muscular dystrophy
- ○ E. Transection of the spinal cord

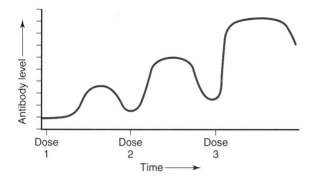

10. The figure above depicts the usual pattern of antibody levels in immunocompetent individuals after the first, second, and third doses of the same vaccine are administered on different dates. Which of the following immunoglobulin isotypes is chiefly responsible for the larger, secondary antibody responses (second and third curves) illustrated in the figure?

○ A. IgA
○ B. IgD
○ C. IgE
○ D. IgG
○ E. IgM

11. A 45-year old woman develops a fever and dyspnea approximately 24-hours post-cholecystectomy for acute gangrenous cholecystitis. Physical examination shows decreased percussion, increased tactile fremitus, and decreased breath sounds in the right lower lobe. The diaphragm is elevated, and there is inspiratory lag on the ipsilateral side. Which of the following is the most likely diagnosis?

○ A. Atelectasis
○ B. Lobar pneumonia
○ C. Lung abscess
○ D. Pulmonary infarction
○ E. Spontaneous pneumothorax

12. Microscopic examination of a surgical specimen taken from a small bowel resection shows varying degrees of pyknosis, karyorrhexis, and karyolysis in enterocytes located on the tips of the intestinal villi. Which of the following conditions is suggested by these findings?

○ A. Anaplasia
○ B. Apoptosis
○ C. Dysplasia
○ D. Inflammation

13. A 52-year-old man who was appropriately treated for *Plasmodium vivax* infection now complains of marked fatigue and notes that his urine has become dark. Urine samples are positive for bilirubin and urobilinogen. Hematologic studies show a hemoglobin concentration of 8.7 g/dL, a hematocrit of 30%, and a total bilirubin concentration of 4.2 mg/dL. The patient's complaints and laboratory findings could best be explained if he were treated with

○ A. chloroquine
○ B. doxycycline
○ C. primaquine
○ D. quinine
○ E. trimethoprim-sulfamethoxazole (TMP-SMX)

14. A 34-year-old woman discovers a lump in her left breast and is diagnosed with metastatic breast cancer. She is told that she has a poor prognosis and will most likely die within 6 months. Her initial reaction is most likely to be

○ A. anger
○ B. denial
○ C. depression
○ D. displacement
○ E. regression

15. A 1-year-old girl has a fever and initially is vomiting and has a generalized cutaneous petechial rash. She develops ecchymosis, mucosal hemorrhaging, hypotension, and cyanosis. Microscopic examination of her blood shows leukocytosis and evidence of disseminated intravascular coagulation. Blood samples cultured on chocolate agar grow an oxidase-positive, nonmotile, gram-negative diplococcus. Vascular damage and most of the other pathologic manifestations of this patient's disease are attributable to the infecting organism's

○ A. adherence to host cells
○ B. extracellular proteases
○ C. lipooligosaccharide endotoxin
○ D. peptidoglycan fragments
○ E. polysaccharide capsule

16. An 8-year-old boy who lives in an old building with flaking paint is suffering from vomiting, abdominal pain, apathy, and pallor. His performance in school has gradually declined. The figure below depicts the biosynthesis of heme. Five of the enzymes are labeled *A–E*. Inhibition of which enzyme would cause this boy's symptoms?

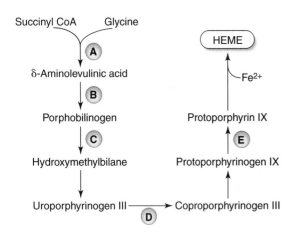

○ A. Enzyme A
○ B. Enzyme B
○ C. Enzyme C
○ D. Enzyme D
○ E. Enzyme E

17. A 62-year-old man who is right-handed says that his right hand shakes when he tries to start his car or open a door. His physician does not observe noticeable shaking when the patient's hands are resting in his lap. When asked to walk, the patient stumbles to the right. He states that he falls frequently. The most likely cause of these findings is a lesion in the

○ A. left internal capsule
○ B. left precentral gyrus
○ C. right caudal medulla
○ D. right cerebellum
○ E. right lateral corticospinal tract

18. A 31-year-old man is brought to the emergency department in an unconscious state. His wife says that he was in good health until 3 days ago, when he suffered a flulike illness that was severe enough to keep him from completing his job of cleaning out an old barn. He is hypotensive. He has a decreased serum albumin level, an increased white blood cell count with a left shift, band forms, and a platelet count that continues to fall. A chest x-ray shows interstitial infiltrate. Within 24 hours, the patient dies. An autopsy shows pulmonary edema. Which of the following agents is the most likely cause of the disease?

○ A. *Brucella suis*
○ B. *Coxiella burnetii*
○ C. Hantavirus
○ D. *Legionella pneumophila*
○ E. *Nocardia asteroides*

19. A 67-year-old woman with Parkinson's disease responds well to treatment with a combination of levodopa and carbidopa. The woman develops gastroesophageal reflux disease (GERD) and is prescribed an appropriate drug for its management. She is instructed to continue taking levodopa and carbidopa. After she starts taking the drug for GERD, she complains that her symptoms of Parkinson's disease have gotten worse. The drug most likely prescribed to treat GERD in this patient was

○ A. atropine
○ B. bethanechol
○ C. cisapride
○ D. famotidine
○ E. metoclopramide

20. A 15-year-old white boy complains of blurred vision, fatigue, and polyuria. He has lost about 3 kg (7 lb) during the past 3 weeks. A random blood glucose level obtained in the emergency department is 586 mg/dL. Laboratory tests show that he has elevated ketones and a pH of 7.1. He has been complaining of nonspecific abdominal pain; mild abdominal tenderness is elicited during the physical examination. He is admitted for diabetic ketoacidosis. Which of the following laboratory tests should be completed as a next step in treating this patient?

○ A. C-peptide and glutamic acid decarboxylase (GAD) titers and fasting glucose tolerance test (GTT)
○ B. C-peptide titer and Hemoccult stool test
○ C. C-peptide, islet cell antibody, and GAD antibody titers
○ D. Fasting GTT, blood urea nitrogen (BUN), and ophthalmologic exam
○ E. Oral GTT, BUN, and ECG

21. A 38-year-old woman with chronic liver disease complains of involuntary, flinging movements of her limbs. She states that other members of her family have had chronic liver disease, dementia, and abnormal body movements. Physical examination shows greenish brown deposits near the limbus of both eyes, an enlarged, firm liver, and splenomegaly. Which of the following laboratory studies would most likely be abnormal in this patient?

○ A. Decreased serum ceruloplasmin
○ B. Increased percent iron saturation
○ C. Increased total iron-binding capacity
○ D. Increased total serum copper

22. A 1-year-old boy is taken to his pediatrician suffering from a fever, chest congestion, rhinorrhea, and a "barking" cough of 3 days' duration. He has no rash, sputum production, or vomiting. Examination shows audible obstructive upper airway sounds typical of laryngeal edema. His throat is erythematous, but his lungs are clear. Bacterial and fungal cultures yield negative results. A virus that reacts with specific anti-HN antibody is isolated. Which of the following viruses is the most likely cause of the disease?

○ A. Influenza A virus
○ B. Influenza B virus
○ C. Parainfluenza virus 1
○ D. Parainfluenza virus 4
○ E. Respiratory syncytial virus

Type of Seizure	Characteristics of Seizure
Type X	Sudden, brief loss of consciousness; ECG shows 3-Hz spike-and-wave pattern.
Type Y	Impaired consciousness; lip-smacking and purposeless behavior; ECG shows discharges in left temporal region, right temporal region, or both regions.
Type Z	Sudden loss of consciousness; loss of postural control; muscle spasms; whole body contraction and relaxation; fecal and urinary incontinence; ECG shows diffuse seizure activity throughout both cerebral hemispheres.

23. The table above describes three types of seizures. Which of the following agents is most likely to be helpful in treating a patient whose mixed seizure disorder is characterized by type X and type Z seizures?

○ A. Carbamazepine
○ B. Clonazepam
○ C. Divalproex sodium
○ D. Ethosuximide
○ E. Phenytoin

24. Blood studies of a 48-year-old man with splenomegaly show elevated blood cell counts, and peripheral blood smears show a spectrum of cell forms ranging from mature polymorphonuclear neutrophils to immature blasts. Bone marrow findings show the presence of the Philadelphia chromosome. The mechanism most likely responsible for the patient's disease is

○ A. aneuploidy
○ B. deletion
○ C. point mutation
○ D. transition
○ E. translocation

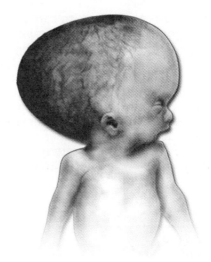

25. The figure shown above is from an in utero sonogram performed at 24-weeks' gestation. The condition of this fetus may be caused by

○ A. failure of the neural tube to close
○ B. maternal toxoplasmosis infection
○ C. premature closure of suture joints in the calvaria
○ D. stenosis of the foramen of Monro
○ E. underdeveloped choroid plexus

26. A 58-year-old man who has smoked 2 packs of cigarettes daily for 30 years has a chronic cough and occasionally produces blood-tinged sputum. X-ray film of the posteroanterior chest shows a mass in the region of the hilum of the left lung. His serum calcium level is 12.5 mg/dL; other laboratory studies are within normal limits. Cytology of the sputum is positive for the presence of malignant cells. The most likely cause of the paraneoplastic syndrome in this patient is

○ A. adenocarcinoma
○ B. bronchial carcinoid tumor
○ C. bronchioalveolar cell carcinoma
○ D. small cell carcinoma
○ E. squamous cell carcinoma

27. A 9-year-old boy is brought to the pediatrician because his mother says he is "out of control." She also says he has a poor attention span and exhibits impulsive behavior, hyperactivity, and occasional aggressiveness at home and in school. The boy has difficulty sitting still even when he is watching television or playing video games. The most likely diagnosis is

○ A. attention deficit hyperactivity disorder (ADHD)
○ B. autistic disorder
○ C. conduct disorder
○ D. oppositional defiant disorder
○ E. separation anxiety disorder

28. A 25-year-old woman has a fever, dysuria, a purulent urethral discharge, asymmetric arthritis, and a rash consisting of scattered erythematous papules. Microscopic examination of the urethral exudate shows the presence of numerous neutrophils and free and phagocytosed gram-negative cocci. Which of the following organisms is the most likely cause of the disease?

○ A. *Chlamydia trachomatis*
○ B. *Haemophilus ducreyi*
○ C. *Mycoplasma genitalium*
○ D. *Neisseria gonorrhoeae*
○ E. *Ureaplasma urealyticum*

29. An afebrile 35-year-old sheepherder who is living in a Basque community in southern Arizona complains of recurrent right upper quadrant pain. The sheepherder says that he and his dog spend their days together tending the sheep. A complete blood cell count shows a marked increase in the percentage of eosinophils. An ultrasound of his liver shows a cystic mass with calcifications in the lining of the cyst. Which of the following most accurately describes the epidemiology of this patient's liver disease?

○ A. The dog ate infected sheep
○ B. The dog is an intermediate host
○ C. The sheep is a definitive host
○ D. The sheepherder ate infected sheep
○ E. The sheepherder is a definitive host

30. If the life span of osteoclasts remains constant with aging but the life span of osteoblasts is progressively shortened, which disease process is most likely to develop?

○ A. Osteoclastoma
○ B. Osteomalacia
○ C. Osteopetrosis
○ D. Osteoporosis
○ E. Scurvy

31. A 2-day-old neonate with respiratory distress syndrome (RDS) has moderately severe hypoxemia. On auscultation, dry inspiratory crackles are heard in the lungs and a continuous harsh murmur is heard over the entire precordium. Which of the following sets of oxygen saturation (SaO_2) values in the cardiac chambers and vessels is most likely present in this patient?

Normal SaO_2 %
  Right atrium (RA) 75
  Right ventricle (RV) 75
  Pulmonary artery (PA) 75
  Pulmonary vein (PV) 95
  Left ventricle (LV) 95
  Aorta (A) 95

	RA	RV	PA	PV	LV	A
○ A.	75	80	80	95	95	95
○ B.	80	80	80	95	95	95
○ C.	75	75	80	95	95	95
○ D.	75	75	75	95	80	80

32. A 46-year-old man sustained severe lacerations in an automobile accident. When examined in the emergency department, he is severely hypovolemic and in hypotensive shock. A drug is administered to induce anesthesia, and isoflurane is used to maintain anesthesia during surgery. During postoperative recovery, the patient suffers from delirium, begins experiencing vivid and frightening dreams, and becomes markedly excited. Which of the following drugs was most likely used to induce anesthesia in this patient?

○ A. Ketamine
○ B. Midazolam
○ C. Nitrous oxide
○ D. Propofol
○ E. Thiopental

33. A 29-year-old woman who recently sustained a head injury after being thrown from a horse is dehydrated, despite having an insatiable thirst (polydipsia). Urine flow measurements confirm that a large volume of urine is being produced (polyuria). Which of the following is the most likely diagnosis?

○ A. Central diabetes insipidus
○ B. Glomerular nephritis
○ C. Nephrogenic diabetes insipidus
○ D. Proximal renal tubular acidosis
○ E. Syndrome of inappropriate antidiuretic hormone (ADH) secretion

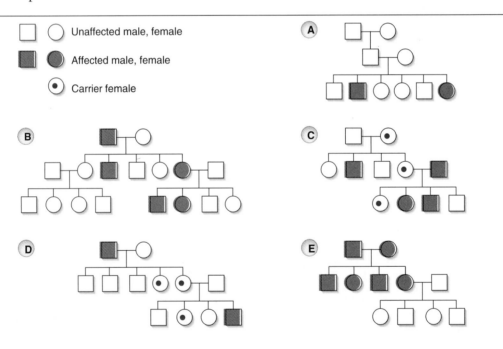

34. Several members of a family are diagnosed with von Willebrand's disease, inherited as an autosomal dominant disorder. After interviewing available unaffected and affected individuals, an epidemiologist is able to draw a pedigree of this family. Which of the pedigree patterns in the figure is consistent with the diagnosis?

○ A. Pattern A
○ B. Pattern B
○ C. Pattern C
○ D. Pattern D
○ E. Pattern E

35. A physician encourages his patients at high risk for negative responses to participate in stress management courses. The physician reminds them that the stressful life event most closely associated with physical and psychiatric illness is

○ A. death of a spouse
○ B. divorce
○ C. marriage
○ D. pregnancy
○ E. retirement

36. A 58-year-old woman with chest palpitations, dizziness, and generalized fatigue is brought to the emergency department. An ECG shows a regular cardiac rhythm with absent P waves. A diagnosis of paroxysmal supraventricular tachycardia (PSVT) is made. Before a drug for PSVT is chosen, the patient mentions that she has been suffering from asthma for at least 15 years and has been undergoing therapy with theophylline, albuterol, and beclomethasone. Shortly after an appropriate drug for PSVT is administered, the patient experiences dyspnea, characterized by wheezing and cough. In light of the patient's medical history, which of the following drugs was most likely administered for the emergency treatment of PSVT?

○ A. Adenosine
○ B. Amiodarone
○ C. Diltiazem
○ D. Lidocaine
○ E. Quinidine

37. A 6-year-old boy who was being treated for otitis media in the pediatric section of a children's hospital acquired a staphylococcal infection. Some staphylococci are phagocytosed by neutrophils (PMNs). About 13 hours later when the PMNs are no longer viable, viable staphylococci are liberated from these cells. Which disease state is suggested by these findings?

○ A. Chédiak-Higashi disease
○ B. Chronic granulomatous disease of childhood
○ C. Chronic inflammation
○ D. Chronic myelogenous leukemia

38. An unmarried 28-year-old woman has recently noticed gaps in her memory. While shopping, several unfamiliar people have called her by another name and talked to her as if they knew her well. She is unable to account for blocks of time and has awakened in bed with unknown men without recalling having invited the men home with her. She denies substance abuse, and there is no organic explanation for her symptoms. Which of the following is the most likely diagnosis?

○ A. Depersonalization disorder
○ B. Dissociative amnesia
○ C. Dissociative fugue
○ D. Dissociative identity disorder
○ E. Posttraumatic stress disorder (PTSD)

39. An 84-year-old man complains of lower back pain and inability to void urine over the past 24 hours. Physical examination shows point tenderness over the lower lumbar vertebrae and an enlarged bladder extending to the level of the umbilicus. The physician suspects metastatic prostate cancer. Which of the following is indicated as the first step in the management of this patient?

○ A. Digital rectal examination
○ B. Prostate-specific antigen (PSA)
○ C. Radionuclide bone scan
○ D. Serum alkaline phosphatase
○ E. Transrectal ultrasound with biopsy

40. A 15-year-old man has extreme difficulty recovering from infections caused by mucosal pathogens. Laboratory studies show a normal plasma IgA level; no IgA is detected in specimens of saliva, feces, and tears. The patient most likely has a defect in

○ A. B cells
○ B. endothelial cells
○ C. epithelial cells
○ D. monocytes and macrophages
○ E. type 2 helper T cells

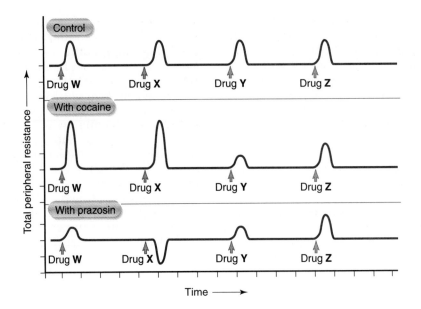

41. The figure above shows changes in total peripheral resistance *(TPR)* that occurred in response to four different drugs (labeled *W*, *X*, *Y*, and *Z*) administered in the same dosage and same order to three hypothetical groups of subjects. The first group *(top panel)* consisted of subjects who were not concurrently taking any other drugs and served as controls. The second group *(middle panel)* consisted of subjects who were concurrently taking cocaine. The third group *(bottom panel)* consisted of subjects who were concurrently taking prazosin. Based on the responses, the identity of drug *Y* is most likely represented by

○ A. acetylcholine
○ B. amphetamine
○ C. angiotensin II
○ D. epinephrine
○ E. norepinephrine

42. Which of the following is the best clinical indicator of significant pulmonary obstruction in patients with asthma?

○ A. Arterial hypoxemia
○ B. Dyspnea
○ C. FEV_1/FVC ratio of less than 75%
○ D. Large anatomic dead space volume
○ E. Rapid respirations

43. An 18-year-old man is hospitalized after being involved in a motorcycle accident. He has flaccid paralysis; deep tendon reflexes in all limbs 24 hours postinjury are absent. Paralytic ileus and loss of bladder function are also noted. The most likely cause of these findings is

○ A. Brown-Séquard's syndrome
○ B. commissural syndrome
○ C. posterior spinal artery bleeding
○ D. spinal shock
○ E. Weber syndrome

44. A 42-year-old woman complains of chronic constipation and progressive weight gain over the past 6 months despite maintaining a pure vegan diet. She takes no prescription or over-the-counter medications. Physical examination shows a pale woman with brittle hair, periorbital puffiness, a symmetrically enlarged, nontender thyroid gland, delayed deep tendon reflexes, and proximal muscle weakness in her lower extremities. Serum creatine kinase level is 350 U/L. Which set of the following sets of thyroid function studies shown below is most compatible with this patient's clinical findings?

	Serum T$_4$	Serum TSH	^{131}I
A.	Low	Low	Low
B.	Low	High	Normal
C.	High	Low	Low
D.	High	Low	High

T_4, Thyroxine; *TSH*, thyroid-stimulating hormone; ^{131}I, radioactive iodine uptake.

45. A 7-month-old infant develops a circumscribed lesion that is vesicular in appearance and contains no purulent exudate. When serous exudate from the lesion is cultured, the growth of staphylococci is noted. The medical records show that the infant has a history of recurrent low-grade infections in which pyogenic organisms cause vesicular, rather than pustular, lesions. Based on this pattern of atypical lesions, the physician should order

○ A. complete blood cell count
○ B. measurement of C3 levels
○ C. measurement of C5, C6, C7, and C8 levels
○ D. measurement of IgA levels
○ E. testing of B cell mitogen response

46. A 17-year-old boy has been engaging in risk-taking behavior by abusing alcohol and drugs, but does so only on weekends. He has also been seen driving at excessive speeds. His physician is concerned and counsels the teenager about his behavior, but the boy disregards the physician's advice and dies 6 months later. Which of the following is the most likely cause of the boy's death?

○ A. AIDS
○ B. Alcohol or drug overdose
○ C. Motor vehicle accident
○ D. Murder
○ E. Suicide

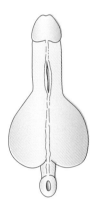

47. A newborn has urine oozing from an opening on the shaft of the penis (see figure above). Which of the following is the most likely explanation for this condition?

○ A. Abnormally high levels of dihydrotestosterone
○ B. Failure of the genital swellings to fuse
○ C. Female pseudohermaphroditism
○ D. Glans hypospadias
○ E. Incomplete fusion of the urethral folds

48. A 30-year-old woman states that she often burns her hands without feeling any pain. Physical examination shows decreased pain and temperature sensation in the upper extremities, atrophy of the intrinsic muscles of the hands, and abnormal deep tendon reflexes in the upper extremities. The pathogenesis of this patient's neurologic problems is most closely associated with which of the following?

○ A. Autoimmune destruction of myelin
○ B. Fluid-filled cavity in the cervical spinal cord
○ C. Superoxide free radical destruction of upper and lower motor neurons
○ D. Tumor in the cervical spinal cord
○ E. Vitamin B_{12} deficiency

49. An otherwise healthy boy has short stature. Although his growth rate and bone age are below the norm for children of the same chronologic age, his growth hormone level is within the normal range. The level of which of the following hormones is most likely to be abnormal?

○ A. Fibroblast growth factor
○ B. Insulin
○ C. Insulin-like growth factor I
○ D. Somatostatin
○ E. Somatotropin

50. A 68-year-old homeless man is in an alcoholic stupor when he is brought to the emergency department. After "drying out," he shows signs of severe retrograde amnesia. He exaggerates wildly about his living conditions, which he describes as luxurious. His in vitro red blood cell transketolase level rises 35% after thiamine diphosphate is added to the culture. A lesion in which of the following is the most likely cause of these findings?

○ A. Amygdaloid nuclei
○ B. Dorsomedial nucleus
○ C. Habenular nuclei
○ D. Nucleus accumbens
○ E. Nucleus basalis of Meynert

ANSWERS AND DISCUSSIONS

1. **E** (Parinaud's syndrome) is correct. Parinaud's syndrome (dorsal midbrain syndrome) is caused by a tumor or infarction in the pretectal region of the brain. It results in paralysis of upward gaze (i.e., patients develop a convergence nystagmus, which is characterized by a slow abduction followed by a quick adduction of the eye when they attempt to look upward). Their pupils react poorly to light but retain some degree of accommodation.

   A (Bell's palsy) is incorrect. Bell's palsy is a unilateral paralysis of the face due to a lesion affecting the facial nerve (CN VII). In severe cases, the eye does not close. The facial nerve innervates structures in the face but not the muscles within the eye or those responsible for its movement. Gaze, convergence, and pupillary dilation are not affected.

   B (cerebellar gaze palsy) is incorrect. The cerebellum helps regulate the timing of extraocular muscle contractions and coordinates compensation for changes in the strength of an extraocular muscle. Damage to the cerebellum can cause the eyes to deviate to the side opposite the lesion (cerebellar gaze palsy). Vertical gaze is not affected.

   C (internuclear ophthalmoplegia) is incorrect. Internuclear ophthalmoplegia results from a lesion in the medial longitudinal fasciculus. This neural pathway, which connects the abducens (CN VI) nucleus on one side with the contralateral oculomotor (CN III) nucleus, coordinates abduction of one eye with adduction of the other and results in a lateral gaze in one direction. Damage to this pathway results in an abnormal lateral gaze, but vertical gaze is not affected.

   D (one-and-a-half syndrome) is incorrect. One-and-a-half syndrome is caused by a relatively large lesion in the medial longitudinal fasciculus and the nucleus of CN VI. As a result, adduction in the ipsilateral eye is limited, but abduction in the contralateral eye is preserved. Vertical gaze is not affected.

2. **D** (sickle cell preparation) is correct. The patient most likely has sickle cell trait, which causes recurrent microscopic hematuria. Although the percentage of sickle hemoglobin in sickle cell trait is only ~40%, with the remainder representing hemoglobin A, the oxygen tension in the renal medulla is low enough to induce sickling of the RBCs in the peritubular capillaries. This results in microinfarctions in the renal medulla and the potential for renal papillary necrosis and loss of both concentration and dilution of urine.

   A (bone marrow examination) is incorrect. The patient most likely has a mild iron deficiency anemia, which is best diagnosed

with a serum ferritin level rather than a bone marrow examination. Furthermore, anemia is not a cause of microhematuria.
B   (cystoscopy) is incorrect. At this point in the patient's work-up, if the sickle cell screen is negative, a cystoscopy may be necessary to determine the cause of the hematuria.
C   (renal biopsy) is incorrect. If the sickle cell screen is negative, a renal biopsy may be necessary to rule out primary renal disease, particularly IgA glomerulonephritis.
E   (no further investigation is necessary) is incorrect. A recurrent history of microhematuria is always cause for concern and should be evaluated.

3. *B*   (glyburide) is correct. The patient's symptoms are consistent with hypoglycemia. Tremors, sweating, elevated blood pressure, and tachycardia are associated with increased sympathetic activity. Dizziness and confusion are due to central nervous system dysfunction. Hypoglycemia is the most common and potentially severe side effect of treatment with oral sulfonylureas, such as glyburide. These agents are believed to act by blocking ATP-dependent K^+ channels, thereby stimulating the release of insulin.

A   (acarbose) is incorrect. Acarbose inhibits α-glucosidase and thereby limits the postprandial rise in the blood glucose level. When given alone, the drug has no associated risk of hypoglycemia.
C   (human insulin) is incorrect. While insulin may cause hypoglycemia, it is a polypeptide and must be given subcutaneously (not orally). Its use in type 2 diabetes mellitus is reserved for patients whose symptoms are not adequately controlled by diet and oral hypoglycemic drugs.
D   (metformin) is incorrect. Since metformin does not stimulate the release of insulin, hypoglycemia has not been associated with its use.
E   (rosiglitazone) is incorrect. Rosiglitazone is a thiazolidinedione that lowers the blood glucose level by improving the target response to insulin without stimulating the secretion of insulin. Hypoglycemia has not been observed when rosiglitazone is used as monotherapy. Troglitazone, another thiazolidinedione, was withdrawn from the market because of liver toxicity. Although clinically significant hepatotoxicity has not yet been observed with rosiglitazone use, periodic liver function tests are recommended in patients treated with rosiglitazone.

4. *B*   (HIV infection) is correct. When a common skin test antigen (such as *Candida* antigen) is used, induration occurs at the test site in individuals who have a normal delayed-type hypersensitivity (DTH) reaction. The lack of a DTH response indicates a possible problem with T helper activity (anergy). In this case, anergy may be due to infection with HIV, so the patient should be tested for HIV.

A (asymptomatic measles virus infection) is incorrect. A person who is 51 years of age (or anyone who was born before 1955) should have naturally acquired immunity to measles. The presence of anergy in this case is therefore unlikely to be due to infection with the measles virus.

C (reaction to cold agglutinins) is incorrect. Cold agglutinins are used to test for infection with *Mycoplasma pneumoniae.* If the patient had been infected with *M. pneumoniae,* he would probably have had symptoms of "walking pneumonia."

D (reactivity to Hib) is incorrect. Reactivity to Hib is dependent on the B cell response (humoral immunity). The ability to mount an anamnestic response to a T cell–independent antigen (Hib) would not explain why the patient is failing to mount a DTH response.

E (response to B cell mitogen) is incorrect. DTH responses are associated with T cells, rather than B cells.

5. **B** (7.37) is correct. An acid-base disturbance is indicated by a base/acid ratio that is above or below physiologic pH (7.40). The disturbance can be either uncompensated, partially compensated, or fully compensated. An uncompensated disturbance (i.e., a "pure" effect) indicates an acute condition in which there is no time for any compensation to develop (e.g., induction of respiratory acidosis by breathholding for 1 minute). A disturbance is considered to be fully compensated if the primary acid-base imbalance is adequately balanced with secondary compensation (the opposing response). For example, if the acid component is too high (primary problem), the base/acid ratio can be restored to near normal by increasing the base component (secondary compensation). Thus, the disturbance in this example is almost fully compensated, as indicated by a base/acid ratio that is almost normal and an acid component that is above normal. Although the base component is not given, it too must also be elevated.

A (7.31) and E (7.50) are incorrect. In both cases, both the pH and acid component lie outside the normal range. Thus, both are too far from normal to be considered fully compensated.

C (7.40) and D (7.43) are incorrect. In both cases, the pH is well within the normal range (7.35–7.45). Thus, evidence of an acid-base disturbance is lacking. Without such a preexisting disturbance, there can be no compensation.

6. **C** (dorsal interossei—palmar interossei) is correct. To hold a dollar bill between any two adjacent digits (2–5), one digit must abduct, while the adjacent digit must adduct to press against its neighbor. The palmar interossei, which insert into the proximal phalanges on the ulnar side of the index finger and the radial sides of the ring and little fingers, adduct digits 2, 4, and 5 (**PAD** = **p**almar **ad**duct). The dorsal interossei, which insert into the proximal phalanges on the radial side of the index finger, on both sides of the middle finger, and on the ulnar side of the ring

finger, abduct digits 2–4 (**DAB** = **d**orsal **ab**duct). The thumb and the fifth digit each has its own abductor. The ulnar nerve innervates all interossei via its deep branch.

A (abductor digiti minimi—dorsal interossei) is incorrect. The dorsal interossei, which insert into the proximal phalanges on the radial side of the index finger, on both sides of the middle finger, and on the ulnar side of the ring finger, abduct digits 2–4 (**DAB** = **d**orsal **ab**duct). Both the palmar and dorsal interossei are necessary for abduction and adduction of digits 2–5. The fifth digit has a palmar interosseous muscle and its own abductor, the abductor digiti minimi. Only the adductor is used in the "dollar bill test." The thumb, with its own abductors and adductor, receives no input from the interossei.

B (adductor pollicis—lumbricals) is incorrect. The adductor pollicis muscle is important in holding the thumb against the index finger. The lumbricals are not involved in the actions of abduction or adduction. The thumb is unique in that it has its own named adductor and abductors. In the fingers, these actions are produced by the palmar and dorsal interossei.

D (lumbricals—palmar interossei) is incorrect. The palmar interossei, which insert into the proximal phalanges on the ulnar side of the index finger and the radial sides of the ring and little fingers, adduct digits 2, 4, and 5 (**PAD** = **p**almar **ad**duct). Both the palmar and dorsal interossei are necessary for abduction and adduction of digits 2–5. The muscles that abduct and adduct those digits would be necessary to hold the fingers against either side of a dollar bill. The thumb has its own abductors and adductor. Lumbricals are not involved in adduction or abduction. Instead, these muscles flex the metacarpophalangeal joints and extend the interphalangeal joints of digits 2–5.

7. *E* (phenylketonuria) is correct. Mental retardation, a musty odor, and hypopigmentation are classic manifestations of PKU. Phenylalanine hydroxylase, which converts phenylalanine to tyrosine, is deficient in this disease. The accumulation of phenylalanine and its metabolites is presumed to be responsible for the mental retardation and musty odor. Since tyrosine is a precursor of melanin, its deficiency will cause hypopigmentation of the skin.

A (alkaptonuria) is incorrect. Alkaptonuria is a defect of tyrosine catabolism. A deficiency of homogentisic acid oxidase (homogentisate 1,2-dioxygenase) causes excretion of homogentisate in the urine. Typical manifestations of alkaptonuria include ochronosis (dark pigmentation of connective tissue) and arthritis. They do not include mental retardation.

B (cystinuria) is incorrect. Cystinuria is characterized by the urinary loss of cystine, lysine, ornithine, and arginine. The loss of the four amino acids is caused by a defect in renal and gastrointestinal transport mechanisms. Cystine precipitation in the kidneys leads to renal stone formation. Cystinuria is not associated with mental retardation.

C (Down syndrome) and D (homocystinuria) are incorrect. Down syndrome and homocystinuria are associated with a variable degree of mental retardation, but they are not associated with hypopigmentation or a musty odor. Down syndrome is a chromosomal disorder. Homocystinuria is usually caused by a defect in cystathionine synthase, the enzyme responsible for converting homocysteine and serine to cystathionine. Homocysteine accumulates and leads to osteoporosis, lens dislocation, and a tendency for vascular thrombosis and mild to moderate mental retardation.

8. *D* (thymidine kinase) is correct. Acyclovir is used in the treatment of HSV infections and varicella-zoster virus (VZV) infections. The drug must be initially phosphorylated by a form of thymidine kinase that is specific to HSV and VZV. It then undergoes nonspecific phosphorylation to acyclovir triphosphate, the active metabolite that inhibits viral DNA polymerase. Mutant HSV strains that lack virus-specific thymidine kinase are resistant to acyclovir.

A (cytosine deaminase) is incorrect. Cytosine deaminase is not required for the activation of acyclovir. This enzyme is required for the activation of flucytosine (an antifungal agent) and is responsible for the reduced bioavailability of cytarabine (an anticancer drug).
B (DNA polymerase) is incorrect. If the HSV lacked DNA polymerase, it could neither multiply nor be affected by foscarnet.
C (reverse transcriptase) is incorrect. Reverse transcriptase (RNA-directed DNA polymerase) is not involved in the action of acyclovir. This enzyme is involved in the replication of HIV. Various nucleoside and nonnucleoside analogues act to inhibit reverse transcriptase and are used in combination therapy for the treatment of HIV infection and AIDS.
E (thymidylate synthase) is incorrect. Thymidylate synthase is not involved in the action of acyclovir. Inhibition of this enzyme does account in part for the antifungal activity of flucytosine and the oncolytic action of fluorouracil.

9. *A* (amyotrophic lateral sclerosis) is correct. This patient's characteristics fit the epidemiologic profile for ALS (also known as Lou Gehrig's disease). ALS tends to strike individuals aged 55 years or older and affects men more often than women. In most cases, the cause is unknown. ALS is characterized by progressive degeneration of the corticospinal tract and the anterior horn cells, which can result in the symptoms described for this patient. Between 5% and 10% of patients with ALS have the familial form of the disease, which is associated with a point mutation on exon 1 of the superoxide dismutase (SOD) gene on chromosome 21.

B (Brown-Séquard's syndrome) is incorrect. Brown-Séquard's syndrome is a result of hemisection of the spinal cord. It involves ipsilateral spastic paralysis, loss of fine touch and proprioception, and loss of contralateral pain and temperature signals below the level of the hemisection.

C (Charcot-Marie-Tooth disease) is incorrect. Charcot-Marie-Tooth disease (also known as hereditary motor and sensory neuropathy or peroneal muscular atrophy) is characterized by muscle weakness and atrophy. However, its effect is limited to the peroneal and distal leg muscles, as opposed to the widespread atrophy reported for this patient.

D (Duchenne muscular dystrophy) is incorrect. Duchenne muscular dystrophy is caused by an X-linked recessive genetic disorder that results in the absence of dystrophin, a protein found in the muscle cell membrane. As with ALS, it is characterized by progressive weakness in all muscles due to the degeneration of proximal muscle fibers. Unlike ALS, it is seen in male neonates rather than adults.

E (transection of the spinal cord) is incorrect. Transection of the spinal cord would cause paralysis caudally from the level of transection.

10. **D** (IgG) is correct. The figure shows the maturation of the immune response. The second and third doses of the vaccine each elicit a rise in IgG antibodies that is faster, higher, and longer-lasting than the rise elicited by the previous dose. IgG is the only immunoglobulin isotype that is increased in the secondary immune response. The development of memory T and B cells is characteristic of this response, which is also called the anamnestic response.

A (IgA), B (IgD), and C (IgE) are incorrect. IgA, IgD, and IgE are generally not induced in serum.

E (IgM) is incorrect. IgM is the first antibody induced after each dose, but it is not produced in increasingly larger amounts with each dose.

11. **A** (atelectasis) is correct. The most common cause of fever occurring within the first 24–36 hours after surgery is atelectasis, which refers to either a collapse of previously inflated lungs or incomplete expansion of the lungs on inspiration. Postoperatively, mucus plugs develop in the terminal bronchioles, allowing resorption of air out of the distal respiratory unit through the pores of Kohn. The physical findings of atelectasis are those of a lung consolidation, mainly decreased percussion and increased tactile fremitus (vibration of the chest wall when the patient speaks). The loss of lung mass results in ipsilateral elevation of the diaphragm and inspiratory lag, because the lung is not expanding properly on inspiration.

B (lobar pneumonia) is incorrect. Postoperative pneumonia usually develops 3–10 days after surgery.

C   (lung abscess) is incorrect. Aspiration of oropharyngeal contents, the most common cause of a lung abscess, does not occur within such a short time (24 h) after surgery. The patient usually has a cough productive of foul-smelling sputum due to the presence of aerobes and anaerobes in the abscess.

D   (pulmonary infarction) is incorrect. Pulmonary embolization usually occurs 5–7 days after surgery. In this patient, there is no history of pleuritic chest pain, which is invariably present in a pulmonary infarction. Most pulmonary emboli originate in the femoral vein.

E   (spontaneous pneumothorax) is incorrect. The physical findings are those of a lung consolidation. In a spontaneous pneumothorax, a portion of the lung collapses, which produces hyperresonance to percussion. Similar to atelectasis, however, a spontaneous pneumothorax shows inspiratory lag, decreased breath sounds, and elevated hemidiaphragm.

12. **B**   (apoptosis) is correct. Apoptosis (programmed cell death) occurs in several stages, which can be identified by light microscopy. During the first stage, pyknotic changes are indicated by the presence of one or more dark-staining masses on the inside of the nuclear membrane. During the second stage (karyorrhexis), nuclear material breaks into fragments. During the third stage (karyolysis), the nucleus breaks up into smaller membrane-bound bodies (apoptotic bodies), each of which contains some nuclear material. Eventually, this apoptotic debris will be scavenged by macrophages and lost to the luminal contents.

A   (anaplasia) is incorrect. Anaplasia is a severe type of dysplasia characterized by marked pleomorphism, extreme hyperchromaticity of the nucleus, and a nucleus/cytoplasm ratio closer to 1.0 than the normal 1:5. It is not characterized by the changes described for this specimen.

C   (dysplasia) is incorrect. Dysplasia is characterized by the loss of uniformity in cell size and a change in the shape and orientation of cells (pleomorphism). It does not result in degradation of the nucleus.

D   (inflammation) is incorrect. Inflammation is characterized by a proliferation of immune cells—neutrophils (PMNs) during the acute phase; lymphocytes, macrophages, and plasma cells during the chronic phase. It is not characterized by the changes described for this specimen.

13. **C**   (primaquine) is correct. Appropriate treatment for the cure of malaria due to *P. vivax* or *P. ovale* would include chloroquine to eradicate the blood schizonts plus primaquine to eradicate the tissue (liver) schizonts. The patient's symptoms and laboratory findings are consistent with primaquine-induced hemolytic anemia (HA) that is likely due to glucose-6-phosphate dehydrogenase (G6PD) deficiency. Drug-induced HA in individuals with G6PD deficiency is attributed to a lack of reduced glutathi-

one secondary to a decreased production of the reduced form of nicotinamide adenine dinucleotide phosphate (NADPH). In the absence of reduced glutathione, oxidizing metabolites (peroxides and other free radicals) of primaquine accumulate within red blood cells, where they convert hemoglobin to methemoglobin and cause Heinz body formation. The red blood cells then lyse and produce HA.

A   (chloroquine) is incorrect. Chloroquine is the drug of choice for eradicating the blood schizonts of all sensitive strains of *P. falciparum, P. malariae, P. ovale,* and *P. vivax.* However, chloroquine use is not associated with drug-induced HA in individuals with G6PD deficiency.
B   (doxycycline) is incorrect. Doxycycline is active against the blood schizonts of all *Plasmodium* species but is reserved for the treatment of chloroquine-resistant *P. falciparum* infection and for the prevention of malaria in individuals who are unable to tolerate mefloquine. Doxycycline treatment is not associated with HA.
D   (quinine) is incorrect. Like doxycycline, quinine is active against blood schizonts but is reserved for the treatment of chloroquine-resistant malaria. While quinine can cause HA in individuals with G6PD deficiency, it would not have been used to treat the patient described, since the patient had *P. vivax* infection, rather than *P. falciparum* infection. Falciparum malaria is the only form of malaria that is chloroquine-resistant.
E   (trimethoprim-sulfamethoxazole) is incorrect. Use of TMP-SMX has been associated with HA in G6PD-deficient patients. However, TMP-SMX is not used to treat malaria. Fansidar, a drug consisting of sulfadoxine (a sulfonamide) and pyrimethamine (a dihydrofolate reductase inhibitor), has been used to treat chloroquine-resistant falciparum malaria. It is ineffective against malariae, vivax, and ovale malaria.

14. **B**   (denial) is correct. The most common defense mechanism used by patients coping with the initial stages of an illness is denial. This mechanism can be initially healthy since it reduces stress and gives the patient time to come to terms with the diagnosis. However, long-term use of denial can be detrimental because it can decrease compliance.

A   (anger) is incorrect. Anger towards health care personnel, family members, or other healthy individuals is not uncommon when someone is coping with illness, especially a terminal illness such as cancer. It is rarely a patient's first reaction.
C   (depression) is incorrect. As an individual accepts the inevitability of an illness, depression is a common reaction. At this point, the physician must ascertain whether the depression represents a normal stage of grieving or is a clinical condition that may need to be treated.
D   (displacement) is incorrect. Displacement refers to the redirecting of a feeling from its original source to an alternative

source. For example, a patient who is angry about having cancer may show increased irritability towards loved ones.

E   (regression) is incorrect. Regression refers to a return to an earlier stage of development in order to cope with stress. For example, when a patient is diagnosed with an illness, it is not uncommon for the patient to temporarily become more dependent upon others. If the behavior persists, it may become problematic.

15. *C*   (lipooligosaccharide endotoxin) is correct. The patient's clinical and laboratory findings are consistent with the diagnosis of septicemia caused by *Neisseria meningitidis* (meningococcemia). The bacterium's lipooligosaccharide (LOS) endotoxin is responsible for the majority of the pathologic manifestations described. This potent endotoxin causes endothelial damage, thrombosis, and disseminated intravascular coagulation.

A   (adherence to host cells) is incorrect. Adherence to host tissue is important for the colonization of *N. meningitidis,* but this process does not contribute to substantial pathologic changes in infected patients.

B   (extracellular proteases) is incorrect. *N. meningitidis* produces an IgA protease, but the role of this enzyme in the pathogenesis of meningococcal disease is unknown.

D   (peptidoglycan fragments) is incorrect. Although peptidoglycan fragments may contribute to the inflammatory process in patients with meningococcal disease, these fragments are not thought to be as important as LOS endotoxin.

E   (polysaccharide capsule) is incorrect. *N. meningitidis* produces a polysaccharide capsule whose characteristics vary from serogroup to serogroup. The main function of the capsule is to inhibit phagocytosis. The capsule is not directly responsible for the pathologic manifestations of meningococcal disease.

16. *B*   (enzyme B) is correct. The clinical manifestations are consistent with the diagnosis of lead poisoning. In the figure, enzyme B is porphobilinogen synthase (also called δ-aminolevulinic acid dehydratase, ALA dehydratase, and ALA dehydrase). This enzyme catalyzes the conversion of δ-aminolevulinic acid (ALA) to porphobilinogen. It is a sulfhydryl enzyme sensitive to the presence of heavy metals. Lead exposure inhibits ALA dehydrogenase, thereby causing ALA to accumulate and be excreted in the urine. In the heme biosynthesis pathway, two other enzymes are sensitive to lead. One is coproporphyrinogen III oxidase, the enzyme that converts coproporphyrinogen III to protoporphyrinogen IX. The other is ferrochelatase (heme synthase), the enzyme that catalyzes the last step in heme biosynthesis, which is the insertion of an Fe^{2+} atom into the center of the porphyrin ring.

A   (enzyme A), C (enzyme C), D (enzyme D), and E (enzyme E) are incorrect. In the figure, enzyme A is ALA synthase, the enzyme that catalyzes the condensation of succinyl CoA with glycine. ALA synthase production is under negative feedback regulation by the pathway's end product, heme. In lead poisoning, the lower heme concentration causes an increase in the production of ALA synthase, and this results in the excess excretion of ALA. Enzyme C is uroporphyrinogen I synthase, the enzyme that converts porphobilinogen to hydroxymethylbilane. Uroporphyrinogen I is then formed from hydroxymethylbilane in the spontaneous cyclization of this compound. If uroporphyrinogen II cosynthase is also present, uroporphyrinogen II (instead of uroporphyrinogen I) is produced from hydroxymethylbilane. Enzyme D is uroporphyrinogen III decarboxylase, and enzyme E is protoporphyrinogen IX oxidase. Enzymes C, D, and E are not sensitive to lead.

17. *D* (right cerebellum) is correct. The fact that the patient's dominant hand shakes when he tries to use keys or turn a doorknob indicates an intention tremor, which is associated with cerebellar damage. The cerebellum affects only voluntary movements; for this reason, the patient does not exhibit a resting tremor, which is induced by damage to the basal ganglia and/or thalamic nuclei influenced by the basal ganglia. Signs of cerebellar damage are usually seen on the same side as the lesion. Signs such as tremor in the right hand and the patient stumbling to the right suggest that the lesion is on the right side of the cerebellum.

A (left internal capsule) is incorrect. The internal capsule contains fibers traveling to and from the cerebral cortex. A lesion in the descending fibers would cause spastic paralysis if it affected descending motor fibers.
B (left precentral gyrus) is incorrect. The precentral gyrus contains the primary motor cortex. Damage to this region would affect output to the upper motor neurons and result in spastic paralysis.
C (right caudal medulla) is incorrect. The right caudal medulla contains corticospinal fibers that have not decussated at the pyramids. A lesion in this region would disrupt upper motor neuron activity and result in spastic paralysis on the right side of the body.
E (right lateral corticospinal tract) is incorrect. The lateral corticospinal tract contains fibers that terminate on the lateral aspect of the anterior horn, which contains neurons that innervate the most distal structures in the limbs. Damage to this tract could cause problems involving the hands. However, the patient's constant falling suggests that the area involved is not limited to one set of limbs.

18. *C* (hantavirus) is correct. The clinical, laboratory, and x-ray findings are consistent with the diagnosis of hantavirus pulmonary syndrome. This disease is caused by a hantavirus, whose reservoirs are rodent feces and urine.

A *(Brucella suis)* is incorrect. *B. suis* infection is usually acquired via contact with the infected tissues or body fluids of pigs. Brucellosis can be ruled out, because it has an insidious onset and course. Signs and symptoms of brucellosis are similar to those of tuberculosis and include fever, night sweats, and weight loss that continues for months.

B *(Coxiella burnetii)* is incorrect. Q fever is caused by *C. burnetii* and is usually acquired via contact with the infected tissues or body fluids of sheep, goats, cattle, or cats. Q fever can be ruled out, because it has a more insidious onset and rarely follows the fulminant and fatal course described.

D *(Legionella pneumophila)* is incorrect. *L. pneumophila* causes legionnaires' disease and Pontiac fever. Either of these diseases can have a sudden onset, and legionnaires' disease can run a fulminant course. The infection is usually acquired via inhalation of contaminated aerosols, and affected individuals are usually over 50 years of age, so the patient described is not in the usual population at risk. In addition, the presence of pulmonary edema and the laboratory findings of a left shift, band forms, and falling platelet count are inconsistent with *L. pneumophila* infection.

E *(Nocardia asteroides)* is incorrect. *N. asteroides* is an opportunistic pathogen that usually affects severely immunocompromised patients, such as those with cancer or AIDS. Although the organism produces pulmonary disease, it has an insidious course and rarely affects immunocompetent individuals.

19. *E* (metoclopramide) is correct. The manifestations of Parkinson's disease are believed to arise from the loss of pigmented neurons in the substantia nigra. This loss causes a decrease in dopamine's inhibitory input to the striatum and also creates a relative increase in acetylcholine's excitatory input to the striatum. In patients with GERD, metoclopramide has beneficial prokinetic and antiemetic activities. Metoclopramide releases acetylcholine from the myenteric plexus of the enteric nervous system and thereby increases the tone of the lower esophageal sphincter. It also blocks dopamine receptors and thereby prevents vomiting. By blocking dopamine receptors in the nigrostriatal dopaminergic pathway, metoclopramide would exacerbate the imbalance of dopamine and acetylcholine input to the striatum and thereby worsen the manifestations of Parkinson's disease.

A (atropine) is incorrect. Atropine would be contraindicated in the treatment of GERD. If it were given to the patient described, it would be more likely to alleviate than to worsen the manifestations of Parkinson's disease, because it would partially correct the imbalance of dopamine and acetylcholine input to the striatum.

B (bethanechol) is incorrect. Bethanechol, a muscarinic agonist, increases the tone of the lower esophageal sphincter but is used less frequently than other agents for the treatment of GERD. As a quaternary compound, it has no central nervous system action and thus would not worsen the manifestations of Parkinson's disease.

C (cisapride) is incorrect. Cisapride, a prokinetic agent, acts in a manner similar to metoclopramide but does not block dopamine receptors. The drug currently has only very limited availability, since its use is associated with QT prolongation (torsade de pointes) leading to fatal ventricular fibrillation.

D (famotidine) is incorrect. Famotidine, a histamine H_2 receptor antagonist, decreases the secretion of gastric acid and is used in the management of mild to moderate GERD.

20. *C* (C-peptide, islet cell antibody, and GAD antibody titers) is correct. This patient has several risk factors for type 1 diabetes mellitus, including race and age. His symptoms of blurred vision, fatigue, polyuria, and weight loss suggest hyperglycemia, where the pancreas fails to produce adequate amounts of insulin. Further studies should include pancreatic function tests: C-peptide, to determine the amount of insulin produced; islet cell antibodies and antibodies to GAD are commonly found in individuals with acute onset type 1 diabetes and reflect an autoimmune process capable of destroying pancreatic tissue.

A (C-peptide and glutamic acid decarboxylase titers and fasting glucose tolerance test) is incorrect. A low C-peptide and elevated GAD antibodies suggest that the pancreas is being destroyed by means of an autoimmune disorder (i.e., type 1 diabetes mellitus). These tests would be useful in a patient with a severe form of the disease or uncontrolled disease, who would be at risk for ketoacidosis. A fasting GTT identifies hyperglycemia or the early stages of type 2 diabetes mellitus, in which pancreatic function is usually preserved. Individuals with borderline or mild case of the disease would have a much lower risk for ketoacidosis.

B (C-peptide titer and Hemoccult stool test) is incorrect. A Hemoccult stool test may be ordered to evaluate the abdominal pain; however, the ketoacidosis may be causing the pain. C-peptide titer is one of several tests used to evaluate the ability of the pancreas to produce insulin. By itself, a C-peptide titer is inadequate to determine whether the patient has type 1 diabetes mellitus or to determine the severity of the disease.

D (fasting GTT, blood urea nitrogen, and ophthalmologic exam) is incorrect. The fasting GTT can identify borderline or early-stage type 2 diabetes mellitus. BUN and ophthalmologic health are monitored regularly in people with this disorder to identify potential complications early. These are useful in patients with borderline or mild disease, who are less likely to develop ketoacidosis. While the latter two tests may also be warranted in patients with type 1 disease on a follow-up visit, the fasting GTT would not provide enough information to verify that the patient has type 1 vs type 2 disease.

E (oral GTT, BUN, and ECG) is incorrect. Patients with a borderline fasting glucose are given an oral GTT to determine whether they have postprandial hypoglycemia and early type 2 diabetes. Patients with diabetes are often monitored with BUN and ECG tests to identify potential complications early, but this 15-year-old patient is an unlikely candidate for coronary artery disease and thus the ECG is unnecessary.

21. *A* (decreased serum ceruloplasmin) is correct. The patient has Wilson's disease (hepatolenticular degeneration), which is inherited as an autosomal recessive trait. The disease is characterized by a defect in the elimination of copper in bile. Copper accumulates in the liver, producing toxic damage to the hepatocytes, starting as acute hepatitis and progressing to chronic hepatitis and cirrhosis. Serum copper levels reflect the amount of copper bound to ceruloplasmin (90%–95% of the total serum copper level) plus free and unbound copper. As expected in any chronic liver disease, protein synthesis is decreased, including synthesis of ceruloplasmin. Hence, the decrease in ceruloplasmin leads to a decrease in the total serum copper level, with a corresponding increase in the circulating level of free copper. The excess copper accumulates in Descemet's membrane of the eyes, producing the Kayser-Fleischer ring. In the brain, copper produces toxic injury in the basal ganglia, particularly in the putamen, where it causes atrophy and visible cavitation. When toxic injury occurs in the subthalamic nucleus, the patient develops hemiballismus (flailing of the limbs). Extrapyramidal signs and dementia also may occur.

    B (increased percent iron saturation) is incorrect. This implies the presence of acquired iron overload disease (hemosiderosis) or hemochromatosis, which is an autosomal recessive disorder. Diseases caused by iron overload are not associated with pigment deposits in the eyes, dementia, or movement disorders.
    C (increased total iron-binding capacity) is incorrect. This reflects increased synthesis of transferrin in the liver, which primarily occurs in iron deficiency anemia. In chronic liver disease, the total iron-binding capacity is decreased due to decreased synthesis of transferrin.
    D (increased total serum copper) is incorrect. The serum ceruloplasmin is decreased in patients with Wilson's disease; total serum copper level is decreased, and the free copper level is increased in serum and urine. Total copper levels are increased in the liver parenchyma.

22. *C* (parainfluenza virus 1) is correct. This is a classic case of croup caused by parainfluenza virus 1. The disease is characterized by laryngeal edema and inflammation that obstruct the airway and cause a dry, "barking" cough. In young children, from 30%–40% of cases of croup are caused by parainfluenza virus type 1, 2, or 3. Type 1 is the most common cause in the United States. The parainfluenza viruses have an envelope protein, called the HN protein, and have both hemagglutinating and neuraminidase activity.

A (influenza A virus) and B (influenza B virus) are incorrect. The influenza A and B viruses occasionally cause croup, but these viruses do not have a combined HN protein. They have distinct H proteins and N proteins.

D (parainfluenza virus 4) is incorrect. Parainfluenza virus 4 causes symptoms of the common cold but is not an etiologic agent of croup.

E (respiratory syncytial virus) is incorrect. Respiratory syncytial virus is an etiologic agent of croup, but it lacks the HN surface protein.

23. *C* (divalproex sodium) is correct. In the table, seizure X is an absence seizure; seizure Y is a complex partial seizure; and seizure Z is a tonic-clonic seizure. Divalproex sodium (a formulation of valproate) is a broad-spectrum antiepileptic agent useful for the treatment of all three types of seizures.

A (carbamazepine) and E (phenytoin) are incorrect. Carbamazepine and phenytoin are useful for the treatment of tonic-clonic and complex partial seizures but ineffective in the treatment of absence seizures.

B (clonazepam) is incorrect. Clonazepam is useful for the treatment of absence seizures but ineffective in the treatment of tonic-clonic and complex partial seizures. Patients develop tolerance for the antiepileptic effect of this drug.

D (ethosuximide) is incorrect. Ethosuximide is considered by many neurologists to be the drug of choice for treating absence seizures. It has no utility in the treatment of tonic-clonic or complex partial seizures.

24. *E* (translocation) is correct. The patient's laboratory findings are consistent with the diagnosis of chronic myelogenous leukemia (CML). The Philadelphia chromosome is the best-known human chromosomal abnormality associated with cancer. In affected patients, chromosome 22 has shortened long arms, part of which are translocated to chromosome 9. This results in the formation of a hybrid *c-abl-bcr* gene that plays a pathogenic role in CML.

A (aneuploidy) is incorrect. Aneuploidy is present if the number of chromosomes is not a multiple of 2; the number may be above or below the normal number of 46. In CML, the number of chromosomes is not changed.

B (deletion) is incorrect. Deletions are mutations in which bases are removed from the normal sequence. Some deletions are huge, affecting large fragments of the chromosome. Deletions are not found in CML.

C (point mutation) and D (transition) are incorrect. A point mutation is a change in a single base pair of the DNA. A transition is a point mutation in which a purine is replaced by another purine or in which a pyrimidine is replaced by another pyrimidine. Transitions and other point mutations are not associated with CML.

25. *B* (maternal toxoplasmosis infection) is correct. *Toxoplasma gondii,* a parasitic contaminant found in infected cat feces and undercooked meat, is the causal pathogen in toxoplasmosis, which causes hydrocephaly. The parasite crosses the placenta, resulting in several destructive changes in the brain, including impaired cerebrospinal fluid (CSF) circulation. All ventricles enlarge if openings (foramina of Magendie and Luschka) from the fourth ventricle are blocked. The hydrocephaly that may result is controlled by implanting a prosthetic shunt.

A   (failure of the neural tube to close) is incorrect. Failure of the neural tube to close affects not only the brain and spinal cord but also overlying tissues. Neural tube defects, which are detectable in utero by elevated levels of alpha-fetoprotein, range from clinically significant defects such as rachischisis to insignificant posterior skin dimples.
C   (premature closure of suture joints in the calvaria) is incorrect. Premature synostosis results in several types of skull deformities, such as scaphocephaly, oxycephaly, or acrocephaly. The type of deformity depends on which sutures close prematurely. In hydrocephaly, increased CSF pressure results in expansion of the brain with concomitant expansion of the calvaria, because suture joints of the calvaria are not yet ossified.
D   (stenosis of the foramen of Monro) is incorrect. Stenosis of the foramen of Monro causes an opening between a lateral ventricle and the third ventricle. It does result in hydrocephaly, but the enlargement is confined to the affected lateral ventricle and not to the entire ventricular system. Narrowing of ventricular foramina results in dilatation in the ventricles proximal to the obstruction.
E   (underdeveloped choroid plexus) is incorrect. Underdevelopment of the choroid plexus implies less-than-normal production of CSF; that would not result in dilatation of the ventricular system unless a blockage has occurred. However, overproduction of CSF can result in hydrocephaly if production of CSF is not balanced by increased absorption.

26. *E* (squamous cell carcinoma) is correct. Any histologic type of neoplasm may produce any of the paraneoplastic syndromes associated with lung cancer, but squamous cell carcinoma is most often associated with hypercalcemia.

A   (adenocarcinoma) and C (bronchioloalveolar cell carcinoma) are incorrect. Adenocarcinoma or bronchioalveolar cell carcinoma may occasionally produce any of the paraneoplastic syndromes associated with carcinoma of the lung, but they are not associated with hypercalcemia.
B   (bronchial carcinoid tumor) is incorrect. A bronchial carcinoid tumor is rarely associated with the production of a paraneoplastic syndrome.

D (small cell carcinoma) is incorrect. Small cell (or oat cell) carcinomas are more likely to be associated with secretion of antidiuretic hormone or adrenocorticotropic hormone.

27. *A* (attention deficit hyperactivity disorder) is correct. Distractibility, poor concentration, impulsivity, and hyperactivity are prominent symptoms of ADHD. The disorder is commonly seen in pediatric practices and is more prevalent in boys than in girls. ADHD is most commonly treated with the drug methylphenidate hydrochloride and/or behavioral therapy approaches (e.g., restructuring the child's environment; rewarding for appropriate behavior).

B (autistic disorder) is incorrect. Autism is a pervasive developmental disorder in which significant impairment is evident in communication, social interaction, and behavior. Repetitive mannerisms (e.g., head banging) and a need for sameness are also common.
C (conduct disorder) is incorrect. A repetitious pattern of antisocial behavior (e.g., lying, stealing, truancy, cruelty to animals) in childhood are all suggestive of a conduct disorder. This disorder is often a precursor to antisocial personality disorder.
D (oppositional defiant disorder) is incorrect. A pervasive pattern of hostile and defiant behavior typifies an oppositional defiant disorder.
E (separation anxiety disorder) is incorrect. Excessive anxiety about separation from home or an individual with whom a child is significantly attached defines separation anxiety disorder. The degree of anxiety exceeds what is expected given the child's developmental level.

28. *D* (Neisseria gonorrhoeae) is correct. The clinical and laboratory findings are consistent with the diagnosis of disseminated gonococcal infection. Dissemination of infection with *N. gonorrhoeae* is seen more frequently in women than in men and develops in 1%–3% of patients who have gonorrhea.

A *(Chlamydia trachomatis)*, C *(Mycoplasma genitalium)*, and E *(Ureaplasma urealyticum)* are incorrect. *C. trachomatis, M. genitalium,* and *U. urealyticum* cause urethritis and other diseases, but these organisms are not cocci and would not typically be found within neutrophils.
B *(Haemophilus ducreyi)* is incorrect. *H. ducreyi* is not a coccus and does not cause urethritis. It causes a genital ulcer called chancroid.

29. *A* (the dog ate infected sheep) is correct. The patient has echinococcosis due to the tapeworm *Echinococcus granulosis* or *E. multilocularis*. In the normal developmental cycle of the *Echinococcus* species, adult worms mate and lay eggs that develop into larvae. The larvae mature into adult worms, and the cycle repeats.

Hosts containing the larval form are called intermediate hosts, while hosts containing the adult worms are called definitive hosts.

B (the dog is an intermediate host) is incorrect. Adult worms in the dog mate and lay eggs. The sheepherder picks up the eggs by petting the dog, then handling his own food and unknowingly ingesting the eggs. The eggs develop into larvae in the sheepherder. The sheepherder then becomes the intermediate host.
C (the sheep is a definitive host) is incorrect. The dog becomes the definitive host.
D (the sheepherder ate infected sheep) is incorrect. The sheep is the intermediate host.
E (the sheepherder is a definitive host) is incorrect. The larvae penetrate the wall of the duodenum, transmigrate across the peritoneum, and penetrate the liver to produce a single cyst *(E. granulosis)* or multiple cysts *(E. multilocularis).* The cysts contain numerous scolices with hooklets representing the heads of future adult worms; however, because the sheepherder is the end-stage of the cycle, adult worms are never produced. Cyst walls often become calcified. Rupture of a cyst often results in anaphylactic shock. Treatment with albendazole and percutaneous drainage or surgery is the treatment of choice.

30. *D* (osteoporosis) is correct. Osteoporosis is a reduction in bone mass, which increases the risk for fracture after minimal trauma. Osteoporosis develops as a result of an imbalance between bone deposition and bone resorption. Women tend to be at greater risk for this condition as they age, because the life span and activity of osteoblasts decreases with the loss of estrogen after menopause. If the loss of osteoblast activity is not accompanied by a change in osteoclast activity, bone loss will continue, resulting in a detectable loss of bone mass over time.

A (osteoclastoma) is incorrect. Osteoclastoma (giant cell neoplasm in bone) is a relatively common benign bone neoplasm and makes up 20% of benign bone neoplasms. It usually arises in the epiphyseal regions of the long bones of the extremities and is characterized by the presence of a large number of osteoclast-like cells. It has no effect on the life span of osteoblasts.
B (osteomalacia) is incorrect. Osteomalacia is characterized by inadequate mineralization of bone matrix. It is associated with vitamin D deficiency, which reduces the rate of absorption of calcium across the lining of the intestines; this then reduces the amount of calcium available to mineralize bone matrix.
C (osteopetrosis) is incorrect. Osteopetrosis is characterized by the production of excessive amounts of bone matrix. Patients with this condition develop brittle bones.
E (scurvy) is incorrect. Scurvy is characterized by the inability of osteoblasts to manufacture normal amounts of bone matrix (collagen). Scurvy is commonly associated with hypovitaminosis C.

31. *C* (RA 75, RV 75, PA 80, PV 95, LV 95, A 95) is correct. The patient has the classic machinery murmur (continuous murmur) of a patent ductus arteriosus (PDA). Because the neonate has hypoxemia (low arterial PO_2) secondary to RDS, the ductus has no stimulus to close. Infants with congenital heart diseases often have shunts between chambers or vessels. The pressure in the chamber or vessel determines the direction of blood flow. When oxygenated blood (SaO_2 95%) is shunted into a chamber or vessel with venous blood (SaO_2 75%), there is a step-up of SaO_2 (~80%) in the venous blood; this is known as a left-to-right shunt. Similarly, when venous blood is shunted into a chamber or vessel with oxygenated blood, there is a step-down of the SaO_2 (~80%) leading to clinical evidence of cyanosis; this is known as a right-to-left shunt. In PDA, blood initially flows from the aorta (where pressure is high), through the patent ductus arteriosus, and into the pulmonary artery (where pressure is low), a left-to-right shunt; hence there is a step-up of the SaO_2 in the pulmonary artery.

A (RA 75, RV 80, PA 80, PV 95, LV 95, A 95) is incorrect. A step-up of SaO_2 in the right ventricle and pulmonary artery is consistent with a ventricular septal defect (VSD, or left-to-right shunt), which is the most common congenital heart disease. If a VSD is left uncorrected, the volume overload in the right side of the heart due to the left-to-right shunt leads to pulmonary hypertension. This is followed by right ventricular hypertrophy and eventual reversal of the shunt (right-to-left), producing clinical evidence of cyanosis, or Eisenmenger's syndrome.

B (RA 80, RV 80, PA 80, PV 95, LV 95, A 95) is incorrect. A step-up of the SaO_2 in the right atrium, right ventricle, and pulmonary artery is consistent with an atrial septal defect (ASD, or left-to-right shunt), which is most often the result of a patent foramen ovale. Eisenmenger's syndrome also may occur in an ASD (refer to the discussion for A).

D (RA 75, RV 75, PA 75, PV 95, LV 80, A 80) is incorrect. A step-down of the SaO_2 in the left ventricle and aorta is consistent with tetralogy of Fallot (right-to-left shunt), which is the most common type of cyanotic congenital heart disease. It consists of an overriding aorta (least common defect), VSD, infravalvular pulmonary stenosis, and right ventricular hypertrophy. The degree of pulmonic stenosis determines the severity of the right-to-left shunt. If the stenosis is not severe, then most of the venous blood enters the pulmonary artery and is oxygenated; hence the patient is often acyanotic. However, when the stenosis is severe, most of the venous blood is shunted through the VSD into the left ventricle (right-to-left shunt), leading to cyanosis. Coexisting PDA and ASD are cardioprotective in a tetralogy. A PDA allows some of the unoxygenated blood in the aorta to reenter the pulmonary artery for oxygenation in the lungs. An ASD allows oxygenated blood from the left atrium to shunt into the right atrium and step-up the SaO_2 in the right side of the heart.

32. *A* (ketamine) is correct. In hypotensive patients, ketamine is useful for inducing anesthesia because it is a cardiovascular stimulant. The drug normally raises blood pressure by increasing cardiac output. During postoperative recovery, 5%–30% of adults suffer from delirium and other symptoms seen in the patient described. Since these adverse effects are rare in children, ketamine is most commonly employed for pediatric surgery. To minimize the adverse effects of ketamine induction, patients should be taken to a recovery room with minimal audiovisual stimulation.

B   (midazolam) is incorrect. Midazolam is a benzodiazepine frequently used for preoperative amnesia or sedation and is less frequently used for induction of anesthesia. Midazolam use is not associated with postanesthetic delirium.

C   (nitrous oxide) is incorrect. Nitrous oxide is used as an adjunct to volatile anesthetic agents for induction and is not associated with delirium upon recovery. Its major adverse effect is diffusional hypoxia, which can be prevented by administering 100% oxygen to the patient for 5–10 minutes after nitrous oxide use is stopped.

D   (propofol) and E (thiopental) are incorrect. Either propofol or thiopental can be used to induce anesthesia. Propofol has an "intrinsic" antiemetic effect and has a shorter recovery time than thiopental. Moreover, propofol does not require inventory logs, since it is not a controlled substance. Because of these major advantages, propofol is the agent most frequently used to induce anesthesia. Use of propofol or thiopental is not associated with postanesthetic delirium.

33. *A* (central diabetes insipidus) is correct. The high urinary output and extreme thirst indicate severe dehydration due to abnormal water processing by the kidney. ADH normally promotes water reabsorption in the kidney, thereby preventing dehydration. However, a head injury such as that sustained by this patient can jar the pituitary stalk and disrupt the normal rate of secretion of antidiuretic hormone (ADH). When ADH levels are too low or its activity cannot be detected properly by the kidney, diuresis (the loss of excessive amounts of watery urine) will occur.

B   (glomerular nephritis) is incorrect. Damage to the glomerulus would interfere with glomerular filtration. The reduced urinary solute load would induce water reabsorption and, consequently, would reduce urinary output.

C   (nephrogenic diabetes insipidus) is incorrect. This type of diabetes insipidus can be caused by renal problems (e.g., a low density of ADH receptors in the collecting ducts).

D   (proximal renal tubular acidosis) is incorrect. Proximal renal tubular acidosis is irrelevant, given the patient's history.

E   (syndrome of inappropriate antidiuretic hormone secretion) is incorrect. Hypersecretion of ADH would result in an excessive water reabsorption rate and possibly result in hypervolemia.

34. *B* (pattern B) is correct. Autosomal dominant disorders affect heterozygotes who have one normal and one abnormal allele. Each child of the affected individual has a 50% chance of being affected. Sons and daughters are affected in equal proportions. Normal (unaffected) children of affected individuals have only normal offspring. Vertical transmission through generations occurs.

A (pattern A) is incorrect. Pattern A depicts autosomal recessive inheritance. In autosomal recessive disorders, clinical manifestations are apparent only in homozygotes. The heterozygous parents are clinically normal. Sons and daughters are affected in equal proportions.

C (pattern C) is incorrect. Pattern C depicts X-linked recessive inheritance. Females are carriers of the trait, and males are affected. A homozygous female may show clinical manifestations if she is the daughter of an affected father and a carrier mother.

D (pattern D) is incorrect. Like pattern C, pattern D depicts X-linked recessive inheritance. All daughters of affected males are carriers, and affected males do not transmit the disease to their sons.

E (pattern E) is incorrect. Like pattern A, pattern E depicts autosomal recessive inheritance. All of the children will be affected by a recessive disorder if both of their parents are affected homozygotes. None of the children will be affected if only one parent is an affected homozygote.

35. *A* (death of a spouse) is correct. In their 1967 study, Dr. Thomas H. Holmes and Dr. Richard H. Rahe interviewed individuals from varying backgrounds to identify recent stressors and rank the amount of readjustment that life events required. A total of 41 major stressors were routinely identified and weighted, leading to the development of the Social Readjustment Rating Scale (SRRS). The death of a spouse was defined as the most stressful life event and ranked as requiring 100 Life-Change Units (LCUs) on a scale where 11 equals the least and 100 equals the most LCUs. Only stressors with sufficient magnitude were identified.

B (divorce) is incorrect. A divorce was defined as the second most stressful event, requiring 73 LCUs, but was ranked considerably below the death of a spouse.

C (marriage) is incorrect. Although marriage is typically viewed as a positive event, the transitions required resulted in marriage being ranked as 7 on the Social Readjustment Rating Scale (SRRS), requiring 50 LCUs.

D (pregnancy) is incorrect. Pregnancy was ranked 12, requiring 40 LCUs.

E (retirement) is incorrect. Retirement was ranked close to marriage, at 10, requiring 45 LCUs.

36. *A* (adenosine) is correct. PSVT is most commonly characterized by atrioventricular (AV) node reentry. Adenosine slows conduction through the AV node and can interrupt reentry pathways and restore normal sinus rhythm in patients with PSVT. Adenosine acts through its own receptor, which is linked to adenylyl cyclase by the inhibitory G protein (G_i). Coupling of the adenosine receptor and G_i causes a decrease in the production of cyclic adenosine monophosphate (cAMP). Adenosine also causes pronounced contraction of bronchiole smooth muscle, which would account for respiratory distress in this patient. Theophylline and other methylxanthines act as competitive adenosine receptor antagonists, and this mechanism is thought to account in part for the effectiveness of theophylline in the management of chronic asthma. In many cases, when adenosine is used for the emergency management of PSVT, the patient's heart will stop briefly (for a few seconds) before it resumes its normal activity.

B (amiodarone) is incorrect. Amiodarone is categorized as a class III antiarrhythmic drug, but it also has class I, II, and IV activity. Amiodarone is reserved for the treatment of life-threatening ventricular arrhythmias that cannot be controlled with class IA or IB drugs.
C (diltiazem) is incorrect. Diltiazem is a class IV antiarrhythmic drug. It has utility in the management of PSVT, but it would not have caused the patient's respiratory distress.
D (lidocaine) is incorrect. Lidocaine is a class IB antiarrhythmic drug. It is not indicated for the management of PSVT. It is reserved for the emergency management of ventricular arrhythmias, especially those arising secondary to myocardial ischemia or infarction.
E (quinidine) is incorrect. Quinidine is a class IA antiarrhythmic drug. It has utility in the management of all types of arrhythmias, including PSVT, but it would not have caused the patient's respiratory distress.

37. *B* (chronic granulomatous disease of childhood) is correct. Chronic granulomatous disease of childhood is associated with a genetic defect that results in the failure of PMNs to produce hydrogen peroxide. As a result, bacteria that enter these cells are not killed by the cell. Instead, when the PMN dies, viable bacteria are released.

A (Chédiak-Higashi disease) is incorrect. Chédiak-Higashi disease is characterized by a lag in the initiation of the fusion of lysosomes with ingested bacteria. In this case, the cell is capable of destroying ingested bacteria (microbicidal defect) but may take longer to do so.
C (chronic inflammation) is incorrect. The term "chronic inflammation" is usually applied to a long-standing infection in connective tissue and it will eventually resolve.

D (chronic myelogenous leukemia) is incorrect. CML is characterized by the appearance of undifferentiated hematopoietic cells in peripheral blood. In contrast, this patient's PMNs are fully functional (i.e., capable of killing phagocytosed bacteria). CML is more likely to occur in adults between the ages of 39 and 60 years of age.

38. **D** (dissociative identity disorder) is correct. The patient's report of multiple apparent strangers calling her by a different name, awareness that there are blocks of time in her life for which she cannot account, and waking up in the company of men she cannot remember having invited home indicate that she is experiencing dissociation (i.e., an organized and cohesive pattern of thinking and behaving for which the memory system is amnestic). This information is suggestive of dissociative identity disorder in which two or more distinct personalities exist within one individual and take control of the person's behavior at varying times.

A (depersonalization disorder) is incorrect. Recurrent alterations in perception or experience in which a sense of reality is temporarily lost or changed suggest depersonalization disorder. The experience of depersonalization is often described as "I knew things were happening, but they didn't seem real."
B (dissociative amnesia) is incorrect. Dissociative amnesia refers to the sudden inability to recall important, personal information secondary to emotional issues. This type of amnesia must be distinguished from neurologic explanations of memory loss.
C (dissociative fugue) is incorrect. Dissociative fugue involves sudden, unexpected travel from home and the creation of a new identity without recall of one's previous identity. Predisposing factors include alcohol abuse, stress, and depression.
E (posttraumatic stress disorder) is incorrect. PTSD occurs when an individual reacts with avoidance and heightened arousal to trauma. Dissociative identity disorder may be related to PTSD secondary to severe childhood abuse.

39. **A** (digital rectal examination) is correct. Prostate cancer is the most common cancer in men. Point tenderness over the vertebral bodies in an elderly patient is highly suggestive of metastatic prostate cancer, especially coupled with clinical evidence of urinary retention. Because prostate cancers develop in the peripheral zone of the prostate, they are palpated easily by digital rectal examination, especially if they have already spread beyond the gland.

B (prostate-specific antigen) is incorrect. Although a serum PSA test is always part of the workup of prostate cancer, a digital rectal examination is accomplished in a few minutes and provides immediate information. Furthermore, PSA is not 100% specific for prostate cancer, because the level is also increased in benign prostatic hyperplasia (BPH). In the absence of vertebral body ten-

derness in this patient, BPH would have been the most likely
cause of urinary retention. BPH develops in the periurethral zone
of the gland; hence enlargement is more likely to cause obstructive uropathy than prostate cancer. Urinary retention secondary to prostate cancer can occur when disease has invaded the
bladder neck and obstructed the ureters. Unlike prostatic acid
phosphatase, a rectal examination does not falsely increase serum
PSA levels.
C   (radionuclide bone scan) is incorrect. A radionuclide bone
scan would be essential for identifying bone metastasis in this patient; however, osteoarthritis and lumbar strain can mimic metastatic cancer in bone.
D   (serum alkaline phosphatase) is incorrect. Prostate cancer is
the most common cause of osteoblastic metastases in men. An osteoblastic response in bone results in increased bone density and
increased serum alkaline phosphatase. An increased serum alkaline phosphatase lacks specificity, however, because it is also elevated in osteoarthritis (due to reactive bone formation) and
cholestatic and metastatic liver disease (due to increased synthesis
by bile duct epithelium).
E   (transrectal ultrasound with biopsy) is incorrect. This is the
confirmatory test for prostate cancer, not the initial screening test.

40. *C*   (epithelial cells) is correct. Epithelial cells are responsible for
production of the secretory factor that protects IgA from degradation as it is transported to the mucosal surface. A defect in epithelial cells would explain the presence of IgA in plasma but not
in body secretions.

A   (B cells) is incorrect. A defect in B cell function would affect
the level of IgA in plasma, as well as in body secretions.
B   (endothelial cells) is incorrect. Endothelial cells are not usually
involved in the elicitation of an IgA response.
D   (monocytes and macrophages) and E (type 2 helper T cells) are
incorrect. The patient's plasma level of IgA was normal. This indicates that T cell help was available if needed for plasma cell development. It also indicates that antigen presentation was
probably not affected.

41. *B*   (amphetamine) is correct. Amphetamine is an indirect-acting
sympathomimetic amine. Along with catecholamines, amphetamine undergoes reuptake into presynaptic adrenergic nerve terminals and then stimulates the release of norepinephrine.
Cocaine is a drug that blocks this reuptake process. Thus, although cocaine would potentiate the effects of direct-acting
sympathomimetic amines, it would block the effects of indirect-
acting sympathomimetic amines, such as amphetamine and
tyramine. Prazosin, an α_1-adrenergic receptor antagonist, would
block the vasoconstrictive effects of both direct-acting and
indirect-acting sympathomimetic amines.

A (acetylcholine) is incorrect. Acetylcholine is a muscarinic receptor agonist that interacts with M_3 receptors on the vascular endothelium and stimulates the production of nitric oxide. This in turn relaxes the smooth muscle and lowers the TPR. The depressor response of acetylcholine would not be affected by cocaine or prazosin. This response is not depicted in the figure.

C (angiotensin II) is incorrect. Angiotensin II interacts with AT_1 receptors and contracts vascular smooth muscle. The pressor response of angiotensin II would not be affected by cocaine or prazosin; however, it would be blocked by losartan, an AT_1 receptor antagonist. Thus, the TPR pattern of angiotensin II would look like that of drug Z in the figure.

D (epinephrine) is incorrect. Epinephrine is a direct-acting adrenergic agonist at α_1, α_2, β_1, and β_2 receptors. Therefore, cocaine would potentiate its pressor response (see the discussion of B). Prazosin would "convert" its pressor response (α_1) to a depressor response (β_2); this phenomenon is called epinephrine reversal. In the figure, drug X is epinephrine.

E (norepinephrine) is incorrect. Norepinephrine is a direct-acting agonist at α_1, α_2, and β_1 receptors. Therefore, cocaine would potentiate its pressor response (refer to the discussion of B), and prazosin would block its pressor response. In the figure, drug W is norepinephrine.

42. C (FEV_1/FVC ratio of less than 75%) is correct. In individuals with chronic obstructive pulmonary diseases (COPD), including asthma, resistance to airflow is increased, which makes it much more difficult to breathe. This difficulty is due to a reduction in the diameter of the airways of the lungs. The most sensitive measure of airway obstruction is the FEV_1/FVC ratio, where FEV_1 is the amount of air that can be exhaled forcefully within 1 second, and FVC (forced vital capacity) is the total amount of air exhaled through a maximal forceful expiration. Airway obstruction is indicated when the FEV_1/FVC ratio falls below 75%.

A (arterial hypoxemia) is incorrect. In individuals with severe airway obstruction, for example, arterial blood can become significantly hypoxemic. However, hypoxemia is not specific to the diagnosis of pulmonary obstruction.

B (dyspnea) is incorrect. Dyspnea is not specific to the diagnosis of pulmonary obstruction. Patients who complain about breathing limitations during exercise or even at rest should be given a pulmonary function test. Normal individuals should be capable of expelling 80%–85% of their vital capacity within 1 second.

D (large anatomic dead space volume) is incorrect. The amount of anatomic dead space does not change, even during a severe asthmatic attack.

E (rapid respirations) is incorrect. In individuals with asthma, constricted airways prohibit rapid expulsion of air. Thus, the respiratory rate in asthmatics tends to be slower than normal.

43. *D* (spinal shock) is correct. Spinal shock is caused by an acute lesion in the corticospinal tract below the foramen magnum. It is characterized by flaccid muscle tone and a lack of tendon reflexes. Spasticity may develop within days to weeks.

A (Brown-Séquard's syndrome) is incorrect. Brown-Séquard's syndrome is caused by hemisection of the spinal cord. It is characterized by ipsilateral symptoms, including spastic paralysis and the loss of postural sense. Contralateral symptoms are limited to a loss of pain and temperature sensations below the level of the lesion. Bilateral symptoms, as reported for this patient, are not associated with this type of lesion.

B (commissural syndrome) is incorrect. Flaccid paralysis is a sign of damage to lower motor neurons. Damage to commissural fibers will affect ascending information, specifically information about pain and temperature below the level of the lesion. No evidence of changes in pain and temperature sensation was reported for this patient.

C (posterior spinal artery bleeding) is incorrect. The posterior spinal arteries supply the dorsal columns, which convey sensory information. The flaccid paralysis reported for this patient indicates a lesion in a lower motor neuron, which would lie in the anterior horn of the spinal cord, and would be supplied by the anterior spinal artery.

E (Weber syndrome) is incorrect. Weber syndrome, which is caused by a lesion in the cerebral peduncle, results in contralateral hemiparesis and ipsilateral oculomotor nerve palsy. It does not involve all four limbs, as is the case with this patient.

44. *B* (low T_4; high TSH; normal ^{131}I) is correct. The patient has primary hypothyroidism, most likely secondary to Hashimoto's thyroiditis. Hashimoto's thyroiditis is an autoimmune thyroiditis with an increase in antimicrosomal and thyroglobulin antibodies. Along with autoimmune destruction of the gland, an autoantibody directed against the TSH receptor inhibits the gland from synthesizing thyroid hormone. The patient exhibits all of the classic signs of hypothyroidism: brittle hair, periorbital puffiness, delayed deep tendon reflexes, and primary myopathy of the proximal muscles of the thigh (note the increase in serum creatine kinase). As expected, serum T_4 levels are decreased because the gland is being destroyed, and serum TSH is increased due to loss of the negative feedback of T_4.

A (low T_4; low TSH; low ^{131}I) is incorrect. These findings are most consistent with secondary hypothyroidism, usually due to hypopituitarism. In children, a craniopharyngioma is the most common cause of hypopituitarism; in adults, a nonfunctioning pituitary adenoma is usually responsible for this condition.

C (high T_4; low TSH; low ^{131}I) is incorrect. These findings are most consistent with a patient whose hyperthyroidism developed from taking an excess amount of thyroid hormone, usually for weight loss. In these patients, the thyroid gland is suppressed and nonpalpable, unlike a gland that produces excessive thyroid hormone. The ^{131}I is decreased, because the gland is inactive and not capable of increasing the uptake of iodine to synthesize thyroid hormone.

D (high T_4; low TSH; high ^{131}I) is incorrect. These findings are consistent with Graves' disease, which is the most common cause of hyperthyroidism. These patients have an autoantibody against the TSH receptor that increases the synthesis of thyroid hormone. Exophthalmos and pretibial myxedema are unique to the disease. Unlike hyperthyroidism due to exogenous intake of excess thyroid hormone, in Graves' disease, the ^{131}I uptake is high, because the gland requires iodine to synthesize T_4 and is diffusely enlarged.

45. *A* (complete blood cell count) is correct. The lack of pus is indicative of an abnormality in the number or function of leukocytes. If the number of leukocytes is found to be normal, then the diagnosis of lazy leukocyte syndrome should be suspected. This syndrome, which is seen in children with repeated low-grade infections, is characterized by the inability of leukocytes to migrate to the site of infection.

B (measurement of C3 levels) and C (measurement of C5, C6, C7, and C8 levels) are incorrect. Individuals who have a C3 deficiency exhibit an increased susceptibility to infections caused by pyogenic organisms. Those who have deficiencies in the terminal complement components (C5, C6, C7, and C8) would be more susceptible to infections with *Neisseria*. However, these increased susceptibilities would not explain the lack of pus in the lesions of the patient described. Therefore, testing for these complement deficiencies would not be helpful.
D (measurement of IgA levels) is incorrect. The measurement of IgA levels would be helpful only if the patient had mucosal infections.
E (testing of B cell mitogen response) is incorrect. Antibody levels would not explain the lack of pus. Therefore, testing of the B cell mitogen response would not be helpful.

46. *C* (motor vehicle accident) is correct. When a 17-year-old boy with a history of risk-taking behaviors (e.g., drinking, using drugs, and driving recklessly) dies within 6 months of seeing his physician, the death is most likely caused by a motor vehicle accident. Motor vehicle accidents are the leading cause of death in the teenage population, with 40% of all deaths related to motor vehicle accidents.

A (AIDS) is incorrect. This patient is at risk for contracting a sexually transmitted disease or contracting HIV. Only one third of sexually active adolescents use condoms, and risk takers are least likely to use protection. However, even if this patient had contracted HIV, he would not have died of the illness in such a short period of time (6 months).

B   (alcohol or drug overdose) is incorrect. Alcohol and drug use are common among adolescents. Surveys suggest 85% of teenagers use alcohol and approximately 15% use drugs. The number of deaths directly related to unplanned alcohol or drug overdose is unclear, but it is thought to be considerably less than deaths caused by accidents, homicides, or suicides. When an adolescent death is associated with alcohol or drug use, it is most commonly linked with a motor vehicle accident or suicide.

D   (murder) is incorrect. Homicide is the second leading cause of death for individuals between the ages of 15 and 25 years. African-American males are at highest risk for homicide.

E   (suicide) is incorrect. Suicide is the third leading cause of death for adolescents, and between 1 and 2 million adolescents attempt suicide yearly. Over the past 10 years, the suicide rate has risen more rapidly in males between the ages of 15 and 24 years than in any other age group.

47. **E**   (incomplete fusion of the urethral folds) is correct. Hypospadias is the most common anomaly of the penis and occurs in about 0.3% of male infants. Of the four types of hypospadias (penile, glandular, penoscrotal, perineal), penile hypospadias occurs most frequently. Inadequate production of androgens or their receptor sites may result in failure of the urogenital folds to fuse, with the external urethral opening occurring on the ventral surface of the penis.

A   (abnormally high levels of dihydrotestosterone) is incorrect. The steroid testosterone causes the wolffian duct to differentiate into male reproductive organs (epididymis, vas deferens, seminal vesicles, scrotum, and penis). Masculinization of the male external genitalia is controlled by 5 α-dihydrotestosterone. A genetic deficiency of the enzyme 5 α-ketosteroid reductase, which converts testosterone to 5 α-dihydrotestosterone, results in the internal anatomy of a male; externally, the individual appears to be a female with a blind vaginal canal and enlarged clitoris.

B   (failure of genital swellings to fuse) is incorrect. In the male, failure of the genital swellings to fuse results in malformation of the scrotal sac, with possible perineal hypospadias.

C   (female pseudohermaphroditism) is incorrect. Female pseudohermaphrodites produce excessive amounts of androgens, causing masculinization of external genitalia. In male pseudohermaphrodism (46,XY), individuals are sex chromatin-negative, resulting in inadequate testosterone production and consequently varying degrees of external genitalia development, such as hypospadias.

D   (glans hypospadias) is incorrect. Hypospadias of the glans penis most likely results from defects in the ectoderm, which is dragged into the glans during development. It does not develop from a failure of the urethral folds to fuse as occurs in penile hypospadias. Regardless of the cause, distal forms of hypospadias account for about 80% of cases.

48. *B* (fluid-filled cavity in the cervical spinal cord) is correct. The patient has syringomyelia, the development of an expanding fluid-filled cavity in the cervical spinal cord. This results in destruction of the crossed lateral spinothalamic tracts (loss of pain and temperature sensation), anterior horn cells (loss of the intrinsic muscles of the hand), and other tracts as the cavity expands. It is often confused with amyotrophic lateral sclerosis (ALS); however, in ALS there are no sensory abnormalities.

A (autoimmune destruction of myelin) is incorrect. Multiple sclerosis (MS) is the most common demyelinating disease. Symptoms of MS include blurry vision (optic neuritis), intention tremors, nystagmus, ataxia, and scanning speech.
C (superoxide free radical destruction of upper and lower motor neurons) is incorrect. This describes the pathogenesis of some cases of ALS where there is a defect in superoxide dismutase on chromosome 21, leading to superoxide free radical damage of upper and lower motor neurons.
D (tumor in the cervical spinal cord) is incorrect. Although a cervical spinal cord tumor potentially could produce the neurologic findings seen in this patient, the sequence of neurologic defects is more compatible with syringomyelia.
E (vitamin B_{12} deficiency) is incorrect. Vitamin B_{12} deficiency is associated with subacute combined degeneration of the spinal cord. The posterior columns and lateral corticospinal tracts are demyelinated, leading to loss of proprioception (posterior column disease) and upper motor neuron signs and symptoms (lateral corticospinal tract).

49. *C* (insulin-like growth factor I) is correct. Insulin-like growth factor I (IGF-I) is the intermediary of several physiologic actions of growth hormone. For example, it promotes the incorporation of sulfate into cartilage and thereby mediates the effects of growth hormone on cartilage cells. Growth hormone has no direct effects on cartilage or bone cells. IGF-I is secreted by the liver and some other tissues in response to stimulation by growth hormone. In some individuals, hepatic unresponsiveness to circulating growth hormone is due to a defect in the growth hormone receptor, and this results in dwarfism. In the patient described, the clinical and laboratory findings are consistent with the diagnosis of Laron-type dwarfism. Children with Laron dwarfism usually have normal to high levels of growth hormone and barely detectable levels of IGF-I. These children are generally resistant to the effects of endogenous and exogenous growth hormone.

A (fibroblast growth factor) is incorrect. The fibroblast growth factor (FGF) family consists of polypeptides that promote angiogenesis and mitogenic activity toward cells of epithelial, mesenchymal, and neural origins. Abnormalities in levels of these polypeptides are not associated with short stature.

B   (insulin) is incorrect. Insulin deficiency may cause growth retardation. However, in this patient, there are no symptoms
suggesting diabetes.

D   (somatostatin) is incorrect. Somatostatins are polypeptides
that act directly on the pituitary somatotrophs to inhibit the release of growth hormone. Somatostatins have been isolated
from the hypothalamus, the endocrine pancreas, and specialized
D cells in the intestine.

E   (somatotropin) is incorrect. Growth hormone is also called somatotropin. The patient has normal levels of somatotropin.

50. **B**   (dorsomedial nucleus) is correct. This patient has Korsakoff's
psychosis, which is characterized by retrograde memory loss, the
inability to form new memories, and a tendency for confabula-
tion (exaggerating) to compensate for these losses. It is caused by
thiamine deficiency and commonly accompanies chronic alcoholism. Thiamine is a coenzyme for transketolase, which participates in the pentose monophosphate pathway of glucose
metabolism. A thiamine deficiency is indicated by a change in
erythrocyte transketolase activity. If enzyme activity increases by
>15% when thiamine diphosphate is added to the culture me-
dium, then the thiamine deficiency is considered significant
enough to indicate Korsakoff's psychosis.

A   (amygdaloid nuclei) is incorrect. The amygdala is a limbic
structure that lies in the dorsomedial portion of the temporal lobe
and is continuous with the parahippocampal uncus. It communicates reciprocally with the hippocampal formation, as well as
the hypothalamus, thalamus, and neocortex. Damage to the
amygdala results in wild, dramatic behaviors and flattened emotions, but not memory loss.

C   (habenular nuclei) is incorrect. The habenula is one of a pair
of small knobs of tissue located at the rostral aspect of the stalk
connecting the pineal gland to the diencephalon. Its nuclei lie un-
derneath it and receive fibers from the stria medullaris thalami,
which originate in the limbic system. The habenular nuclei allow
the limbic system to influence activity in the reticular formation. Thus, damage to the habenular nuclei may disrupt normal
patterns of alertness, but not memory.

D   (nucleus accumbens) is incorrect. The nucleus accumbens is
situated between two basal ganglia: the caudate nucleus and
the putamen. Damage to this structure may disrupt the flow of information through the basal ganglia and prevent them from
modulating motor signals before they descend through the corticospinal tract. Slight, uncontrollable tremors (as are seen with
Parkinson's disease) may develop. However, memory and learning
are not under their control.

E   (nucleus basalis of Meynert) is incorrect. The nucleus basalis of
Meynert lies within the basal forebrain and extends cholinergic
fibers to the cerebral cortex, hippocampus, and amygdala. Recent
evidence suggests that it may play a role in Alzheimer's disease,
but not Korsakoff's psychosis.

Test 7

TEST 7

DIRECTIONS: Each numbered item or incomplete statement is followed by options arranged in alphabetical or logical order. Select the best answer to each question. Some options may be partially correct, but there is only **ONE BEST** answer.

1. A 50-year-old man who has been taking phenelzine for 2 months is brought to the emergency department. His blood pressure is 245/175 mm Hg, and he has exaggerated sympathetic nervous system symptoms associated with an acute hypertensive crisis. He says that he began experiencing these symptoms shortly after he drank red wine and ate gefilte fish and aged cheese. The patient's hypertensive crisis was most likely caused by the ability of phenelzine to inhibit

- A. aromatic amino acid decarboxylase
- B. catechol-*O*-methyltransferase
- C. monoamine oxidase A
- D. monoamine oxidase B
- E. tyrosine hydroxylase

2. A 60-year-old woman complains of persistent breathing difficulties. Her laboratory studies show:

pH	7.36
[H$^+$]	44 nmol/L
PaCO$_2$	55 mm Hg
[HCO$_3^-$]	30 mmol/L

Which of the following is the most likely diagnosis?

- A. Combined metabolic acidosis and respiratory acidosis
- B. Primary respiratory acidosis, secondary metabolic alkalosis, full pH compensation
- C. Primary respiratory acidosis, secondary metabolic alkalosis, partial pH compensation
- D. Pure metabolic acidosis without pH compensation
- E. Pure respiratory acidosis

3. A 55-year-old man complains of a painful lump in his neck and has enlarged lymph nodes just behind the sternocleidomastoid muscle in the posterior triangle. A biopsy specimen confirms that the nodes are malignant. After surgery to remove the nodes, the lateral angle of the man's scapula drags downward and the superior angle is elevated. Which of the following nerves has been severed?

- A. Accessory
- B. Dorsal scapular
- C. Great auricular
- D. Phrenic
- E. Posterior auricular

4. A local physician conducting a study on smoking cessation divides the subjects into four groups. One group is given bupropion hydrochloride; one is given nicotine patches; one receives behavioral techniques for smoking cessation; and one acts as a control group and is given a placebo medication. To determine whether the percentage of men and women who quit smoking in each group is significantly different, which of the following statistical tests should be used?

○ A. Analysis of variance (ANOVA)
○ B. Chi-square test
○ C. Correlation
○ D. Independent *t* test
○ E. Paired *t* test

5. A 40-year-old man has a lesion on his forearm. Based on the characteristics of the lesion, a presumptive diagnosis of squamous cell carcinoma is made. Subsequent microscopic examination of biopsy material from the lesion shows the presence of yeasts with broad-based buds and bud scars. The most likely diagnosis is

○ A. blastomycosis
○ B. coccidioidomycosis
○ C. mycetoma
○ D. primary dermatophytic lesion
○ E. secondarily infected squamous cell carcinoma

6. A 22-year-old woman complains of fatigue and frequent nosebleeds. Physical examination shows generalized petechiae and ecchymoses, generalized lymphadenopathy, and hepatosplenomegaly. The peripheral smear shows hypergranular blast cells containing numerous Auer rods. Laboratory studies show:

Hemoglobin	7.0 g/dL
Leukocyte count	50,000/mm^3
Platelet count	10,000/mm^3
Prothrombin time	30 sec
Partial thromboplastin time (activated, aPTT)	65 sec
D-dimer assay	Positive

Treatment with retinoic acid is initiated. Which of the following is the rationale for treating the patient's hematologic disorder with this agent?

○ A. Destroys the blast cells
○ B. Enhances cellular immunity
○ C. Increases maturation of the blast cells
○ D. Prevents infection associated with bone marrow suppression
○ E. Prevents intravascular coagulation

7. A 72-year-old man who is right-handed suddenly develops paralysis in his right arm. He is alert, afebrile, and understands questions but has great difficulty communicating his answers verbally. He has most likely had a stroke that involves the

○ A. left cerebral cortex
○ B. right arcuate fasciculus
○ C. right internal capsule
○ D. right precentral gyrus
○ E. superior temporal gyrus

8. A 31-year-old woman with aortic valve disease develops atrial fibrillation. She is initially treated with digoxin and warfarin and is later treated with quinidine. The efficacy of warfarin in the management of this patient is attributed to its ability to

○ A. activate plasminogen that is bound to fibrin, thereby catalyzing the conversion of plasminogen to plasmin
○ B. bind to antithrombin III (AT-III) and act catalytically to facilitate the interaction of AT-III with activated clotting factors
○ C. bind to inactive plasminogen, thereby catalyzing the conversion of plasminogen to active plasmin
○ D. inhibit cyclooxygenase-1, thereby preventing the formation of thromboxane
○ E. inhibit vitamin K epoxide reductase, thereby preventing the formation of inactive clotting factors

9. An 8-year-old boy of African-American descent is diagnosed with homozygous sickle cell anemia. In which area of the body will the abnormal blood cells resulting from this condition be destroyed by erythrophagocytosis?

○ A. Cord of Billroth in the spleen
○ B. Hematopoietic cord of bone marrow
○ C. Marginal zone of the spleen
○ D. Medullary region of the thymus
○ E. Paratrabecular sinus in a lymph node

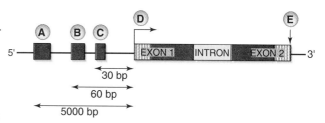

10. The figure above shows a fragment of eukaryotic DNA. Base pairs *(bp)* are marked, but the figure is not drawn to scale. Dotted areas of exon 1 and exon 2 depict untranslated regions of the gene. In a series of experiments, investigators will delete various sites (labeled *A, B, C, D,* and *E*) to determine how each deletion affects mRNA synthesis in vitro. Deletion of which one of the sites is most likely to completely abolish mRNA synthesis because of an inability to correctly position RNA polymerase II?

○ A. Site A
○ B. Site B
○ C. Site C
○ D. Site D
○ E. Site E

11. A 65-year-old woman has a fever, stiff neck, headache, and other signs of meningitis. A nonencapsulated organism, motile at room temperature, is isolated from a cerebrospinal fluid sample. The organism is facultatively intracellular and catalase-positive. It hydrolyzes esculin and produces an oxygen-sensitive β-hemolysin. Which of the following organisms is the most likely cause of the disease?

○ A. *Cryptococcus neoformans*
○ B. *Listeria monocytogenes*
○ C. *Staphylococcus aureus*
○ D. *Streptococcus pneumoniae*
○ E. *Toxoplasma gondii*

12. A 62-year-old man with small cell carcinoma of the lung complains of a headache and visual disturbances. An MRI of the head shows cerebral edema but no evidence of metastatic disease. There is no evidence of pitting edema or volume depletion. The serum Na^+ level is 110 mEq/L. Assuming the patient has a normal salt and water intake, which of the following is the most appropriate nonpharmacologic treatment for this patient?

	Na^+ Intake	H_2O Intake
A.	Decrease	Decrease
B.	Decrease	No change
C.	Increase	Increase
D.	No change	Decrease
E.	No change	No change

13. During a physical examination of a 12-year-old girl complaining of leg pain, the physician evaluates the lower motor neurons by using the knee jerk reflex test. If no lesions are present, the process of reciprocal inhibition should be normal. Which of the following events mediates this process?

A. Antagonistic extensor is inhibited by supraspinal connections

B. Extensors are directly inhibited by the flexors

C. Inhibitory interneuron is activated by the Ia afferent and inhibits flexors

D. Ia afferent releases a neurotransmitter that triggers flexors and another that inhibits extensors

E. Neurotransmitter that excites the flexors inhibits the extensors

14. Although biotin deficiency due to a poor dietary intake is rare, some of the clinical manifestations of this deficiency have been observed in patients treated with high-dose antibiotics on a long-term basis. The activity of which of the following enzymes in fatty acid biosynthesis is affected by a deficiency of biotin?

A. Acetyl-CoA carboxylase

B. Acyl-CoA dehydrogenase

C. Fatty acid synthase

D. Fatty acid thiokinase

E. Propionyl-CoA carboxylase

15. A 63-year-old man with Parkinson's disease has a history of chronic constipation, cognitive impairment, and recurrent cystitis in association with prostatic hypertrophy. Which antiparkinsonian drug would be most likely to exacerbate the patient's pre-existing problems?

A. Amantadine

B. Benztropine

C. Bromocriptine

D. Levodopa

E. Selegiline

16. An 18-year-old woman sees her family physician because she is hoarse, has difficulty swallowing, and has been suffering from a sore throat, fever, easy fatigability, and myalgia for 1 week. Examination shows enlarged tonsils, cervical lymphadenopathy, and splenomegaly. Bacterial cultures yield negative results, and a viral etiologic agent is suspected. A white blood cell count shows lymphocytosis, and a serum agglutination test is positive for heterophile antibodies. The most likely etiologic agent of the disease is

A. adenovirus

B. cytomegalovirus

C. Epstein-Barr virus

D. influenza B virus

E. rubella virus

17. A patient with hypoxia breathes 100% O_2 for several minutes, and his PAO_2/PaO_2 gradient decreases from 35 mm Hg to 30 mm Hg. Which abnormality best explains the cause of the original hypoxia?

A. Anatomic shunt blood flow

B. Hypoventilation

C. Pharmacologic depression of brainstem neurons

D. Pulmonary diffusion impairment

E. Ventilation/perfusion mismatch

18. A 48-year-old woman with lung cancer has been told by her physician that she most likely has only a few weeks to live and that no further treatment can be offered. She is experiencing excruciating pain that cannot be alleviated by pain medications. She asks her physician to inject her with a lethal substance. The ethical guidelines of the American Medical Association state that the physician should do which of the following?

- ○ A. Comply with the patient's request if the physician feels the patient is competent
- ○ B. Inform the patient's family of the request and, if the family agrees, comply with the request
- ○ C. Not comply with the patient's request, but attempt to work with the patient and family to maintain the highest quality of life
- ○ D. Not comply with the patient's request, but request a psychiatric evaluation and place the patient on a suicide watch
- ○ E. Seek psychiatric consultation and, if the patient is deemed competent, comply with the request

19. A 28-year-old man is hospitalized for hypotensive shock. Gram-negative diplococci are observed on a gram-stained blood film. The patient's medical records indicate that he has been hospitalized for disseminated gonococcal infection on three prior occasions. In addition to ordering a blood culture, the physician should order which of the following?

- ○ A. Lymphocyte proliferation test
- ○ B. Measurement of C3 levels
- ○ C. Measurement of C5, C6, C7, and C8 levels
- ○ D. Measurement of immunoglobulin levels
- ○ E. Measurement of mucosal IgA levels

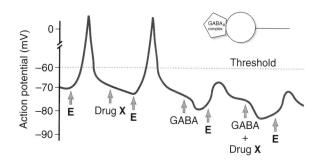

20. The figure above depicts an intracellular electrophysiologic recording taken from a hypothetical neuron containing only a GABA$_A$-receptor complex. In the figure, E = excitation by direct excitatory stimulation; *drug X* is a drug administered alone; *GABA* = gamma-aminobutyric acid administered alone; and *GABA + drug X* = drug X administered in the presence of GABA. Based on the behavior of drug X in the absence and presence of GABA, which agent is most likely to be drug X?

- ○ A. Baclofen
- ○ B. Buspirone
- ○ C. Hydroxyzine
- ○ D. Midazolam
- ○ E. Morphine

21. A febrile 68-year-old woman with a 40-year history of smoking cigarettes complains of fatigue and weight loss. Physical examination shows generalized nontender lymphadenopathy, hepatosplenomegaly, and petechiae and ecchymoses scattered over the entire body. Laboratory studies show:

Hemoglobin	8.7 g/dL
Leukocyte count	95,000/mm^3
Platelet count	60,000/mm^3
Total serum protein concentration	4.5 g/dL

The peripheral smear contains predominantly mature-appearing lymphocytes, many of which have a smudged appearance. A blood culture is positive for *Streptococcus pneumoniae*. A serum protein electrophoresis shows a flat gamma-globulin peak. The pathogenesis for this patient's hematologic condition is most closely associated with which of the following?

- ○ A. B-cell malignancy arising from the bone marrow
- ○ B. Hypogammaglobulinemia related to sepsis
- ○ C. Lymphoid leukemoid reaction secondary to sepsis
- ○ D. Metastatic lung cancer associated with smoking cigarettes
- ○ E. T-cell malignancy arising from lymph nodes

22. A 7-year-old child from a poor family has purpura and ecchymoses in the oral mucosa and skin, subperiosteal hematomas, and blood in several joints after minimal trauma. The child has a history of impaired wound healing. Which of the following should be considered when making a differential diagnosis?

- ○ A. Failure to maintain fully differentiated epithelia
- ○ B. Inadequate mineralization of cancellous bone
- ○ C. Increased intracellular levels of p53
- ○ D. Lack of prolyl and lysyl hydroxylase activity

23. A 48-year-old man reports experiencing tinnitus in his right ear, which has become progressively worse during the past 6 months. He says that the sounds are louder on the right side than on the left. He has also noticed a decreased sense of taste in the anterior portion of his tongue. Findings upon physical examination are within normal limits. Which of the following is the most likely diagnosis?

- ○ A. Acoustic neuroma
- ○ B. Lacunar stroke in the internal capsule
- ○ C. Lesion in the caudal medulla
- ○ D. Lesion in the mesencephalic tegmentum
- ○ E. Lesion in the tectum

24. A 13-year-old boy has a 3-week history of weight loss and complains of excessive thirst and urination. Type 1 diabetes mellitus is suspected. Testing of blood samples is most likely to show

- ○ A. increased erythrocyte sedimentation rate
- ○ B. increased serum creatinine level
- ○ C. presence of anti–pancreatic amyloid antibodies
- ○ D. presence of anti–pancreatic islet cell antibodies
- ○ E. presence of anti–streptolysin O antibodies

25. A 52-year-old woman with rheumatoid arthritis is treated on a long-term basis with a nonsteroidal anti-inflammatory drug (NSAID) and auranofin. When the treatment is no longer effective, her physician decides to stop auranofin treatment and institute therapy with an alternative drug whose mechanism of action is similar to that of trimethoprim. Before therapy with the alternative drug is started, a complete blood cell count (CBC) is taken and liver function tests are performed. The patient is told that these tests will be repeated every 6–8 weeks and a liver biopsy will be performed every 2–3 years while she is undergoing treatment with this alternative drug. The alternative drug is most likely

○ A. azathioprine
○ B. hydroxychloroquine
○ C. methotrexate
○ D. penicillamine
○ E. sulfasalazine

26. After several weeks of severe depression, tearfulness, and difficulty concentrating, a 27-year-old woman seeks therapy. The therapist explains to her that depression coincides with a tendency to view life events negatively. The patient is told that treatment will be aimed at developing healthier, more rational beliefs. This therapist is using which of the following types of therapy?

○ A. Behavioral
○ B. Cognitive
○ C. Family systems
○ D. Psychodynamic
○ E. Supportive

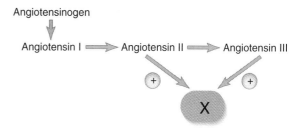

27. Angiography in a 60-year-old hypertensive man shows the presence of stenosis of a major renal artery. To compensate for decreased blood perfusion of the affected kidney, he produces an excess of the compound labeled X in the figure above. Which of the following best characterizes compound X?

○ A. It causes arteriolar vasoconstriction
○ B. It is produced by juxtaglomerular cells of the kidney
○ C. It is secreted in response to infusions rich in Na^+
○ D. It is under tight control of adrenocorticotropic hormone (ACTH)
○ E. It promotes sodium retention and potassium excretion in the distal tubules of nephrons

28. The fundamental benefit of applying positive end-expiratory pressure (PEEP) to an elderly patient with a large closing volume is that PEEP

○ A. increases area available for gas exchange by opening closed alveoli
○ B. increases compliance, making it easier to breathe
○ C. promotes an increase in pulmonary blood flow
○ D. significantly increases the PAO_2 when the patient is breathing air
○ E. stimulates breathing by tonically activating pulmonary stretch receptors

29. During a subclavian venipuncture, the cannula is inserted into the patient's neck just superior to the clavicle. Which of the following is the relative position of the subclavian vein in the root of the neck?

○ A. Anterior to medial end of clavicle
○ B. Anterior to scalenus anterior muscle
○ C. Just posterior to internal jugular vein
○ D. Posterior to scalenus anterior muscle
○ E. Posterior to subclavian artery

30. A 72-year-old man with a 20-year history of osteoarthritis of the hips and knees develops urinary retention secondary to benign prostatic hyperplasia. A transurethral resection of the prostate is performed to relieve the obstruction. Shortly after the procedure, the patient begins bleeding profusely from the penis. Coagulation studies show the following:

Partial thromboplastin time (activated, aPPT)	38 seconds
Prothrombin time (PT)	14 seconds
Bleeding time (BT)	>15 minutes
Platelet count	350,000 mm^3
D-dimer assay	Negative

Which of the following mechanisms is most likely responsible for this patient's bleeding disorder?

○ A. Circulating anticoagulant
○ B. Coagulation factor deficiency
○ C. Platelet function disorder
○ D. Secondary fibrinolytic disorder

31. A 1-year-old child develops watery diarrhea accompanied by vomiting and a fever. Bacteriologic cultures yield negative results, but a virus from the family *Reoviridae* is isolated from a fecal specimen. Which of the following viruses is the most likely cause of the disease?

○ A. Astrovirus
○ B. Coltivirus
○ C. Hepatitis E virus
○ D. Norwalk virus
○ E. Rotavirus

32. A 10-year-old boy is irritable and complains of severe abdominal pain and headache. Physical examination shows evidence of muscle weakness, including wristdrop of the left hand. Laboratory studies show microcytic anemia with basophilic stippling and an elevated level of free erythrocyte protoporphyrin. The most likely cause of this patient's symptoms and an appropriate treatment would be

○ A. acetaminophen poisoning; treatment with acetylcysteine
○ B. arsenic poisoning; treatment with dimercaprol
○ C. iron poisoning; treatment with deferoxamine
○ D. lead poisoning; treatment with calcium disodium edetate
○ E. mercury poisoning; treatment with succimer

33. A male physician discovers that a colleague in his practice is drinking alcohol every day during office hours. The physician talks to his colleague about the drinking, but the colleague minimizes his use of alcohol and denies a need for treatment, but does state that the concern is appreciated. Which of the following is the most appropriate next step for the concerned physician?

○ A. Coerce the colleague to seek help by threatening to inform the colleague's patients of the alcohol use
○ B. Contact the colleague's family and encourage the family to deal with the problem
○ C. Continue to monitor the colleague's behavior and report the alcohol use if other signs of impairment occur
○ D. Nothing more, since the physician has completed his duty by discussing the matter with the colleague
○ E. Report the colleague to the appropriate authorities to allow for an investigation

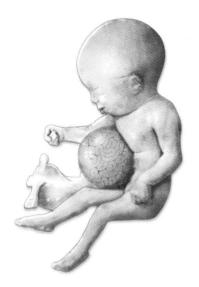

34. An ultrasound examination of a 28-year-old woman at 30 weeks' gestation shows an abdominal mass protruding from the fetus (see the figure above). Which of the following is the most likely diagnosis of this mass?

○ A. Complete exstrophy of the bladder
○ B. Gastroschisis
○ C. Meckel's diverticulum
○ D. Omphalocele
○ E. Umbilical hernia

35. A 35-year-old pharmacist complains of recurrent episodes of forgetfulness and tiredness. Physical examination is essentially unremarkable. Laboratory studies show a serum glucose level of 20 mg/dL. Additional studies on the same serum sample show a high serum insulin level and a low C-peptide level. Based on these findings, which of the following is the most likely diagnosis?

○ A. Benign tumor involving β-islet cells in the pancreas
○ B. Ectopic secretion of an insulin-like factor
○ C. Malignant tumor involving α-islet cells in the pancreas
○ D. Surreptitiously injected human insulin

36. Upon awakening one morning, a 62-year-old man, who is right-handed, is unable to use that hand. He recently experienced conjugate deviation of the eyes to the left and paralysis of voluntary gaze to the right. Five days later, his eye movements returned to normal. This man has most likely had a stroke involving the

○ A. left frontal cortex
○ B. left mesencephalic tegmentum
○ C. left occipital cortex
○ D. right lateral geniculate nucleus
○ E. right occipital cortex

37. A 9-month-old girl is brought to the emergency room in a coma. Initial examination shows hepatomegaly and hypotonia. An analysis of blood samples shows elevated levels of muscle and liver enzymes and decreased levels of glucose. Samples taken after 24 hours of fasting show an increase in the level of free fatty acids, but no ketone bodies are detected. Fatty changes are seen in liver and muscle biopsy specimens. The disease is most likely the result of

○ A. carnitine deficiency
○ B. decrease in citrate production
○ C. decrease in malonyl CoA production
○ D. lipoprotein lipase deficiency

38. A 40-year-old man has a fever, chills, headache, malaise, myalgia, chest pain, and a dry to slightly productive cough. As his condition becomes progressively worse, he develops symptoms of delirium and confusion. By the time he is admitted to the hospital, he has multisystem failure secondary to bilateral bronchopneumonia. Bronchial washings examined microscopically and cultured show high concentrations of bacteria growing within alveolar macrophages. A motile, gram-negative, highly fastidious bacterium is isolated on charcoal-yeast extract (CYE) agar that has been supplemented with cysteine. The patient later dies of respiratory failure. Which of the following organisms is the most likely cause of the disease?

○ A. *Haemophilus influenzae*
○ B. *Klebsiella pneumoniae*
○ C. *Legionella pneumophila*
○ D. *Mycobacterium tuberculosis*
○ E. *Pseudomonas aeruginosa*

39. A chromosomal analysis of various tissues taken from a woman shows XO, XX, and XXX. Cells from every tissue type contain 44 autosomes. It is assumed that a single abnormal division accounts for all of these aberrations. The division process that would account for these chromosome numbers is

○ A. meiotic anaphase lagging
○ B. meiotic nondisjunction
○ C. mitotic anaphase lagging
○ D. mitotic deletion
○ E. mitotic nondisjunction

40. The mother of an atopic 8-year-old boy notices that her son's face and legs began to swell over the past few days. She assumes that the boy is having a reaction to something he ate, so she immediately takes him to the emergency department. Physical examination shows a normotensive child with generalized pitting edema. Laboratory studies include a normal complete blood cell count and a urinalysis showing a positive dipstick reaction to protein and a sediment containing numerous fatty casts. Electron microscopy of the glomeruli in this patient would most likely demonstrate

○ A. fusion of the podocytes
○ B. intramembranous electron-dense deposits
○ C. mesangial electron-dense deposits
○ D. subendothelial electron-dense deposits
○ E. subepithelial electron-dense deposits

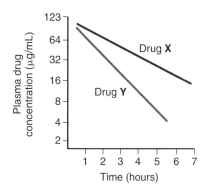

41. Drug X and drug Y are agents that are therapeutically effective at the same steady-state plasma concentration (Cp_{ss}). The graph above depicts the elimination curves of these drugs after the same dose of each of them is given at the same time via an intravenous bolus. A patient is given an intravenous loading dose of each drug and is then given an oral maintenance dose. Which of the following best describes the relationship between the oral maintenance dose of drug X and the oral maintenance dose of drug Y, assuming the oral bioavailability (F) of each is 1.0?

○ A. At Cp_{ss}, the maintenance dose administered every half-life would be equal for drug X and drug Y
○ B. At Cp_{ss}, the maintenance dose administered every half-life would be greater for drug X than for drug Y
○ C. At Cp_{ss}, the maintenance dose administered every half-life would be less for drug X than for drug Y
○ D. The relationship between the maintenance doses of drugs X and Y cannot be determined from the information supplied

42. To calculate the maximum tubular transport rate (T_{max}, in mg/min) accurately for any substance, whether actively secreted or reabsorbed, the physician must be sure that the

○ A. highest capacity nephrons are saturated with the substance
○ B. lowest capacity nephrons are saturated with the substance
○ C. plasma and urine concentrations of the substance are easily measured
○ D. renal plasma threshold for the substance is not exceeded
○ E. substance is bound to plasma proteins

43. A 45-year-old woman with a history of mitral stenosis and chronic arrhythmia dies suddenly at her home. At autopsy, a wedge-shaped hemorrhagic lesion is seen at the periphery of the temporal lobe. The mechanism for the temporal lobe lesion is most closely associated with which of the following conditions?

○ A. Atherosclerosis of the internal carotid artery
○ B. Embolic occlusion of a cerebral artery
○ C. Intracerebral hematoma
○ D. Neoplastic transformation of astrocytes
○ E. Rupture of a congenital aneurysm

44. A 72-year-old man has had fatigue, back pain, and several episodes of fever during the day and at night. A diagnosis of multiple myeloma is suspected. Which of the following results is most likely to be found on serum protein electrophoresis?

○ A. Broad, short peak between the alpha and gamma globulin fractions
○ B. Increased amount of specific IgA antibodies
○ C. Large albumin peak
○ D. Large complement peak
○ E. Narrow, tall spike in the gamma globulin fraction

45. A 33-year-old woman is stabbed in the chest during a robbery. The knife cut through the intercostal musculature and entered the right upper lobe of the lung, but missed the heart, aorta, superior vena cava, and major bronchial vessels. Which of the following is most likely an immediate consequence of such a wound?

○ A. The affected lobe will collapse and remain collapsed, even though the chest wall continues to move
○ B. The chest wall will spring out somewhat, but the affected lobe will not collapse
○ C. The lung lobe will collapse, but the chest wall will remain at its functional residual capacity (FRC) position
○ D. The wound will quickly seal itself, thereby allowing the collapsed lung to expand automatically
○ E. Rhythmic breathing will stop abruptly, and the patient will die of asphyxiation without immediate medical care

46. A 41-year-old woman is convinced she has cancer and has visited several physicians asking to be examined to determine if she has the disease. The physicians complete thorough evaluations, all of which confirm that the woman does not have the disease. This patient is most likely demonstrating

○ A. conversion disorder
○ B. factitious disorder
○ C. hypochondriasis
○ D. phobia
○ E. somatization disorder

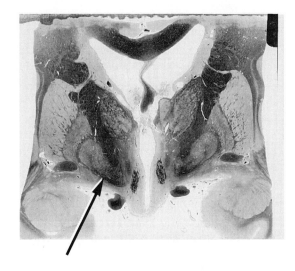

47. A 78-year-old man has a lesion in the structure located at the tip of the arrow in the figure above. Which of the following conditions is his physician most likely to find?

○ A. Bitemporal hemianopia
○ B. Decreased GABAergic output to the thalamus
○ C. Decreased olfactory sensitivity
○ D. Increased vocal and oral tendencies
○ E. Sham rage

48. An 8-year-old boy is brought to the emergency department because of vomiting and convulsions. His urine has a fruity odor and is found to contain an elevated level of ketone bodies. Neurologic studies show central nervous system defects. Despite intensive treatment, the boy dies after several days. The disease most likely resulted from a deficiency of

○ A. arginase
○ B. branched-chain α-keto acid dehydrogenase complex
○ C. cystathionine synthase
○ D. homogentisic acid oxidase
○ E. phenylalanine hydroxylase

49. A 24-year-old professional weight lifter develops sudden onset of abdominal pain while bench-pressing 550 pounds. Within 10 minutes of the onset of pain, he becomes hypotensive and collapses. During emergency surgery, the surgeon finds clotted and unclotted blood filling the peritoneal cavity. Which of the following best explains the likely origin of the patient's intraabdominal bleeding?

○ A. Ruptured abdominal aortic aneurysm
○ B. Ruptured cavernous hemangioma of the liver
○ C. Ruptured liver cell (hepatic) adenoma
○ D. Ruptured splenic artery aneurysm

50. Which of the following drugs is active against *Bacteroides fragilis* and *Clostridium difficile* but is inactive against *Chlamydia trachomatis*, beta-lactamase-positive *Haemophilus influenzae*, and methicillin-resistant *Staphylococcus aureus*?

○ A. Amoxicillin
○ B. Imipenem
○ C. Metronidazole
○ D. Oxacillin
○ E. Vancomycin

1. **C** (monoamine oxidase A) is correct. Phenelzine is an agent that irreversibly inhibits monoamine oxidase A (MAO-A) and monoamine oxidase B (MAO-B). When an MAO-A inhibitor interacts with foods that contain tyramine, it can cause an acute hypertensive crisis. The reaction typically occurs from 30 minutes to 2 hours after the patient ingests foods such as fermented beverages and aged cheeses (hence, the term "cheese effect" for this reaction). MAO-A in the gastrointestinal tract and liver normally inactivates tyramine. Inhibition of MAO-A allows tyramine to enter the bloodstream and function as an indirect-acting sympathomimetic amine. In addition, inhibition of MAO-A causes levels of norepinephrine in the presynaptic nerve terminals to increase, so there is more norepinephrine to be released by tyramine. The result is a rapid increase in blood pressure.

A (aromatic amino acid decarboxylase) is incorrect. Aromatic amino acid decarboxylase (also called dopa decarboxylase) is the enzyme that converts dopa to dopamine. Carbidopa is an inhibitor of this enzyme in peripheral tissues. When carbidopa is given in combination with levodopa, the effect of levodopa in brain tissue is increased.
B (catechol-*O*-methyltransferase) is incorrect. Catechol-*O*-methyltransferase (COMT) is the enzyme that inactivates norepinephrine and dopamine. Tolcapone is a reversible inhibitor of this enzyme. When tolcapone is given in combination with levodopa and carbidopa, high plasma levels of levodopa are sustained.
D (monoamine oxidase B) is incorrect. MAO-B is the enzyme that oxidatively deaminates dopamine. This enzyme is selectively inhibited by selegiline when it is administered in dosages used to treat patients with Parkinson's disease. Selegiline is used alone for its "neuroprotective" effect or is used in combination with levodopa to increase its central "buffering capacity."
E (tyrosine hydroxylase) is incorrect. Tyrosine hydroxylase is the rate-limiting enzyme in the synthesis of norepinephrine and epinephrine. This enzyme is inhibited by α-methyltyrosine, an agent that has been used in experimental studies to produce a chemical sympathectomy.

2. **B** (primary respiratory acidosis, secondary metabolic alkalosis, full pH compensation) is correct. The acid and base components are both higher than normal (normal $PaCO_2$ = 35–45 mm Hg; normal HCO_3^- = 22–28 mmol/L); thus an acid-base imbalance must exist. The pH is within normal limits; thus the compensation must be complete. Since the pH is slightly acidic compared to physiologic pH, an alkaline condition (i.e., pH >7.4)

must have been responsible for compensation (i.e., to bring the acid-base disturbance closer to neutral). Thus the primary condition is respiratory acidosis, because both the $PaCO_2$ and HCO_3^- concentrations are elevated; the compensatory process has created a secondary alkalosis—specifically a metabolic alkalosis since the HCO_3^- concentration has been reduced to an almost normal level.

A (combined metabolic acidosis and respiratory acidosis) is incorrect. Metabolic acidosis is characterized by a low pH and low HCO_3^- concentration. Respiratory acidosis is also characterized by a low pH, but elevated $PaCO_2$ concentration. If the two conditions were present simultaneously, the low HCO_3^- and the high $PaCO_2$ values would result in a very low arterial pH with no opportunity for compensation.
C (primary respiratory acidosis, secondary metabolic alkalosis, partial pH compensation) is incorrect. These laboratory studies show a primary respiratory acidosis with secondary metabolic alkalosis. Since the pH is within the normal range, the compensation is complete, not partial.
D (pure metabolic acidosis without pH compensation) is incorrect. Pure metabolic acidosis would be characterized by low values for pH and HCO_3^- and $PaCO_2$ concentrations. In this case, however, both the HCO_3^- and $PaCO_2$ concentrations are elevated.
E (pure respiratory acidosis) is incorrect. Respiratory acidosis is characterized by elevated $PaCO_2$ and HCO_3^- and reduced H^+ concentrations. In this case, both the HCO_3^- and H^+ concentrations have returned to near-normal values, but the $PaCO_2$ concentration is still fairly elevated. This suggests that some "correction" has been made in these values. Therefore, a pure respiratory acidosis without compensation can be ruled out.

3. *A* (accessory) is correct. The spinal accessory nerve, which travels through the posterior triangle of the neck, supplies the upper fibers of the trapezius muscle, which is solely responsible for the elevation of the lateral angle of the scapula. If the accessory nerve is injured, the lateral angle of the scapula is dragged downward by the weight of the free limb, having nothing to support it. The levator scapula and rhomboid muscles, which are located between the medial border of the scapula and the spine, become overstretched and contract more strongly to produce elevation of the superior angle of the scapula.

B (dorsal scapular) is incorrect. The dorsal scapular nerve (C5) innervates the rhomboid muscles, which participate in retraction and downward rotation of the scapula. Injury to this nerve would affect retraction and downward rotation of the scapula.
C (great auricular) is incorrect. The great auricular nerve (C2–C3) is a sensory nerve to the skin over the parotid gland, mastoid process, and back of the auricle. Injury to this nerve would cause only sensory losses.

D (phrenic) is incorrect. The phrenic nerve (C3–C5) is a motor nerve to the diaphragm. Injury to this nerve results in paralysis of half of the diaphragm.

E (posterior auricular) is incorrect. The posterior auricular nerve, a branch of the facial nerve (CN VII), innervates the posterior auricular and occipital muscles. Injury to this nerve would not affect the movements of the scapula.

4. *B* (chi-square test) is correct. A chi-square test assesses for differences between frequencies in a sample. Because the researcher wants to contrast overall percentages of nonsmokers in each group, this statistical method would be best. A chi-square test is useful when nominal data must be analyzed (e.g., race, gender).

A (analysis of variance) is incorrect. The ANOVA test is used to compare two or more groups. If the researcher wants to compare the number of cigarettes smoked during a week for all four groups, an ANOVA test would be appropriate.

C (correlation) is incorrect. To determine whether a relationship is present between two variables, a correlation coefficient is obtained. A correlation demonstrates the direction and strength of a relationship but not the cause and effect. If the researcher wants to know if weight gain is related to the number of cigarettes smoked, a correlation would provide this information.

D (independent *t* test) is incorrect. In an independent *t* test, the means for two distinct groups are assessed for differences. If the researcher wants to compare the number of cigarettes smoked weekly by the group given bupropion hydrochloride with the control group, a *t* test could be conducted.

E (paired *t* test) is incorrect. A paired *t* test examines pretest and posttest differences between means for a sample. If the researcher wants to examine the number of cigarettes smoked before and after an intervention for one group, this test would be utilized.

5. *A* (blastomycosis) is correct. The finding of yeasts with broad-based buds and bud scars strongly suggests the diagnosis of disseminated blastomycosis. Before the advent of AIDS, this finding alone would have been considered definitive. The biopsy material can be cultured to confirm the presence of *Blastomyces dermatitidis*, a dimorphic organism. It is thought to occur in the soil, possibly from bird droppings high in nitrogen content, which promote the growth of *Blastomyces*. Blastomycosis occurs worldwide, but most cases are found in the United States along the Mississippi, Ohio, and Tennessee river valleys and near the Smoky and Blue Ridge mountains. Most cases occur in males between the ages of 30 and 50 years.

B (coccidioidomycosis) is incorrect. Coccidioidomycosis most commonly disseminates to the bone, not to the skin. If the cause of the patient's lesion had been *Coccidioides immitis*, spherules would have been seen in the biopsy material.

C (mycetoma) is incorrect. Mycetomas can be caused by numerous bacteria, including *Actinomadura, Actinomyces, Nocardia,* and *Streptomyces*. Although mycetomas sometimes look like squamous cell carcinomas, the microscopic findings in this case rule out the diagnosis of a mycetoma.

D (primary dermatophytic lesion) is incorrect. If the lesion had been caused by a dermatophyte (such as a *Trichophyton* or *Epidermophyton* species), it would not have resembled a squamous cell carcinoma, and microscopic examination would have shown the presence of filamentous forms and microconidia.

E (secondarily infected squamous cell carcinoma) is incorrect. The presence of gram-positive cocci would be expected in a secondarily infected site on the arm.

6. *C* (increases maturation of the blast cells) is correct. The patient has acute promyelocytic (progranulocytic) leukemia (FAB classification M3). Unique characteristics associated with this form of leukemia include a high incidence of disseminated intravascular coagulation, or DIC (which is present in this patient), a t(15; 17) translocation, abnormal retinoic acid metabolism, and an excellent response to treatment with retinoic acid, which matures the promyelocytes.

A (destroys the blast cells), B (enhances cellular immunity), D (prevents infection associated with bone marrow suppression), and E (prevents intravascular coagulation) are incorrect. Substances released from the granules of the promyelocytes activate the coagulation cascade, leading to intravascular coagulation. D-dimers are fibrin monomers found in a fibrin clot that have been cross-linked by factor XIII (fibrin-stabilizing factor). Their presence indicates that intravascular coagulation has occurred. Refer to the discussion for C.

7. *A* (left cerebral cortex) is correct. A lesion affecting the left cerebral cortex, including Brodmann's areas 44 and 45, will disrupt Broca's area (speech production area) and make it difficult for the patient to respond verbally. If it also affects Brodmann's area 4 (the primary motor cortex), the lesion will also disrupt motor activity in the arm. Since many descending corticospinal fibers cross at the level of the pyramids, changes in motor activity would be expected in the contralateral (right) arm.

B (right arcuate fasciculus) is incorrect. The arcuate fasciculus runs between Wernicke's area (Brodmann's area 22, which includes the auditory comprehension center) and Broca's area (Brodmann's area 45, the speech production area). It does not include Brodmann's area 4 (the primary motor cortex). Thus, a lesion in the arcuate fasciculus would affect the patient's ability to respond verbally to questions but would not affect motor activity in the arm.

C (right internal capsule) is incorrect. The internal capsule is a bundle of fibers that passes between the thalamus and the cortex. Damage to this structure would block sensory input from the midbrain, brain stem, and spinal cord, as well as motor output to those structures. Thus, damage to the right internal capsule would cause the left-sided paralysis seen in this patient. It would also cause cranial nerve damage and/or abnormal somatosensory activity, neither of which is apparent in this patient. Furthermore, it would not cause the communication problems experienced by this patient.

D   (right precentral gyrus) is incorrect. Although a lesion in the right precentral gyrus (which contains the motor cortex) could cause left arm paralysis, it would not account for the patient's communication problems.

E   (superior temporal gyrus) is incorrect. The superior temporal gyrus contains Wernicke's area, which governs the interpretation of speech. Since the patient can understand questions asked of him, Wernicke's area may not be involved.

8. *E*   (inhibit vitamin K epoxide reductase, thereby preventing the formation of inactive clotting factors) is correct. Clotting factors II (prothrombin), VII, IX, and X are formed by posttranslational carboxylation. Reduced vitamin K is required for this reaction, and vitamin K epoxide reductase catalyzes the conversion of oxidized vitamin K to reduced vitamin K. Warfarin is an anticoagulant that acts by inhibiting this enzyme and thereby preventing the formation of vitamin K–dependent clotting factors. The prothrombin clotting time is a measurement of the anticoagulant effect of warfarin. The effects of warfarin can be reversed by the administration of phytonadione (vitamin K_1).

A   (activate plasminogen that is bound to fibrin, thereby catalyzing the conversion of plasminogen to plasmin) is incorrect. This is a description of the mechanism of action of alteplase, a thrombolytic drug that is a recombinant form of tissue plasminogen activator (t-PA). By preferentially activating plasminogen that is bound to fibrin, t-PA confines thrombolysis to the formed thrombus. The effects of alteplase can be reversed by the administration of aminocaproic acid, a drug that inhibits plasminogen activation.

B   (bind to antithrombin III and act catalytically to facilitate the interaction of AT-III with activated clotting factors) is incorrect. This is a description of the mechanism of action of heparin, an anticoagulant that is given parenterally. The activated partial thromboplastin time (aPTT) is a measurement of the anticoagulant effect of heparin. The effects of heparin can be reversed by the administration of protamine sulfate.

C   (bind to inactive plasminogen, thereby catalyzing the conversion of plasminogen to active plasmin) is incorrect. This is a description of the mechanism of action of streptokinase and urokinase. These "clot busters" bind to plasminogen and cause a conformational change in the complex that facilitates the cleavage of plasminogen to plasmin. The effects of these thrombolytic drugs can be reversed by aminocaproic acid, a drug that inhibits plasminogen activation.

D   (inhibit cyclooxygenase-1, thereby preventing the formation of thromboxane) is incorrect. This is a description of the mechanism of action of acetylsalicylic acid (ASA, or aspirin). Cyclooxygenase-1 (COX-1) is irreversibly inhibited by ASA and is reversibly inhibited by most other "typical" nonsteroidal anti-inflammatory drugs (NSAIDs). Inhibition of COX-1 prevents thromboxane A_2 formation in platelets and thereby inhibits platelet hemostasis. The primary of effect of ASA is manifested as an increase in bleeding time. Selective COX-2 inhibitors (celecoxib and fofecoxib) and nonacetylated salicylates do not affect platelet hemostasis.

9. *A*   (cord of Billroth in the spleen) is correct. The cords of Billroth are oblong aggregations of lymphatic tissue that lie between venous sinusoids in the red pulp of the spleen. Blood entering the spleen from the circulatory system passes through the cords of Billroth, where the formed elements of blood encounter macrophages that reside in these cords. The macrophages destroy damaged erythrocytes, including the sickle-shaped cells in this patient. Because of this activity, splenomegaly is a common finding in patients with sickle cell anemia of African-American descent.

B   (hematopoietic cord of bone marrow) is incorrect. The hematopoietic cords of the bone marrow are the areas in which erythrocytopoiesis occurs (not erythrophagocytosis).
C   (marginal zone of the spleen) is incorrect. The marginal zone lies between the red pulp and white pulp of the spleen. Although it contains macrophages, the primary activity in this region is the presentation of antigens to T cells and B cells by dendritic cells in an attempt to trigger an immune response.
D   (medullary region of the thymus) is incorrect. The primary function of the thymus is to produce immunocompetent T cells. The medulla of the thymus contains mature T cells, which leave the thymus via venules and efferent lymphatic vessels to populate other lymphoid organs (e.g., the lymph nodes and spleen). Phagocytosis is not carried out by red blood cells.
E   (paratrabecular sinus in a lymph node) is incorrect. The supcapsular, medullary, and paratrabecular sinuses of the lymph node are bridged by phagocytic cells. These sinuses contain lymph, not blood.

10. *C*   (site C) is correct. Site C, called the TATA box, is a short consensus sequence that starts about 30 base pairs (bp) upstream from the cap site (the transcription start site). The TATA box is important because it correctly positions RNA polymerase II.

A   (site A) is incorrect. Site A is an enhancer sequence. Enhancer sequences increase the transcription of neighboring genes. In most cases, they are located several thousand bp upstream from the gene. Rarely, they are found downstream from the gene.
B   (site B) is incorrect. Site B, called the CAAT box, is found about

60 bp upstream from a transcription start site and is a consensus region in many genes. Its function is not well understood.
D   (site D) is incorrect. Site D is called the cap site or the transcription start site. RNA polymerase II binds to promoter sites and begins mRNA synthesis at the transcription start site. The eukaryotic mRNA cap consists of 7-methylguanylate residue, attached by a triphosphate 5′-5′ linkage to the terminal nucleotide of the primary mRNA transcript.
E   (site E) is incorrect. Site E, called the polyA tail, is added by the poly A polymerase, one A at a time, to the 3′ end of the transcript. The polyA tail is usually about 200 nucleotides long.

11. **B** *(Listeria monocytogenes)* is correct. The clinical and laboratory findings are consistent with meningitis caused by *L. monocytogenes.* This gram-positive bacterium grows in macrophages and epithelial cells and produces listeriolysin O, an oxygen-sensitive hemolysin. Most *Listeria* infections occur in neonates and elderly individuals.

A   *(Cryptococcus neoformans)* and D *(Streptococcus pneumoniae)* are incorrect. *C. neoformans* and *S. pneumoniae* can cause infections of the central nervous system (CNS). However, *C. neoformans* is an encapsulated yeast, and *S. pneumoniae* is an encapsulated bacterium that is a coccus.
C   *(Staphylococcus aureus)* is incorrect. *S. aureus,* a rare cause of CNS infection, is a nonmotile coccus.
E   *(Toxoplasma gondii)* is incorrect. *T. gondii* can infect the CNS, but it is a strictly intracellular sporozoan parasite.

12. **D** (no change in Na^+; decrease H_2O intake) is correct. The patient has the syndrome of inappropriate antidiuretic hormone (ADH), or SIADH, due to ectopic secretion of ADH by a primary lung cancer (small cell carcinoma). ADH is normally involved in the reabsorption of electrolyte free water in the collecting tubules of the kidneys, which concentrates the urine. Therefore, an excess of ADH results in increased reabsorption of water, which enters the extracellular fluid (ECF) compartment and produces a dilutional hyponatremia. Hyponatremia then establishes an osmotic gradient favoring the movement of water into the intracellular fluid (ICF) compartment, which produces cerebral edema. Because pure water is added to both the ECF and ICF compartments, the best nonpharmacologic treatment is water restriction.

A   (decrease Na^+ and H_2O intake) is incorrect. The hyponatremia is related to the addition of pure water to the ECF and not to a loss of sodium.
B   (decrease Na^+; no change in H_2O intake) and C (increase both Na^+ and H_2O intake) are incorrect. Refer to the discussion for D.
E   (no change in either Na^+ or H_2O intake) is incorrect. Water must be restricted in the patient. Refer to the discussion for D.

13. *C* (inhibitory interneuron is activated by the Ia afferent and inhibits flexors) is correct. Inhibitory interneurons, which lie within the spinal cord, "convert" excitatory Ia afferent input into inhibitory output by releasing an inhibitory neurotransmitter (usually GABA) to bind with its receptors on the alpha motor neuron that innervates the antagonistic flexor.

A (antagonistic extensor is inhibited by supraspinal connections) is incorrect. Although there is supraspinal control over reflexes, reciprocal inhibition occurs through local spinal reflex mechanisms.

B (extensors are directly inhibited by the flexors) is incorrect. There is no direct connection between extensors and flexors.

D (Ia afferent releases a neurotransmitter that triggers flexors and another that inhibits extensors) is incorrect. A single neuron does not release two neurotransmitters with opposing effects in response to a single set of environmental conditions.

E (neurotransmitter that excites the flexors inhibits the extensors) is incorrect. An excitatory neurotransmitter will excite virtually all neurons carrying its receptors, and an inhibitory neurotransmitter will inhibit nearly all neurons carrying its receptors.

14. *A* (acetyl-CoA carboxylase) is correct. In fatty acid biosynthesis, acetyl-CoA carboxylase catalyzes the rate-limiting step, which is the conversion of acetyl CoA to malonyl CoA. This is a typical adenosine triphosphate–dependent carboxylation, with enzyme-bound biotin serving as a carrier of the carboxyl group. Acetyl-CoA carboxylase is regulated by both rapid- and slow-acting mechanisms. Short-term control involves allosteric activation by citrate, as well as covalent modification. Long-term control involves changes in the concentration of the enzyme.

B (acyl-CoA dehydrogenase) is incorrect. Acyl-CoA dehydrogenase catalyzes the first step in β-oxidation of fatty acids. It does not require biotin.

C (fatty acid synthase) is incorrect. The fatty acid synthase complex has a phosphopantetheine, a prosthetic group of acyl carrier protein (ACP). The fatty acid synthase complex does not require biotin.

D (fatty acid thiokinase) is incorrect. Fatty acid thiokinase (also called acyl-CoA synthetase) catalyzes the formation of a thioester linkage between the carboxyl group of a fatty acid and the sulfhydryl group of CoA. This activation is a necessary step for β-oxidation of fatty acids. It does not require biotin.

E (propionyl-CoA carboxylase) is incorrect. Propionyl-CoA carboxylase requires biotin, but it does not take part in fatty acid synthesis. It functions in a pathway from propionyl CoA to succinyl CoA. This pathway is involved in the oxidation of fatty acids that have an odd number of carbon atoms. The pathway also serves as a point of entry into the Krebs cycle for some of the carbon atoms of methionine, isoleucine, and valine.

15. **B** (benztropine) is correct. Benztropine is an antimuscarinic agent that is useful in the treatment of Parkinson's disease, particularly in patients with an early manifestation such as tremor or rigidity. The drug helps restore the balance of input of dopamine and acetylcholine to the striatum. Like other drugs that block muscarinic receptors (including diphenhydramine and trihexyphenidyl), benztropine can cause the following adverse effects: dry mouth, blurred vision, and constipation; impaired cognition, which is due to blockade of central muscarinic receptors in the hippocampus; and urinary retention, which would further predispose this patient to cystitis.

A (amantadine) is incorrect. Amantadine is useful in the treatment of Parkinson's disease, particularly in patients with an early manifestation such as bradykinesia or rigidity. The drug acts to stimulate dopamine release or block dopamine reuptake. Amantadine has some antimuscarinic activity but less than that of benztropine. Therefore, it would be less likely than benztropine to exacerbate the patient's preexisting problems.
C (bromocriptine) is incorrect. Bromocriptine, pergolide, pramipexole, and ropinirole are examples of dopamine receptor agonists. These drugs are useful in treating the early stages of Parkinson's disease. In addition, they are useful in treating the later stages, when other agents that require the presence of intact presynaptic nerve terminals (agents such as levodopa, amantadine, and selegiline) lose their effectiveness. The dopamine receptor agonists would not exacerbate the patient's preexisting problems.
D (levodopa) is incorrect. Levodopa is a prodrug whose clinically active metabolite, dopamine, does not cross the blood-brain barrier. Levodopa is the cornerstone drug in the clinical management of Parkinson's disease. Its use would not exacerbate the patient's preexisting problems.
E (selegiline) is incorrect. Selegiline is a selective inhibitor of monoamine oxidase B (MAO-B) that can be used alone or in combination with levodopa to treat Parkinson's disease. When used alone, selegiline has been found to have a neuroprotective effect, which slows progression of the disease and thus delays the need to begin concurrent treatment with levodopa or another antiparkinsonian drug. As an adjunct agent, selegiline is useful for treating patients who exhibit the "wearing off" response to treatment with levodopa and carbidopa. Selegiline would not exacerbate the patient's preexisting problems.

16. **C** (Epstein-Barr virus) is correct. The clinical and laboratory findings are consistent with the diagnosis of infectious mononucleosis caused by the Epstein-Barr virus (EBV). The virus is transmitted from person to person via contact with saliva. EBV is a member of the family *Herpesviridae* and the subfamily *Gammaherpesvirinae*. The primary targets of viruses in this subfamily

are B cells and epithelial cells. EBV establishes a latent infection in B cells, and the T cell response to B cell infection contributes to the clinical manifestations of the disease.

A (adenovirus) and D (influenza B virus) are incorrect. Adenoviruses are a common cause of pharyngitis, and some of the patient's symptoms resemble the symptoms of influenza. However, heterophile antibodies are not found in association with adenoviruses or influenza B virus.
B (cytomegalovirus) is incorrect. Cytomegalovirus (CMV) is a cause of infectious mononucleosis, but heterophile antibodies are not found in association with CMV.
E (rubella virus) is incorrect. Rubella virus causes rubella (German measles), a disease with a characteristic rash. The patient's clinical manifestations are not consistent with the diagnosis of rubella.

17. A (anatomic shunt blood flow) is correct. The fact that breathing pure O_2 for several minutes had little effect on the difference between arterial and arteriolar PO_2 suggests that as quickly as O_2 entered arterial blood, it was "diluted" with oxygen-poor venous blood. This would be most likely to happen in the presence of an arteriovenous shunt.

B (hypoventilation) is incorrect. Hypoventilation, for whatever cause (e.g., chronic airway obstructions, neuromuscular diseases, or pharmacologic depression of central respiratory neurons), reduces alveolar PO_2, which leads to a reduction in blood oxygenation. However, if this patient had been hypoventilating, exposure to 100% O_2 would have increased PAO_2 and reduced the PAO_2/PaO_2 gradient substantially.
C (pharmacologic depression of brainstem neurons) is incorrect. Depression of the brainstem neurons descending from central respiratory centers could induce hypoventilation with low PAO_2 and low PaO_2. Oxygenation would not increase these oxygen partial pressures by very much, but the PAO_2/PaO_2 gradient would still be near normal, because there is no barrier to gas exchange within the lungs.
D (pulmonary diffusion impairment) is incorrect. Pulmonary diffusion can be impaired by thickening of the respiratory membranes, since this would impede the flux of oxygen across alveolar walls. The result would be a serious mismatch between alveolar and blood oxygen tensions. However, exposure to 100% O_2 would have reduced the PAO_2/PaO_2 gradient significantly.
E (ventilation/perfusion mismatch) is incorrect. Ventilation/perfusion mismatching does lead to arterial hypoxemia, but it is usually not suspected until the three other potential causes of hypoxemia (i.e., hyperventilation, thickened respiratory membranes, and anatomic shunts) have been ruled out. Oxygenation typically improves the PAO_2/PaO_2 gradient substantially.

18. *C* (not comply with the patient's request, but attempt to work with the patient and family to maintain the highest quality of life) is correct. Although the patient's condition is terminal, her pain medications are not alleviating the pain; therefore, she has requested that the physician administer a lethal injection, but the physician cannot comply. The American Medical Association does not support active euthanasia. The physician can only offer treatments that are likely to decrease suffering and maintain quality of life.

A (comply with the patient's request if the physician feels the patient is competent) is incorrect. Regardless of the patient's competence, euthanasia cannot be offered.
B (inform the patient's family of the request and, if the family agrees, comply with the request) is incorrect. The patient has made a confidential request that should not be discussed with family members. Even if the family concurred with the patient's request, the physician cannot offer euthanasia.
D (not comply with the patient's request, but request a psychiatric evaluation and place the patient on a suicide watch) is incorrect. Placing the patient on a suicide watch would be unnecessary unless there is additional evidence of a comorbid depression or active thoughts of suicide. The patient's request is most likely linked to the degree of suffering and is not an active desire to die.
E (seek psychiatric consultation and, if the patient is deemed competent, comply with the request) is incorrect. Psychiatric consultation might prove useful if a comorbid depression is present; however, the absence of psychologic problems would not allow the physician to comply with the patient's request.

19. *C* (measurement of C5, C6, C7, and C8 levels) is correct. Individuals who have deficiencies in the terminal complement components have a difficult time handling diseases caused by *Neisseria*. Measurement of C5, C6, C7, and C8 levels would confirm that a complement deficiency is present.

A (lymphocyte proliferation test) is incorrect. Lymphocyte function would not be affected by deficiencies associated with the case described.
B (measurement of C3 levels) is incorrect. A deficiency in C3 levels would increase a person's susceptibility to diseases caused by encapsulated organisms. Although some individuals have reported *Neisseria gonorrhoeae* to have a loosely associated capsule, the organism's serum sensitivity or resistance is attributable to its lipooligosaccharide.
D (measurement of immunoglobulin levels) is incorrect. Immunoglobulin measurements would reveal the presence of hypogammaglobulinemia. Although this condition could certainly lead to hypotensive shock, the history of repeated bouts of gonococcal disease is inconsistent with the diagnosis of hypotensive shock due to hypogammaglobulinemia.

E   (measurement of mucosal IgA levels) is incorrect. IgA deficiency is related to an increased incidence of colitis, but has not been linked to disseminated gonorrhea.

20. *D* (midazolam) is correct. The GABA$_A$-receptor complex is a multimeric protein complex consisting of five subunits: an α subunit (the GABA-binding site); a β subunit (the barbiturate-binding site); a γ subunit (the benzodiazepine-binding site); and two other subunits that are uncharacterized. The subunits together form the Cl$^-$ channel, through which GABA exerts its inhibitory activity by hyperpolarizing the cell after Cl$^-$ influx. When benzodiazepines (including midazolam) and barbiturates bind to their receptors, they facilitate (potentiate) GABA-mediated neuronal inhibition. The benzodiazepines do this by increasing the frequency of GABA-gated Cl$^-$ channel openings. In contrast, the barbiturates do this by increasing the duration of GABA-gated Cl$^-$ channel openings (a mnemonic device is to think of barbiturates as barbiDURATES).

A   (baclofen) is incorrect. Baclofen is a spasmolytic agent that acts as a GABA agonist at the GABA$_B$-receptor complex. This complex is linked to the K$^+$ channel. Activation of the GABA receptor by baclofen increases K$^+$ conductance and thereby hyperpolarizes the cell.
B   (buspirone) is incorrect. Buspirone is a nonsedating anxiolytic drug whose therapeutic effect is attributed to its action as a partial agonist at serotonin 5-HT$_{1a}$ receptors. Buspirone would have no effect on the GABA$_A$-receptor complex.
C   (hydroxyzine) is incorrect. Hydroxyzine is a histamine H$_1$ receptor antagonist. It would have no effect on the GABA$_A$-receptor complex.
E   (morphine) is incorrect. Morphine produces its pharmacologic effects by acting as an agonist at the opioid mu (μ) receptor. It would have no effect on the GABA$_A$-receptor complex.

21. *A* (B-cell malignancy arising from the bone marrow) is correct. The patient has chronic lymphocytic leukemia (CLL). CLL is the most common leukemia; in patients 60 years of age, it is the most common leukemia and the most common cause of generalized lymphadenopathy. Like all leukemias, it arises from stem cells in the bone marrow and can metastasize throughout the body, typically to the lymph nodes, liver, and spleen. Because the B cells are neoplastic, they cannot be antigenically stimulated to produce plasma cells, hence the high incidence of hypogammaglobulinemia and infection in CLL patients.

B   (hypogammaglobulinemia related to sepsis) is incorrect. In this patient, hypogammaglobulinemia did not produce this patient's hematologic condition; however, it is most likely responsible for her sepsis.
C   (lymphoid leukemoid reaction secondary to sepsis) is incorrect. The patient does not have an exaggerated, benign proliferation of lymphocytes (leukemoid reaction) in response to an

infection. In patients with sepsis, expected findings do not include hepatosplenomegaly, generalized nontender lymphadenopathy, lymphocytosis, and hypogammaglobulinemia. These patients have tender lymphadenopathy and neutrophilic leukocytosis.

D (metastatic lung cancer associated with smoking cigarettes) is incorrect. Although smoking has been implicated in causing leukemia, the clinical and laboratory findings in this patient are totally inconsistent with metastatic lung cancer.

E (T-cell malignancy arising from lymph nodes) is incorrect. T-cell leukemias are uncommon, usually metastasize to skin, have lytic lesions in bone, and are not associated with hypogammaglobulinemia.

22. **D** (lack of prolyl and lysyl hydroxylase activity) is correct. Ascorbic acid is a cofactor in the catalysis of procollagen hydroxylation. Inadequate hydroxylation of procollagen results in inadequate cross-linking of collagen fibers, and consequently in weak collagen fibers or an inadequate number of normal collagen fibers. This defect causes weakened capillary and venule walls, which results in the leakage of blood and leads to purpura and ecchymosis. It also results in weakened mucosa, which allows oral ulcers to develop. Sharpey's fibers, which attach the periosteum to bone, will also weaken, resulting in subperiosteal hemorrhages.

A (failure to maintain fully differentiated epithelia) is incorrect. Epithelial differentiation is an important function of vitamin A. A deficiency in this vitamin can be ruled out in this patient, because his symptoms are not consistent with this problem. Much of the damage observed in the patient (particularly the ecchymoses and purpura) indicates the presence of leaky small blood vessels and suggests that the entire depth of the blood vessel wall has been breached—the endothelium as well as connective tissue surrounding these vessels. Vitamin A deficiency would not be responsible for this type of damage.

B (inadequate mineralization of cancellous bone) is incorrect. The absorption of calcium from the intestine and its uptake into bone is diminished in individuals with hypovitaminosis D. Inadequate mineralization of bone can result in rickets (distortion of muscle-associated bones) or osteomalacia (softening of bone). Neither of these conditions was reported for this patient.

C (increased intracellular levels of p53) is incorrect. The intracellular protein p53 accumulates in the cell in response to DNA damage (e.g., as a result of exposure to mutagenic agents or ionizing radiation). This type of exposure was not reported for this patient. p53 causes the cell to arrest in the G_1 phase of the cell cycle, which gives the cell time to attempt to repair the damage before entering the S phase (when DNA is synthesized).

23. *A* (acoustic neuroma) is correct. An acoustic neuroma is a tumor that develops from Schwann cells, commonly in the vestibular division of the vestibulocochlear nerve (CN VIII). It can grow into the cerebellopontine angle, where it may compromise the facial nerve (CN VII) and sensory axons in the cochlear division of CN VIII. Early symptoms of this condition include hearing loss and tinnitus. Sounds seem louder on the affected side because the stapedial reflex is compromised. This reflex causes the stapes in each ear to contract in response to a sudden or loud noise. Contraction causes the remaining ossicles to stiffen and changes the transmission of vibrations. Since CN VII also detects sensation in the anterior two thirds of the tongue, damage to this nerve can also compromise the sense of taste.

B (lacunar stroke in the internal capsule) is incorrect. The internal capsule contains fibers traveling to and from the cerebral cortex. Fibers carrying auditory signals leave the medial geniculate nucleus and form the auditory radiations (a retrolenticular portion of the internal capsule) on their way to the primary auditory cortex in the temporal lobe. A lacunar stroke would not affect the facial nerve and thus would not result in changes in the stapedial reflex and sense of taste.

C (lesion in the caudal medulla) is incorrect. Auditory fibers in CN VIII enter the brain stem and CN III fibers exit the brain stem at the rostral end of the medulla (specifically, the pontomedullary junction), not the caudal end. Therefore, a lesion in the caudal end of the medulla would not affect hearing in either ear or alter the stapedial reflex. It also would not affect the sense of taste, since the relay neurons involved in this sensation lie in the gustatory portion of the nucleus solitarius, which is in the rostral medulla.

D (lesion in the mesencephalic tegmentum) is incorrect. The tegmentum is the posterior segment of the mesencephalon (midbrain). Auditory fibers contain information from both ears once they pass the level of the superior olivary nucleus, which lies at the caudal end of the midbrain. Thus, a lesion in the more rostral structure would affect hearing in both ears. A lesion in the rostral midbrain would not involve the pontomedullary border or CN VII (which projects from that border). Since CN VII would be spared, the stapedial reflex and sense of taste would not be affected.

E (lesion in the tectum) is incorrect. The tectum (the uppermost portion of the midbrain) contains two pairs of colliculi—the superior colliculi, which contain fibers carrying visual information; and the inferior colliculi, which contain auditory fibers carrying information from both ears. A lesion in the tectum would affect hearing in both ears. A lesion in this area would not affect CN VII; thus, the stapedial reflex and sense of taste would not be altered.

24. ***D*** (presence of anti–pancreatic islet cell antibodies) is correct. Anti–pancreatic islet cell antibodies are found in type 1 diabetes mellitus. These antibodies contribute to the destruction of islet cells and thereby reduce the amount of insulin that is secreted by the pancreas. Unlike type 1 diabetes mellitus, which is caused by insulin deficiency, type 2 diabetes mellitus is caused by target tissue resistance to insulin.

A (increased erythrocyte sedimentation rate) and B (increased serum creatinine level) are incorrect. Type 1 diabetes mellitus does not cause changes in the erythrocyte sedimentation rate or serum creatinine level.
C (presence of anti–pancreatic amyloid antibodies) and E (presence of anti–streptolysin O antibodies) are incorrect. Anti–pancreatic amyloid antibodies are found in patients with islet cell tumors. Anti–streptolysin O antibodies are directed against an exotoxin produced by *Streptococcus pyogenes* and are found in patients with streptococcal disease. Neither of these types of antibodies is found in patients with diabetes mellitus.

25. ***C*** (methotrexate) is correct. All of the drugs listed are considered to be slow-acting antirheumatic drugs (SAARDs) or disease-modifying antirheumatic drugs (DMARDs) and are employed in the advanced ("step 2") treatment of rheumatoid arthritis (RA). Methotrexate is preferred by most rheumatologists because it is considered to be the most efficacious step 2 drug. Like trimethoprim, methotrexate acts by inhibiting dihydrofolate reductase and thereby preventing the synthesis of purines and pyrimidines. Hematologic toxicity and hepatic toxicity are the adverse effects of greatest concern when methotrexate is used to treat RA.

A (azathioprine) is incorrect. Azathioprine is a prodrug that is converted to 6-mercaptopurine (6-MP). The 6-MP is then converted by hypoxanthine phosphoribosyltransferase to 6-thioinosinic acid, an agent that inhibits purine synthesis. Since 6-MP is inactivated by xanthine oxidase, the dose of azathioprine must be reduced in patients who are concurrently treated with allopurinol (a purine analogue). Azathioprine use is associated with hematologic toxicity, and a CBC must be monitored in patients who are treated with this drug.
B (hydroxychloroquine) is incorrect. Hydroxychloroquine is used to treat malaria as well as advanced RA. Its mechanism of action in the management of RA is not fully understood but may involve inhibition of the release or synthesis of inflammatory mediators (such as prostaglandins) and cytokines (such as interleukin-1). Routine blood tests are not required with hydroxychloroquine treatment.
D (penicillamine) is incorrect. Penicillamine is used in the treatment of a variety of conditions. It effectively chelates copper and is therefore the drug of choice for treating Wilson's disease. It effectively chelates organic mercury, lead, and arsenic and is use-

ful for the treatment of intoxication with these heavy metals. When penicillamine is used to treat advanced RA, its efficacy is thought to be due to the drug's recruitment of T helper cells. Penicillamine use is associated with hematologic toxicity, and a CBC should be performed every 6–12 weeks in patients taking the drug. E (sulfasalazine) is incorrect. In the colon, bacteria break down sulfasalazine to form 5-aminosalicylic acid (5-ASA) plus sulfapyridine. The 5-ASA moiety is responsible for the drug's beneficial effects in the management of inflammatory bowel diseases, such as ulcerative colitis. The sulfapyridine moiety is thought to be responsible for the drug's beneficial effects in the treatment of RA. Sulfasalazine use is associated with hematologic toxicity, and a CBC must be monitored in patients who are treated with this drug.

26. *B* (cognitive) is correct. Cognitive therapy is based on the concept that how an individual thinks largely determines the individual's feelings and behaviors. A cognitive therapist teaches patients to identify and evaluate maladaptive thoughts and to form healthy alternatives.

A (behavioral) is incorrect. Behavioral therapy is based on learning principles. This approach focuses on changing a patient's activities and interactions by altering reinforcement contingencies.
C (family systems) is incorrect. In a family systems approach, disorders are viewed as serving a function within a family. For example, depression might be a way of decreasing marital conflict and thus increasing the likelihood of maintaining a better relationship.
D (psychodynamic) is incorrect. Psychodynamic therapy is aimed at increasing a patient's insight into the unconscious bases behind their current conflicts and behaviors.
E (supportive) is incorrect. Supportive listening and empathy are emphasized in supportive therapy. No interpretations or direct suggestions are made in this type of treatment.

27. *E* (it promotes sodium retention and potassium excretion in the distal tubules of nephrons) is correct. Decreased blood perfusion of the kidney causes secretion of renin from the juxtaglomerular cells. This activates the angiotensinogen cascade and results in aldosterone secretion. Compound X represents aldosterone. Aldosterone acts primarily on the distal tubules of nephrons, where it promotes sodium retention and potassium excretion.

A (it causes arteriolar vasoconstriction) is incorrect. Aldosterone does not cause arteriolar vasoconstriction; however, it is caused by angiotensin II.
B (it is produced by juxtaglomerular cells of the kidney) is incorrect. Renin, an enzyme that converts angiotensinogen to angiotensin I, is produced and secreted by juxtaglomerular cells of

the kidney in response to a decrease in blood volume, arterial pressure, or Na^+ load.

C (it is secreted in response to infusions rich in Na^+) is incorrect. Aldosterone is released in response to hyperkalemia. This regulatory action by potassium appears to act independently of the renin-angiotensin system.

D (it is under tight control of adrenocorticotropic hormone) is incorrect. Abnormal levels of ACTH, such as those seen in patients with Cushing syndrome, do not affect plasma aldosterone levels. Thus, ACTH plays only a minor role in aldosterone release.

28. *A* (increases area available for gas exchange by opening closed alveoli) is correct. The lung is subject to the effects of gravity. The sheer weight of the lung, particularly when the subject is standing, causes the average alveolus at the base of the lung to become very small or even collapse; this is in contrast to alveoli in the apex, which stretch open. As aging occurs, more and more of the basal alveoli collapse, making it impossible for gas exchange to take place within this region of the lung. To overcome this situation, positive pressure may be applied during expiration. In this procedure, a special valve directs exhaled air through a tube submerged under water. If the tube is 10-cm deep, the end-expiratory pressure will be +10-cm H_2O. Thus, PEEP helps open closed basal alveoli and prevents other alveoli from collapsing. This simple procedure increases the functional residual capacity (FRC), recruits more lung units, increases the area available for gas exchange, and greatly improves oxygenation of the blood.

B (increases compliance, making it easier to breathe) is incorrect. Compliance is an inherent characteristic of lung tissue. The pressure with which air is "forced" through the airways has no effect on the ability of pulmonary tissue to expand and recoil.

C (promotes an increase in pulmonary blood flow) is incorrect. When PEEP is administered appropriately, it should have little or no effect on pulmonary blood flow. Pulmonary blood flow is based on resistance within the pulmonary vessels. If the pressure used in the administration of PEEP is too high, however, it can overinflate the alveoli, causing them to press against the pulmonary capillaries and collapse. This would increase pulmonary vascular resistance and result in stress (afterload) on the right ventricle.

D (significantly increases the PAO_2 when the patient is breathing air) is incorrect. If the patient is breathing air, the alveolar PO_2 will not change because the ambient PO_2 has not changed. PEEP does not change PAO_2 levels.

E (stimulates breathing by tonically activating pulmonary stretch receptors) is incorrect. It is possible for pulmonary stretch receptors to be activated during inflation, but if this were to happen, an inspiratory inhibitory reflex would be activated.

29. *B*   (anterior to scalenus anterior muscle) is correct. The subclavian vein crosses the root of the neck between the scalenus anterior muscle and the clavicle. Situated anterior to the scalenus anterior muscle, it extends laterally from the scalenus anterior to arch over the first rib. At the lateral border of the first rib, it becomes the axillary vein.

The scalenus anterior muscle is an important anatomic landmark because of its relationship with a number of structures in the neck. The phrenic nerve, which forms on the anterior surface of the scalenus anterior from C3, C4, and C5 off the cervical plexus, crosses posterior to the subclavian vein on its way into the thoracic cavity to innervate the diaphragm. The subclavian artery and the roots of the brachial plexus are posterior to the scalenus anterior. Branches of the thyrocervical trunk cross to the posterior triangle of the neck anterior to the scalenus anterior.

A   (anterior to medial end of clavicle) is incorrect. The subclavian vein arises from the brachiocephalic vein posterior (not anterior) to the medial end of the clavicle, just before the brachiocephalic vein descends through the superior thoracic aperture.

C   (just posterior to internal jugular vein) is incorrect. The internal jugular vein courses for most of its length in the neck deep to the sternocleidomastoid muscle. In the root of the neck and between the two heads of the sternocleidomastoid, the internal jugular vein unites with the subclavian vein to form the brachiocephalic vein. Thus, the internal jugular vein does not lie anterior to the subclavian vein; instead, it connects to the subclavian vein from a superior position.

D   (posterior to scalenus anterior muscle) is incorrect. The subclavian vein lies anterior to this muscle. The subclavian artery enters the posterior triangle by crossing the root of the neck between the scalenus anterior and scalenus medius. Likewise, the roots (contributions) to the brachial plexus enter the posterior triangle between the scalenus anterior and scalenus medius.

E   (posterior to subclavian artery) is incorrect. The subclavian vein courses anterior to the subclavian artery. This vein and artery are separated from each other in the root of the neck by the scalenus anterior muscle. The roots of the brachial plexus lie posterior to the subclavian artery in the root of the neck.

30. *C*   (platelet function disorder) is correct. The patient has a qualitative platelet disorder most likely associated with the use of nonsteroidal anti-inflammatory drugs (NSAIDs) for his chronic osteoarthritis. NSAIDs block platelet cyclooxygenase, which prevents the synthesis of thromboxane A_2 (TXA_2). Normally, TXA_2 is a potent platelet aggregator and vasoconstrictor of small vessels. It is primarily responsible for producing a temporary hemostatic plug composed of platelets that stop bleeding in injured small vessels. Hence, blocking the synthesis of TXA_2 in this patient causes severe bleeding from small vessels that lack

platelet plugs. The best test of platelet function is indicated by BT, which evaluates small vessel and platelet function up to the formation of the platelet plug. The BT is prolonged in this patient. The aPTT evaluates the intrinsic coagulation system down to the formation of a fibrin clot, which includes the following factors (in sequence of activation): XII, XI, IX, VIII, X, V, II (prothrombin), and I (fibrinogen). The PT evaluates the extrinsic coagulation system down to the formation of a fibrin clot, which includes the following factors (in sequence of activation): VII, X, V, II, and I. The platelet count is a quantitative measurement of platelets; however, it does not evaluate platelet function. The most appropriate treatment for this patient is infusion with a few units of platelets, which are functionally capable of forming platelet plugs and participating in the formation of fibrin clots.

A (circulating anticoagulant) is incorrect. Circulating anticoagulants are antibodies that inhibit specific coagulation factors (e.g., antibodies against factor VIII), thus simulating a coagulation factor deficiency. Normal PTT and PT exclude circulating anticoagulants as a cause of the bleeding.
B (coagulation factor deficiency) is incorrect. The PTT and PT in this patient are both normal.
D (secondary fibrinolytic disorder) is incorrect. The D-dimer assay is negative, and the PT and PTT are both normal in this patient. Secondary fibrinolysis refers to activation of the fibrinolytic system (activation of plasminogen produces plasmin) as a compensatory mechanism to destroy fibrin clots in intravascular coagulation. Plasmin destroys fibrin, fibrinogen, and many of the coagulation factors; therefore, it prolongs the PT and PTT. D-dimers are fibrin monomers in a fibrin clot that have been cross-linked by factor XIII (fibrin-stabilizing factor). Their presence indicates that intravascular coagulation has occurred.

31. *E* (rotavirus) is correct. Of the viruses listed, rotaviruses are the only ones that cause gastroenteritis and are also members of the family *Reoviridae*. Rotavirus disease usually occurs during the winter months, is typically seen in children under the age of 2 years, and is transmitted via the fecal-oral route. Like all reoviruses, rotaviruses are double-stranded, segmented RNA viruses.

A (astrovirus) and D (Norwalk virus) are incorrect. Astroviruses and Norwalk virus cause gastroenteritis. However, astroviruses are members of the family *Astroviridae,* and Norwalk virus is a member of the family *Caliciviridae.* Both families consist of single-stranded, positive-sense, nonsegmented RNA viruses.
B (coltivirus) and C (hepatitis E virus) are incorrect. Coltiviruses and hepatitis E virus do not cause gastroenteritis. A coltivirus causes Colorado tick fever, and hepatitis E virus causes a liver infection that is similar to the one caused by hepatitis A virus. Coltiviruses are members of the family *Reoviridae,* and hepatitis E virus

is a member of the family *Caliciviridae*. The genomes of these families are described above.

32. **D** (lead poisoning; treatment with calcium disodium edetate) is correct. The patient's clinical and laboratory findings are consistent with lead intoxication. Chelation therapy with calcium disodium edetate (edetate calcium disodium; EDTA) is the preferred treatment in patients who have severe gastrointestinal symptoms ("lead colic"). Alternatively, therapy with succimer, dimercaprol, or penicillamine may be given.

A (acetaminophen poisoning; treatment with acetylcysteine) is incorrect. When acetaminophen is metabolized, a potentially toxic intermediate is formed. This intermediate is usually inactivated by conjugation with glutathione, but it begins to accumulate when endogenous stores of glutathione are depleted. Free radicals formed from acetaminophen metabolism then cause lipid peroxidation of hepatic membranes and lead to hepatic necrosis. Early manifestations of intoxication with acetaminophen include mild gastrointestinal complaints. Later manifestations include hepatic failure and encephalopathy. Death sometimes ensues. Acetylcysteine, a reducing agent, is the antidote for acetaminophen intoxication.
B (arsenic poisoning; treatment with dimercaprol) is incorrect. Symptoms of intoxication with arsenic may include gastroenteritis, leukopenia, anemia, Aldrich-Mees lines, alopecia, neuropathy, and encephalopathy. Chelation therapy would consist of dimercaprol, succimer, or penicillamine.
C (iron poisoning; treatment with deferoxamine) is incorrect. Early manifestations of acute intoxication with iron include abdominal pain, hematemesis, and bloody diarrhea. Later manifestations may include shock (which occurs secondary to the loss of fluid and blood into the gastrointestinal tract) and hepatic failure. Chelation therapy would include the administration of deferoxamine.
E (mercury poisoning; treatment with succimer) is incorrect. Manifestations associated with mercury intoxication vary, depending on the form of mercury to which the patient is exposed. Intoxication with elemental (metallic) mercury may cause tremor, gingivostomatitis, and neuropsychiatric disturbances, such as fatigue, memory loss, shyness, depression, and irritability. Intoxication with inorganic mercury may cause acute hemorrhagic gastroenteritis, renal failure, and acrodynia ("pink disease"). Intoxication with organic mercury (methylmercury) may cause paresthesias, ataxia, dysarthria, and other disorders of the central nervous system. Chelation therapy is as follows: succimer or penicillamine for elemental mercury; dimercaprol or succimer for inorganic mercury; and succimer (but not dimercaprol) for organic mercury.

33. *E* (report the colleague to the appropriate authorities to allow for an investigation) is correct. Legal requirements regarding impaired physicians vary from state to state. Ethically, the physician must report the colleague's behavior to the appropriate authorities (e.g., licensing board, hospital administration) because the use of alcohol during office hours is placing patients at risk. The physician's use of alcohol while working also suggests alcohol dependence.

A (coerce the colleague to seek help by threatening to inform the colleague's patients of the alcohol use) is incorrect. Reporting the alcohol use to patients would create additional problems. The impaired physician should be relieved of his medical duties until substance abuse treatment can be sought.
B (contact the colleague's family and encourage the family to deal with the problem) is incorrect. Although in some cases contacting the family may be helpful, in other cases, the family may be enabling the substance use or may be unable to deter the drinking. Therefore, contacting the family is not sufficient.
C (continue to monitor the colleague's behavior and report the alcohol use if other signs of impairment occur) is incorrect. There is already enough evidence to warrant reporting the physician if he does not immediately seek treatment. Consuming alcohol while providing medical care is unethical.
D (nothing more, since the physician has completed his duty by discussing the matter with the colleague) is incorrect. Simply having a conversation with an impaired physician about substance use is not sufficient.

34. *D* (omphalocele) is correct. Ultrasound examination of the woman done at 30 weeks' gestation shows an abdominal mass protruding from the ventral body wall of the fetus, diagnosed as an omphalocele. An omphalocele is the result of gastrointestinal structures herniating through an unclosed umbilical ring. An amniotic membrane covers the herniated organs that do not retract normally into the abdominal cavity during the 10th week of development. The incidence of omphalocele is about 1 in 5000 births, of which 50% are usually stillborn. If no other defects are present, immediate surgical repair is recommended.

A (complete exstrophy of the bladder) is incorrect. Extrophy of the urinary bladder results from incomplete closure of the anterior abdominal wall inferiorly. The muscles and connective tissue over the bladder are absent. This severe anomaly occurs in about 1 in 25,000 births. When exstrophy of the bladder involves the penis, the condition is known as epispadias.
B (gastroschisis) is incorrect. Failure of the lateral folds to close results in a near median plane defect, usually on the right side, in the ventral abdominal wall. Abdominal viscera protrude into the amniotic cavity without involving the umbilical cord, resulting in a condition called gastroschisis. The defect occurs in about 1 in

10,000 births and is more common in males than females. Gastroschisis is not associated with chromosomal abnormalities.

C (Meckel's diverticulum) is incorrect. A Meckel's (ileal) diverticulum is the persistence of the vitelline (yolk) stalk. It occurs in 2% the–4% of the population. Typically, it appears as a fingerlike diverticulum, a few centimeters long, that arises about 50 cm from the ileocecal junction. Meckel's diverticulum is of clinical significance because it can become inflamed and mimic appendicitis or contain ectopic tissues (e.g., gastric, pancreatic), which can cause ulceration. Surgical management is indicated when a patient develops clinical symptoms.

E (umbilical hernia) is incorrect. In a patient with an umbilical hernia, the herniation is covered by skin and subcutaneous tissue. The defect in the ventral abdominal wall usually occurs along the linea alba and reaches maximum size about 1 month after birth. Umbilical hernias constitute about 14% of all hernias.

35. *D* (surreptitiously injected human insulin) is correct. Normally, β-islet cells first synthesize preproinsulin in the rough endoplasmic reticulin. Preproinsulin then is delivered to the Golgi apparatus, where proteolytic reactions generate insulin and a cleavage peptide called C peptide. Hence, C peptide is a marker for endogenous synthesis of insulin. In this case, the patient has been injecting himself with insulin. This increases the serum insulin level; however, serum C peptide is decreased due to suppression of the β-islet cells by the exogenously administered insulin.

A (benign tumor involving β-islet cells in the pancreas) is incorrect. Insulinomas are benign tumors of the β-islet cells that synthesize excess insulin, resulting in severe fasting hypoglycemia. As expected, these patients have increased serum insulin and C-peptide levels, indicating that β-islet cells are synthesizing the insulin.

B (ectopic secretion of an insulin-like factor) is incorrect. This lowers both the serum insulin and the C-peptide levels due to hypoglycemia suppressing the β-islet cells from synthesizing insulin.

C (malignant tumor involving α-islet cells in the pancreas) is incorrect. This describes a glucagonoma, which produces hyperglycemia by stimulating gluconeogenesis.

36. *A* (left frontal cortex) is correct. This man most likely has had a stroke affecting the left frontal cortex, specifically the precentral gyrus and the frontal eye field. The precentral gyrus contains much of the primary motor cortex. It gives rise to the corticospinal tract, which projects contralaterally below the medullary pyramids. Damage to fibers in this projection could be responsible for the right-sided paralysis. Damage to fibers descending from the frontal eye fields could interrupt transmission to the horizontal and vertical gaze centers; however, a few days after the lesion occurs, adjacent cortical eye fields (e.g., parietal centers) will take over that function.

B   (left mesencephalic tegmentum) is incorrect. The mesencephalic tegmentum lies anterior to the fourth ventricle and contains the reticular formation, the nuclei and tracts of several cranial nerves, and pathways ascending from the spinal cord. Damage to this structure could affect horizontal gaze if it occurred within the abducens nuclei (CN VI) and tracts. It would not have a significant effect on descending motor signals.

C   (left occipital cortex) and E (right occipital cortex) are incorrect. The occipital lobe contains the visual cortex, which receives signals originating from photoreceptors in the retina. Damage to this structure would interfere with vision, not eye movement.

D   (right lateral geniculate nucleus) is incorrect. The right lateral geniculate body of the thalamus receives crossed nasal fibers and uncrossed temporal retinal ganglion cell axons. Because it contains sensory fibers, damage to this structure would not interfere with motor function, even in the eyes.

37.   A   (carnitine deficiency) is correct. β-Oxidation of long-chain fatty acids takes place in mitochondria. Long-chain fatty acids must be transported across the mitochondrial inner membrane by L-carnitine. In carnitine shuttle defects, long-chain fatty acids accumulate in the cytoplasm, causing the fatty changes seen in biopsy specimens. Tissues that utilize long-chain fatty acids as an energy source switch to glucose, and this leads to hypoglycemia. Ketone bodies are produced in mitochondria from long-chain fatty acids. The absence of these fatty acids in mitochondria prevents ketone formation.

B   (decrease in citrate production) is incorrect. Citrate transports the acetyl portion of acetyl CoA from mitochondria to the cytoplasm. This is the first step in de novo synthesis of fatty acids. When citrate production is decreased, acetyl CoA will accumulate in mitochondria and be converted to ketone bodies.

C   (decrease in malonyl CoA production) is incorrect. Malonyl CoA is an intermediate in de novo synthesis of fatty acids. Malonyl CoA inhibits the carnitine shuttle, preventing newly synthesized fatty acid from being degraded in mitochondrial β-oxidation.

D   (lipoprotein lipase deficiency) is incorrect. Familial lipoprotein lipase deficiency (type I hyperlipidemia) leads to massive hyperchylomicronemia.

38.   C   (*Legionella pneumophila*) is correct. The clinical and laboratory findings are consistent with the diagnosis of legionnaires' disease, a form of pneumonia that is transmitted by aerosols and has an incubation period of 2–10 days. Most cases of legionnaires' disease are caused by *L. pneumophila*. This highly fastidious bacterium is a facultatively intracellular parasite that is able to grow within unactivated macrophages by inhibiting lysosome fusion with phagosomes.

A *(Haemophilus influenzae)*, B *(Klebsiella pneumoniae)*, and E *(Pseudomonas aeruginosa)* are incorrect. *H. influenzae*, *K. pneumoniae*, and *P. aeruginosa* are all organisms that can cause pneumonia. However, they are all extracellular pathogens.

D *(Mycobacterium tuberculosis)* is incorrect. *M. tuberculosis* is a facultatively intracellular parasite that causes pneumonia. However, *M. tuberculosis* is cytologically gram-positive.

39. *E* (mitotic nondisjunction) is correct. Changes in the chromosomal constitution of a cell indicate that a mitotic event has occurred. Mitotic nondisjunction is the failure of sister chromatids to separate during anaphase. This process is responsible for a cell containing an extra chromosome.

A (meiotic anaphase lagging) and C (mitotic anaphase lagging) are incorrect. Anaphase lagging is the failure of a chromatid to move as quickly as the other chromatids during anaphase. This results in that chromatid (chromosome) being excluded from a daughter cell and in a cell with fewer (not extra) chromosomes.

B (meiotic nondisjunction) is incorrect. Meiotic nondisjunction is the failure of chromatids to separate during meiosis. It results in all cells having the same chromosomal constitution.

D (mitotic deletion) is incorrect. Mitotic deletion is the loss of part of a chromosome during mitosis. It does not change the number of chromosomes in the cell.

40. *A* (fusion of the podocytes) is correct. The patient has the classic findings of nephrotic syndrome, which, in children, is usually due to lipoid nephrosis (minimal change disease). Preceding upper respiratory tract infection, atopy, nonsteroidal anti-inflammatory drugs, and Hodgkin's disease all have been implicated in the pathogenesis of the disease. The gold standard for diagnosis of nephrotic syndrome is a 24-hour urine protein level >3.5 g (<150 mg/24 h). In lipoid nephrosis, a T-cell immune reaction against visceral epithelial cells causes loss of the negative charge of the glomerular basement membrane (called polyanion loss), which results in a selective loss of albumin in the urine. Because the plasma albumin concentration is responsible for 80% of the oncotic pressure, hypoalbuminemia results in leakage of a protein-poor transudate from the vascular compartment into the interstitial tissue (pitting edema) and body cavities (ascites). Furthermore, hypoalbuminemia stimulates increased liver synthesis of cholesterol and subsequent hypercholesterolemia (type II hyperlipoproteinemia). Cholesterol leaks into the urine, producing fatty casts that polarize and often show "Maltese crosses." Lipid stains are positive in the glomeruli and renal tubular cells; however, no proliferative or glomerular basement membrane changes are seen in the glomeruli. Immunofluorescent stains are negative. Electron microscopy shows fusion of the podocytes, which is a universal finding in any nephrotic syndrome. Lipoid nephrosis is not considered an

immunocomplex-mediated disease, since no electron-dense deposits are found in the glomeruli. Children respond extremely well to steroid therapy.

B (intramembranous electron-dense deposits) is incorrect. These findings are consistent with type II membranoproliferative glomerulonephritis ("dense deposit" disease), which produces nephrotic syndrome. An autoantibody against C_3, called the C_3 nephritic factor, causes continual activation of the alternative pathway, leading to low complement levels.

C (mesangial electron-dense deposits) is incorrect. These findings are consistent with IgA glomerulonephritis (Berger's disease), which is the most common type of glomerulonephritis. Children have recurrent macrohematuria (usually following respiratory infections), whereas adults have recurrent microhematuria.

D (subendothelial electron-dense deposits) is incorrect. These findings are seen in type IV proliferative glomerulonephritis in patients with systemic lupus erythematosus and in type I membranoproliferative glomerulonephritis.

E (subepithelial electron-dense deposits) is incorrect. These findings are seen in poststreptococcal glomerulonephritis and diffuse membranous glomerulonephritis, which is the most common cause of nephrotic syndrome in adults.

41. *A* (at Cp_{ss}, the maintenance dose administered every half-life would be equal for drug X and drug Y) is correct. Under conditions in which the dosing interval is equal to the half-life ($t_{1/2}$) of a drug, the maintenance dose (MD) is equal to one-half the loading dose (LD) corrected for bioavailability (F). That is, $MD = (LD/2) \times (1/F)$. Recall that the equation for calculating the LD of a given drug is as follows: $LD = Cp_{ss} \times V_d$, where V_d is the volume of distribution. The V_d is calculated as the intravenous bolus dose divided by the Cp_0, where Cp_0 is the plasma drug concentration at time zero. Because drug X and drug Y were given in the same intravenous bolus dose and have the same Cp_0, they have the same V_d. Since both drugs have the same V_d and Cp_{ss}, their loading doses would be identical. With identical loading doses and identical oral bioavailabilities, their MD given every $t_{1/2}$ would be identical. Note that in cases in which the dosing interval is not equal to the $t_{1/2}$ of the drug, the formula for determining the maintenance dose is as follows: $MD = Cp_{ss} \times CL \times$ dosing interval, where CL is the clearance. The CL of a given drug is as follows: $CL = 0.7 \times V_d/t_{1/2}$. As indicated above, the V_d for both drugs is the same. However, because the graph shows that drug X has a longer $t_{1/2}$ than drug Y, the CL for drug X would be less than that for drug Y. Consequently, maintenance with drug X would require less frequent administration than would maintenance with drug Y.

B, C, and D are incorrect. Refer to the explanation for A.

42. *A* (highest capacity nephrons are saturated with the substance) is correct. The maximum rate at which a substance is reabsorbed from the renal tubule or secreted into it is most accurately calculated when receptors for that substance are saturated maximally in every nephron. The highest-capacity nephrons contain the greatest number of transporters for the substance. Therefore, an accurate calculation of maximum transport requires complete saturation of these nephrons.

   B (lowest capacity nephrons are saturated with the substance) is incorrect. Receptors in the lowest capacity nephrons are saturated most quickly and are likely to become saturated before all the higher capacity nephrons. Thus, using the low-capacity nephrons to calculate maximum transport rates would result in underestimating transport maximum (Tm).
   C (plasma and urine concentrations of the substance are easily measured) is incorrect. To perform the calculation, it is necessary to know the plasma and urine concentrations of the substance, but this does not guarantee the accuracy of the calculation. The plasma concentration will indicate when transporters for the substance in the highest capacity nephrons become saturated, but it does not indicate whether the kidney is completely saturated with that substance. The urine concentration of the substance does not indicate the degree of saturation either.
   D (renal plasma threshold for the substance is not exceeded) is incorrect. If the renal plasma threshold is not exceeded, not even the low capacity nephrons are saturated.
   E (substance is bound to plasma proteins) is incorrect. The rate of transport is based on the transport of free (not bound) substance.

43. *B* (embolic occlusion of a cerebral artery) is correct. Patients with mitral stenosis develop left atrial dilatation and produce thrombi due to stasis of blood in the chamber. Furthermore, left atrial dilatation predisposes to atrial fibrillation. The combination of a thrombus in the left atrium and atrial fibrillation results in multisystem embolic disease with infarctions. When emboli from the heart disseminate to the brain, they usually enter the middle cerebral artery. Occlusion of the artery results in wedge-shaped infarction extending to the periphery of the brain. When the embolus dissolves, reperfusion of the infarcted area causes a hemorrhagic infarction. An infarction in the brain is an example of liquefactive (not coagulative) necrosis.

   A (atherosclerosis of the internal carotid artery) is incorrect. An atherosclerotic stroke is usually due to a platelet thrombus overlying an atherosclerotic plaque near the bifurcation of the internal carotid artery. This produces a pale infarction of the ipsilateral brain that extends to the periphery of the brain. However, unlike an embolic stroke, reperfusion is less likely to occur, so the infarct remains pale due to the lack of blood flow to the area.

C (intracerebral hematoma) is incorrect. Intracerebral hematomas usually are caused by hypertension. Long-standing hypertension leads to the formation of Charcot-Bouchard macroaneurysms of the lenticulostriate vessels, which supply the putamen and thalamus. When these aneurysms rupture, they produce an intracerebral hematoma (not an infarction), most commonly in the basal ganglia area of the brain. Other areas where hematomas can form in a hypertensive bleed are the pons and cerebellar hemispheres.

D (neoplastic transformation of astrocytes) is incorrect. Astrocytomas are neoplasms arising from astrocytes. Low-grade astrocytomas (grades I and II) are benign; high-grade astrocytomas (e.g., glioblastoma multiforme) are malignant. Glioblastoma multiforme is the most common primary brain tumor found in adults and is characterized by hemorrhagic necrosis. The frontal lobes usually are involved, and the tumor frequently extends across the corpus callosum to the contralateral lobe.

E (rupture of a congenital aneurysm) is incorrect. Congenital aneurysms in the brain usually develop at the junction of the anterior communicating artery with the anterior cerebral artery or the posterior communicating artery with the posterior cerebral artery. Loss of internal elastic lamina and smooth muscle at the branching points of the vessel occurs, predisposing to berry aneurysm formation. When these rupture, the blood usually enters the subarachnoid space, causing a severe occipital headache and loss of consciousness.

44. *E* (narrow, tall spike in the gamma globulin fraction) is correct. Multiple myeloma results in a large increase of a specific clone of cells producing a single type of immunoglobulin, which bands in the gamma globulin region.

A (broad, short peak between the alpha and gamma globulin fractions), C (large albumin peak), and D (large complement peak) are incorrect. In patients with multiple myeloma, there is no increase in proteins banding between the alpha and gamma globulin fractions. There is also no increase in proteins banding where albumin or complement bands in electrophoresis.

B (increased amount of specific IgA antibodies) is incorrect. Multiple myeloma results in a sharp increase in IgM antibodies, not IgA antibodies.

45. *A* (the affected lobe will collapse and remain collapsed, even though the chest wall continues to move) is correct. The lung and chest wall are mechanically coupled through the serous fluid layer that lies between the visceral and parietal walls of the pleural cavity. This fluid allows the lungs and chest wall to glide over each other, but negative intrapleural pressure prevents their separation (as seen with two glass plates that are "joined" by a thin layer of water). By cutting through the intercostal muscles, the parietal layer of the pleural cavity is pierced, allowing air to enter, breaking the seal and disrupting mechanical coupling between the chest wall and lung. The affected lobe will

recoil inward until it reaches its low equilibrium volume, and the chest will spring outward. Since the upper cervical spine was not severed, rhythmic breathing should continue because the phrenic nerve is still intact and, thus, diaphragmatic movement is expected to be normal.

B   (the chest wall will spring out somewhat, but the affected lobe will not collapse) is incorrect. Violation of the integrity of the intrapleural space permits air to enter and break this seal, thereby disrupting the mechanical coupling between the chest wall and lung. In such cases, the affected lobe of the lung recoils inward until it reaches its low equilibrium volume, and the chest wall springs outward.
C   (the lung lobe will collapse, but the chest wall will remain at its functional residual capacity position) is incorrect. The wound violated the pleural membrane, thereby uncoupling the chest wall and lung. This allows the lung to recoil inward and the chest wall to expand outward. Thus, the chest wall will not remain in the position it maintains when the FRC is normal.
D   (the wound will quickly seal itself, thereby allowing the collapsed lung to expand automatically) is incorrect. The collapsed lobe will reexpand only if positive pressure is applied at the mouth or negative pressure is applied around the lung.
E   (rhythmic breathing will stop abruptly, and the patient will die from asphyxiation without immediate medical care) is incorrect. Rhythmic breathing will continue, because the upper cervical spinal cord was not severed. This indicates that the phrenic nerve is probably still intact; thus diaphragmatic activity will remain normal. However, chest motion will not reexpand the collapsed lobe because of the loss of mechanical coupling between the lung and the chest wall.

46. *C*   (hypochondriasis) is correct. Hypochondriasis refers to a preoccupation with disease. Individuals with this disorder do not have a medical illness but truly believe that they do. They focus on any perceived signs of disease and will "shop" for a physician who can adequately diagnose their illness. A patient who remains convinced of the presence of disease, despite being reassured by many physicians that there is no disease, demonstrates hypochondriasis.

A   (conversion disorder) is incorrect. In conversion disorder, an individual develops pseudoneurologic symptoms in response to stress. The process occurs at an unconscious level, and the prognosis is generally good once the stressor is identified and addressed. For example, a woman who wants to leave her husband to be with someone else might develop a paralysis, which keeps her from "walking away" from the marriage.
B   (factitious disorder) is incorrect. In a factitious disorder, an individual wants to assume a sick role and deliberately produces symptoms to accomplish this goal. Additional external incentives are not motivating the behavior.

D (phobia) is incorrect. A phobia is a morbid fear of a specific object or situation. For example, an extreme fear of heights would be considered a phobia.

E (somatization disorder) is incorrect. Individuals with somatization disorder report multiple somatic complaints across various organ systems (e.g., gastrointestinal, cardiovascular, neurologic). This chronic disorder usually begins before age 30, and the prognosis is guarded.

47. *B* (decreased GABAergic output to the thalamus) is correct. The arrow in the figure is pointing to the ansa lenticularis, which is one of two sets of fibers that connect the internal globus pallidus and the thalamus. Axons projecting from the globus pallidus produce the inhibitory neurotransmitter GABA, and act on the thalamic ventrolateral and ventroanterior nuclei, which project to the motor and premotor areas of the cerebral cortex. Thus, the lesion in this figure would interfere with the ability of the thalamic nuclei to modulate cortical motor signals.

A (bitemporal hemianopia) is incorrect. Bitemporal hemianopia is the inability to see objects in the temporal visual fields in both eyes. This condition may occur as a result of a lesion of the optic chiasm, not the ansa lenticularis (shown).

C (decreased olfactory sensitivity) is incorrect. The olfactory nerve (CN I) extends from receptors within the nasal epithelium directly to the olfactory bulb and from there to the anterior portion of the cerebrum. It does not pass through the diencephalon, as shown in the illustration.

D (increased vocal and oral tendencies) is incorrect. Increased vocal and oral tendencies occur as a result of a temporal lobectomy, which causes the Klüver-Bucy syndrome. Patients with this syndrome tend to pick up objects and examine them with their mouths. They also tend to exhibit psychic blindness and hypermetamorphosis (increased exploratory behavior).

E (sham rage) is incorrect. Sham rage is indicated in decorticate animals by tail lashing, limb jerking, clawing, biting, and several autonomic responses, including sweating, piloerection, urination, defecation, and increased blood pressure. It is also associated with lesions in the limbic system. In this figure, neither the cerebral cortex nor any limbic structures show injury.

48. *B* (branched-chain α-keto acid dehydrogenase complex) is correct. The patient's manifestations are consistent with the diagnosis of maple syrup urine disease. Patients with this disease have a deficiency of the branched-chain α-keto acid dehydrogenase complex, which impairs their catabolism of leucine, isoleucine, and valine.

A (arginase) is incorrect. A deficiency of arginase disrupts the urea cycle and causes argininemia and hyperammonemia.

C (cystathionine synthase) is incorrect. A deficiency of cystathionine synthase impairs the catabolism of methionine and causes homocystinuria.

D (homogentisic acid oxidase) is incorrect. A deficiency of homogentisic acid oxidase (homogentisate 1,2-dioxygenase) impairs the catabolism of tyrosine and causes alkaptonuria.

E (phenylalanine hydroxylase) is incorrect. A deficiency of phenylalanine hydroxylase impairs the catabolism of phenylalanine and causes phenylketonuria (PKU).

49. *C* (ruptured liver cell adenoma) is correct. Professional weight lifters commonly use anabolic steroids to increase muscle mass and strength. One of the complications of anabolic steroids is the development of liver cell (hepatic) adenomas, which are benign tumors arising from hepatocytes. These tumors tend to rupture and produce intraperitoneal hemorrhage. Women taking estrogen-containing medications are subject to the same complication.

A (ruptured abdominal aortic aneurysm) is incorrect. The most common mechanism for producing these aneurysms is atherosclerosis. Most abdominal aortic aneurysms occur in men over 50 years of age.

B (ruptured cavernous hemangioma of the liver) is incorrect. Cavernous hemangiomas are the most common benign tumor of the liver. Although large cavernous hemangiomas can rupture, the clinical scenario in this case involving a professional weight lifter shifts the differential to a liver cell adenoma as the more likely cause of the intra-abdominal bleeding.

D (ruptured splenic artery aneurysm) is incorrect. Splenic artery aneurysms are the second most common intra-abdominal aneurysm. They are more commonly found in women and often rupture during pregnancy.

50. *C* (metronidazole) is correct. Metronidazole is active against most obligate anaerobes, including *B. fragilis* and *C. difficile*. It is considered the drug of choice for treating antibiotic-induced pseudomembranous colitis (which occurs secondary to proliferation of *C. difficile*), many anaerobic bacterial infections, and numerous anaerobic parasitic infections (including amebiasis, giardiasis, and trichomoniasis). Metronidazole is inactive against obligate aerobes, including *S. aureus* and *H. influenzae*. It is also inactive against *C. trachomatis*.

A (amoxicillin) is incorrect. Amoxicillin is an extended-spectrum aminopenicillin. When given alone, it is sensitive to beta-lactamases. Thus, it must be given in combination with a beta-lactamase inhibitor, such as clavulanic acid, to be useful in the treatment of infections caused by beta-lactamase-positive *H. influenzae*. When given alone or in combination with clavulanic acid, amoxicillin has no activity against the other organisms listed in the question.

B   (imipenem) is incorrect. Imipenem is active against *B. fragilis* and beta-lactamase-positive *H. influenzae*. Although imipenem is a broad-spectrum drug, it is inactive against all of the other organisms listed in the question.

D   (oxacillin) is incorrect. Oxacillin is a beta-lactamase-resistant penicillin. It is active only against gram-positive aerobic bacteria. No beta-lactam antibiotic would have activity against methicillin-resistant *S. aureus* (MRSA). Thus, oxacillin would be ineffective against all of the organisms listed in the question.

E   (vancomycin) is incorrect. Vancomycin is active against gram-positive bacteria, including many anaerobes. Although it is active against most *Bacteroides* species, it is inactive against *B. fragilis*. It is active against *C. difficile* and is used as an alternative to metronidazole for the treatment of antibiotic-induced pseudomembranous colitis (refer to the discussion of C). Vancomycin is the drug of choice for treating infections caused by MRSA. It has no activity against *C. trachomatis*.